Clinical Topics
in Addiction

Clinical Topics in Addiction

Edited by Ed Day

RCPsych Publications

© The Royal College of Psychiatrists 2007

RCPsych Publications is an imprint of the Royal College of Psychiatrists, 17 Belgrave Square, London SW1X 8PG, UK
http://www.rcpsych.ac.uk

British Library Cataloguing-in-Publication Data.
A catalogue record for this book is available from the British Library.

ISBN 978-1-904671-50-3

Distributed in North America by Balogh International Inc.

The views presented in this book do not necessarily reflect those of the Royal College of Psychiatrists, and the publishers are not responsible for any error of omission or fact. The Royal College of Psychiatrists is a registered charity (no. 228636).

Printed in Great Britain by Henry Ling Limited, The Dorset Press, Dorchester.

Contents

Tables

Boxes

Figures

Contributors

Mohammed T. Abou-Saleh Section of Addictive Behaviour, Division of Mental Health, St George's, University of London, London

Sangeeta Ambegaokar Orchard House, Leamington Spa, Warwickshire

David Best Queen Elizabeth Psychiatric Hospital, Edgbaston, Birmingham

Sanjoo Chengappa Section of Addictive Behaviour, Division of Mental Health, St George's, University of London, London

Alex Copello University of Birmingham School of Psychology, and Birmingham and Solihull Mental Health NHS Trust

Glenice Cox St Andrews, Wells, Somerset

Ilana B. Crome Academic Psychiatry Unit, Keele University Medical School (Harplands Campus), Stoke-on-Trent

Ian Cumming Her Majesty's Prison Belmarsh, Thamesmead, London

Ed Day University of Birmingham, Department of Psychiatry, Birmingham

Colin Drummond Section of Addictive Behaviour, Division of Mental Health, St George's, University of London, London

Paul Egleston Rampton Hoospital, Retford, Nottinghamshire

Sanju George Bridge Community Drug Team, Birmingham and Solihull Mental Health NHS Trust, Larch Croft, Chelmsley Wood, Birmingham

Hamid Ghodse International Centre for Drug Policy, St George's, University of London, London

Quazi Haque Priory Secure Services, Farmfield Hospital, Charlwood, Surrey

Adam Huxley Birmingham and Solihull Mental Health NHS Trust

Olawale Lagundoye Sheffield Care Trust, The Fitzwilliam Centre, Sheffield

Anne Lingford-Hughes Psychopharmacology Unit, University of Bristol, Bristol

Jason Luty   South Essex Partnership NHS Foundation Trust and Cambridge and Peterborough Mental Health NHS Trust, Community Drug and Alcohol Team, Taylor Centre, Southend-on-Sea

Claire McIntosh   Community Alcohol and Drug Service, Bannockburn Hospital, Stirling, Stirlingshire

Charles McMahon   Renfrew Substance Abuse Resource, Paisley, Renfrewshire

Vijaya Murali   Azaadi Community Drug Team, Birmingham and Solihull Mental Health NHS Trust, Birmingham

Tracey Myton   Pennine Care NHS Trust, Rochdale Substance Misuse Service, Rochdale

David Nutt   Psychopharmacology Unit, University of Bristol, Bristol

John Potokar   Psychopharmacology Unit, University of Bristol, Bristol

Duncan Raistrick   Leeds Addiction Unit, Leeds

Hagen Rampes   Barnet and Haringey Mental Health Trust, Edgware

Bruce Ritson   Alcohol Problems Service, Royal Edinburgh Hospital, Edinburgh

Nicholas Seivewright   The Fitzwilliam Centre, Sheffield

Iain Smith   Gartnavel Royal Hospital, Glasgow

Peter Snowden   Meadow Lodge Secure Unit, Priory Hospitals, Widnes

John Strang   King's College London, Institute of Psychiatry, National Addiction Centre, London

Harith Swadi   115 Memorial Avenue, Christchurch 8053, New Zealand. samitara@xtra.co.nz

Janet Treasure   Department of Academic Psychiatry, Guy's Hospital, London

Sarah Welch   Countrywide Specialist Substance Misuse Service, Gloucester

Kim Wolff   King's College London, Institute of Psychiatry, National Addiction Centre, London

Nat Wright   HMP Leeds Health Care Department, 2 Gloucester Terrace, Leeds

Foreword

In his preface, Ed Day highlights that this book originated in articles written in the peer-reviewed psychiatry literature for a generic audience of consultant psychiatrists. This stimulated me to think whether the book will serve as a useful tool for my generic psychiatry colleagues. Our paths frequently cross as in our daily professional lives we constantly encounter problems relating to problematic drug or alcohol use. I am convinced that this book is a 'must have' for every consultant psychiatrist. However, the value of this book is for a much wider audience. I reflected upon how it would feel to be a junior doctor considering a career in addiction psychiatry. Would this book reassure me that it is possible to pursue a fulfilling career in providing professional, evidence-based clinical care to people whose drug use has become a problem to themselves, their families and wider society? Without doubt I am sure that it does have the potential to fulfil such a function. There are few books that offer both a wide scope (breadth) and an exhaustive reservoir of knowledge (depth) by combining the current evidence base with diverse expert clinical knowledge and experience. This book has managed to achieve these aims in a style that is readable, engaging, yet authoritative

There is another readership, however, to whom I would unreservedly recommend this book, namely that of my own professional people-group, primary care clinicians. One of the chapters alludes to the recent growth in primary-care-based drug treatment and another points out that, although psychiatry services for those with mental ill-health and drug dependence are largely separate, in primary care such comorbid conditions are managed by the same clinician. If primary care has traditionally offered the drug treatment field strengths of pragmatism and integrated clinical care for those with comorbid conditions, then there is much that we can receive in return from our colleagues in specialist addiction psychiatry services. This book offers us an authoritative collection of the evidence, and I would like it to sit on the bookshelves of all my primary care colleagues who have clinical responsibility for those who use drugs in a problematic fashion.

I feel sure that other primary care clinicians sometimes feel beleaguered as I do by the homogenising sense of reducing drug treatment to pharmacological provision for large numbers of opiate users. Well, this book can support us as we seek to develop our professional knowledge, experience and self-esteem. We may not agree with all that is said in it – our professional cultures are perhaps too diverse for such an ideal. Yet I am reminded of the words of Mahatma Gandhi, who wrote 'I do not want my house to be walled in on all sides and my windows to be stuffed. I want the cultures of all the lands to be blown about my house as freely as possible. But I refuse to be blown off my feet by any'. So let the culture of our secondary care colleagues blow around us and take us on a journey. Initially, it will take us back in time to learn about how drug treatment services have developed in the UK. The journey gathers pace as we are taken into less familiar areas of clinical care and learn about a plant that grows on the banks of the Red Sea and has a stimulant action. Then there are accounts of mushrooms that grow across the world and have hallucinogenic properties. We will also be encouraged to think afresh about the interplay between problematic drug use and mental ill health. Authoritative overviews of psychological interventions are provided, as well as the current evidence base pertaining to pharmacological interventions. Fresh consideration of the common class A drugs encountered in clinical practice leads on to an authoritative critique that reflects on the complex link between intoxication, criminal activity and liability. The journey ends with a delightful chapter that offers a rarity in a clinical textbook, namely a good bedtime read! We are treated to an overview of the influence of substance use in popular literature. Linger for a while at the journey's end, as one has the sense that the conclusion is essentially humanitarian. It is people, not cases, who struggle with problems encountered by excessive drug or alcohol use and it is our great gain as clinicians to have privileged access into people's lives! If this book can facilitate access in a way that is more sensitive yet more confident, then the drug treatment field will be the richer.

Nat Wright
Clinical Director for Substance Misuse, Her Majesty's Prison, and
GP advisor, Department of Health, Offender Health Unit

Preface

There have been huge changes in the treatment of addictive behaviours in the past 30 years. The steady development of a scientific evidence base and fluctuating levels of political interest in the topic have led to an evolving and increasingly complex treatment system in the UK and other wealthy countries.

This book has been complied from articles written for the journal *Advances in Psychiatric Treatment*, a key resource to support continuing professional development in psychiatry. The journal first appeared in September 1994, and has focused on topics such as physical methods of treatment, psychosocial treatments, sub-specialties of psychiatry (such as addiction psychiatry) and issues concerning the management of clinical services. The aim has always been to publish useful articles for trained consultant psychiatrists who may, however, have completed their training some years before. It has assumed that readers are familiar with conventional basic terminology and have considerable clinical experience, but may have no expert knowledge in the subject of a particular article.

This book is made up of 20 articles that have appeared in *APT* over the past 10 years, and two newly commissioned chapters. Several articles have been extensively updated by the original author to take into account new developments in the field. Each chapter therefore provides continuing medical education with an emphasis on the practical implications of the subject. They are factual, lucid and informative, with clear information and techniques that can be used in everyday practice. The book is written by practising clinicians for practising clinicians. It highlights and references up-to-date evidence, but its main aim is to synthesise this into information that is useful in clinical practice. Thus, this book has much to offer the specialist, but also the general psychiatrist, psychiatric nurse or general practitioner who is interested in the area.

The book covers 'mainstream' areas within the substance misuse treatment field, but also broadens its scope to less commonly discussed, but no less important, topics. Chapters 1 and 6, by Jason Luty, provide an analysis of the evidence supporting the range of pharmacological and non-pharmacological approaches to drug and alcohol misuse in enough detail to comfortably guide non-specialists managing individuals with such problems. In addition, Duncan Raistrick (chapter 7) gives an extended account of alcohol detoxification, a skill that doctors or nurses practising in all branches of medicine should be acquainted with.

Chapter 2 gives a potted history of the drug treatment system in the UK, highlighting the rapid process of evolution seen in the past 10 years. Chapters 3, 4 and 5 explore the implications of using psychostimulant and hallucinogenic drugs, including khat and magic mushrooms. Nicotine dependence is an extremely common problem, particularly among individuals under the care of psychiatric services, and in chapter 8, Jason Luty explores the evidence for a variety of effective management strategies. By contrast, gambling addiction is a smaller, but growing, problem in the UK, and Sanju George and Vijaya Murali highlight issues surrounding its management in chapter 9.

Chapters 10 and 11 cover the issue of laboratory testing for alcohol and drugs in detail. Clinicians from all specialties may encounter the need for objective testing, particularly in medico-legal work, and it is therefore important to understand the benefits and limitations of the available technologies. The challenging topic of comorbidity of psychiatric illness and substance misuse is covered in detail in chapters 12–15. Ilana Crome and Tracey Myton give a broad overview of the range of pharmacological strategies available for managing these problems (chapter 12), and Mohammed Abou-Saleh (chapter 13) describes the psychosocial context. The most commonly encountered psychiatric problems in users of drugs and alcohol are depression and anxiety, and each is given a chapter. Claire McIntosh and Bruce Ritson (chapter 14) describe the management of depression complicated by substance misuse, and Anne Lingford-Hughes, John Potokar and David Nutt (chapter 15) cover anxiety.

Although great strides have been made in developing pharmacotherapies for addictive behaviours, psychological interventions remain the mainstay of treatment in many cases. Effective interventions are reviewed and described by Adam Huxley and Alex Copello in chapter 16, and motivational interviewing is explored in detail in chapter 17. Motivational interviewing has developed rapidly in terms of theory and evidence for effectiveness in the past 10 years, and has become an essential skill in many areas of psychiatry and behaviour modification.

Addiction in special populations is covered by chapters 18 and 19. Harith Swadi and Sangeeta Ambegaokar give an overview of the unique problems of treating substance misuse problems in adolescents, whereas Sanju George and I focus on pregnancy. There is a strong link between addiction and crime, and two aspects of this relationship and explored in chapters 20 and 21. Medico-legal aspects of intoxication are covered by Quazi Haque and Ian Cumming in chapter 20, and in chapter 21 Peter Snowden reviews violence and substance misuse from the perspective of a forensic psychiatrist.

The final chapter explores what can be learnt from the rich and growing literature about users' subjective perceptions of a variety of psychoactive substances.

Overall, the book aims to be both stimulating and practically useful, and should be a valuable resource in a world where use and misuse of a variety of psychoactive substances is increasing.

Ed Day
Senior Lecturer in Addiction Psychiatry,
Department of Psychiatry, University of Birmingham, Birmingham

CHAPTER 1

What works in drug addiction?

Jason Luty

Summary   Treatment of illicit drug dependence typically involves a combination of pharmacotherapy and psychosocial interventions. Efficacy research supports methadone maintenance in opiate dependence. There is less evidence to support the use of buprenorphine (an opiate receptor partial agonist), lofexidine (an α_2-adrenoreceptor agonist) and naltrexone (an opiate receptor antagonist). Evidence for the effectiveness of detoxification, which is one of the most widely used treatments, is poor. Of the psychosocial interventions, reasonable evidence exists for the effectiveness of motivational interviewing. Other psychosocial treatments have rarely been compared with no or minimal contact conditions in randomised trials, and their reported effectiveness is often weak. Residential treatments are not demonstrably more effective than community programmes.

Substance dependence, or 'addiction', is diagnosed taking several factors into consideration (Box 1.1). Substance misuse refers to the non-therapeutic use of drugs in a manner that is potentially harmful, but does not meet criteria for dependence.

Many trials report significant benefits of addiction treatments (National Consensus Development Panel, 1998), and guidelines for drug addiction treatment have been published by the Department of Health (1999). However, only 20% of participants report abstinence from all illicit substances for at least 1 year, despite receiving treatment. Furthermore, drop-out rates

---

Box 1.1   Diagnostic features for substance dependence

Three or more of the following should have been present in the previous year:
- a compulsion to take the substance
- escalation of amount used
- a withdrawal syndrome following reduction in use
- tolerance
- neglect of other activities in favour of substance use (salience)
- persistent use despite evidence of harm

---

of nearly 50% are common. It is notable that only half of patients with other chronic disorders (such as hypertension or diabetes) fully adhere to medication schedules, and high drop-out rates are common with many forms of psychotherapy.

Trials of treatment for drug addiction are liable to all the common methodological flaws seen in clinical trials in psychiatry, including failure to use intention-to-treat analysis, failure to randomise results, lack of socio-demographically matched control groups and confounding due to unplanned variations in contact with treatment services. A US government report concluded that 'results derived from self-selected patients who remain in treatment optimistically skew findings in favour of effectiveness' (National Research Council, 2002).

There is no consensus on outcome measures of trials of addiction treatments. Urine (and saliva) analysis can provide objective measures of drug use. However, many trials report subjective ratings, such as scores on the Addiction Severity Index (McLellan et al, 1980), a 45 min semi-structured interview based on psychosocial functioning and drug use. Meta-analysis results are often expressed as an effect size: the difference in mean scores divided by the pooled standard deviation. This statistical technique allows the direct comparison of the results of trials that have used different outcome measures. A trial comparing 50–100 users and controls is usually sufficient to identify a treatment with a modest effect size (conventionally 0.25–0.5) that is likely to be clinically significant.

Pharmacotherapy for drug dependence

There are no effective medications for treating stimulant dependence, despite trials of several agents (Bruce, 2000; de Lima et al, 2002; see also chapter 3, this volume). Hence, most research involves treatment of opiate dependence. Commonly used agents are summarised in Table 1.1.

Prescribed maintenance treatment

Maintenance treatment involves the prolonged prescription of a drug with no intention to reduce the dose, whereas detoxification is any treatment intended to produce abstinence from use of drugs (including prescribed drugs).

Methadone and buprenorphine are both long-acting opioid agonists or partial agonists that are used to prevent withdrawal symptoms in opioid addicts. Persistent use leads to cross-tolerance and reduces the reinforcement effects of illicit opiates. Ward et al (1999) have produced an excellent short review of methadone treatment.

An influential meeting of experts in the USA concluded that the safety and efficacy of methadone maintenance treatment 'has been unequivocally established' (National Consensus Development Panel, 1998). Many studies

Table 1.1   Drugs used in opioid dependence

Medication	Action	Typical daily dose
Methadone	Opioid agonist	20–100 mg orally
Buprenorphine	Partial agonist	8–24 mg sublingually
Naltrexone	Opioid agonist	50 mg orally
Lofexidine	α_2-adrenergic agonist	0.8–2.4 mg orally

have shown the advantages of methadone maintenance in reducing drug use, criminality and blood-borne virus infection and improving general health and social status. The median death rate for addicted individuals maintained on methadone is 30% of that for those who are not in treatment. Urine analysis from one sample of 435 methadone maintenance clients showed that almost half were able to quit daily heroin after 12 months (Simpson *et al*, 1997). The average number of 'crime-days' fell from 11 per month to 4. Two large cohort studies suggest that the odds of HIV infection were five times greater among those who were not in methadone maintenance treatment than among those who were (Ward *et al*, 1999).

A classic double-blind study involved 100 heroin addicts in Hong Kong, who were randomised to methadone maintenance or methadone detoxification at 1 mg/day (Newman & Whitehill, 1979). Retention rates were 60% in the maintenance group and 5% in the detoxification group. Urine analysis at 2-year follow-up indicated that 70% of participants in the maintenance group had abstained from illicit opiate use in the previous month. Similar results have been obtained with buprenorphine (Kakko *et al*, 2003).

Methadone doses above 60 mg/day are often required to prevent heroin use. However, it is important to note that initial methadone doses should be less than 40 mg/day to prevent accidental overdose by individuals who have not developed a high tolerance to opiates. One study concluded that patients who receive daily doses of less than 60 mg of methadone have nearly five times the risk of dropping out of treatment than those who receive doses of 80 mg or more (Capelhorn & Bell, 1991). A double-blind trial of 193 intravenous opiate addicts revealed that 53% of the urine samples after 30 weeks were heroin-positive in those randomised to 80–100 mg methadone, compared with 62% of those on 40–50 mg (Strain *et al*, 1999).

Contingency management in methadone maintenance and cocaine treatment

Contingency management techniques make clinic privileges or even continued prescribing available pending objective evidence of abstinence from illicit drugs (see chapter 16).

McCarthy & Borders (1985) reported a controlled trial of 69 individuals in methadone maintenance programmes who were randomised so that for half of them prescribing would be discontinued after 4 consecutive months with one or more opioid-positive urine result. Intention-to-treat analysis indicated that 48% of the participants in the trial sample were drug-free at 1 year compared with 31% in the more liberal control group. Unfortunately, aversive control techniques (such as reduction of methadone) led some individuals to leave treatment. Positive control techniques are reported by Stitzer *et al* (1992) in a study of 53 individuals in methadone maintenance who were randomly assigned to contingent or non-contingent take-home privileges: up to three take-home doses per week were permitted following 2 consecutive weeks of drug-free urine samples. The contingent group produced more individuals with at least 4 consecutive weeks of abstinence (32% *v*. 8%) over the 6-month trial.

Comparable results are reported in a randomised controlled trial of opiate and cocaine addicts in which clean urine samples were rewarded with vouchers that could be exchanged for retail goods (Higgins *et al*, 1994; Preston *et al*, 2000).

Opioid detoxification

Medical detoxification relies on the use of agents, including methadone, buprenorphine, lofexidine or clonidine, in relatively short courses to suppress withdrawal symptoms. The daily dose of methadone can comfortably be reduced at rates of 1 mg/week in the community or 5 mg/day in in-patients. Detoxification is widely used, and it is perhaps surprising to find that it is one of the least effective treatments for drug addiction.

A major problem with opioid detoxification is the rate of relapse. A US follow-up study of 10 000 opiate addicts (the Drug Abuse Reporting Program; Simpson & Friend, 1988) found that individuals entering out-patient detoxification had almost half the abstinence rate at discharge of those who received other types of treatment (12% *v*. 18–21%). The results for Newman & Whitehill's (1979) randomised controlled trial of methadone maintenance described above indicated that detoxification had poor outcomes. The expert National Consensus Development Panel (1998) concluded that 'although the drug-free state represents an optimal treatment goal, research has demonstrated that the state cannot be achieved or sustained by the majority of persons dependent on opiates'.

Other agents used in the treatment of opioid dependence

Clonidine and lofexidine are α_2-adrenoreceptor agonists that reduce somatic symptoms of opioid withdrawal. Opioid detoxification with these agents can be achieved in 5–7 days. However, neither agent can suppress symptoms such as craving, lethargy, insomnia, restlessness and muscle aches. Adverse effects include sedation and hypotension, although these are less common with lofexidine.

A systematic Cochrane review of 10 studies comparing α_2-agonists and methadone detoxification over 10 days found no difference in efficacy, although more clients remained in contact with treatment services following methadone detoxification (Gowing et al, 2002). Kleber et al (1985) reported a trial involving 49 individuals on methadone maintenance randomised to out-patient detoxification with clonidine or reducing doses of methadone over 30 days. Forty per cent completed the detoxification process, of whom one-third were abstinent at 6-month follow-up. An equivalent proportion had returned to methadone maintenance. There was no significant difference in outcome between the groups.

Buprenorphine is a partial opioid agonist and partial antagonist that is given sublingually. It might have a lower risk of overdose than methadone and produce less severe dependence, allowing a smoother withdrawal than methadone. A meta-analysis identified five randomised clinical trials, involving 540 participants over 16–26 weeks. This showed that buprenorphine was comparable with methadone in preventing illicit drug use, although it was more expensive (Barnett et al, 2001). Around 50% of urine tests were positive for illicit opiates. Doses of 8–12 mg/day of buprenorphine have been shown to be as effective as 60–90 mg of methadone (Schottenfeld et al, 1997). The risk that oral buprenorphine will be injected is greater than that for oral methadone, and to deter this a combination of buprenorphine with naloxone has recently been marketed in the UK under the trade name Suboxone (the naloxone nullifies the buprenorphine only when injected).

Naltrexone is an opioid antagonist that produces no psychoactive effects or dependence. Naltrexone completely blocks the effects of opiates and acts as an 'insurance policy' against opiate use. It can precipitate acute withdrawal and should only be used following abstinence from all opioids (including methadone). Treatment can be given daily or three times per week. Unfortunately, naltrexone has not proven effective in treatment settings (Kirchmayer et al, 2002), although peculiarly, some investigators appear to have viewed it as a direct alternative to methadone rather than as an approach that can enable a completely opiate-free state. For example, in one trial only 15 of 300 participants chose naltrexone instead of detoxification or methadone maintenance, and of those 15, only three continued naltrexone for more than 2 months (Fram et al, 1989).

L-alpha-acetylmethadol (LAAM) is a long-acting opiate agonist like methadone. It is not available in the UK, following reports of cardio-toxicity.

Ultra-rapid opiate detoxification

Ultra-rapid opiate detoxification involves administration of opiate antagonists (naloxone and naltrexone) to opiate-dependent individuals under general anaesthesia. This leads to an acute withdrawal. No large-scale controlled trials of this procedure have been published (O'Connor & Kosten, 1998). Concerns about safety, expense and effectiveness also limit its usefulness. In the UK, ultra-rapid opiate detoxification was the subject of a General Medical Council investigation following the death of a patient during recovery, and the anaesthetist involved was struck off the medical register (Bedenoch, 2002). It seems unlikely that there will be any enthusiasm for ultra-rapid opiate detoxification among clinicians in the foreseeable future, although less drastic measures involving sedation rather than anaesthesia are not so controversial.

Injectable opioid treatment

Heroin is available to addicts in the UK from licensed specialists. Parenteral methadone is also available, with licensing not required. Hartnoll *et al* (1980) reported a 12-month follow-up trial of intravenous heroin *v.* oral methadone in 96 heroin-addicted individuals in London. Those on heroin maintenance were twice as likely to remain in treatment (74% *v.* 29%). However, the proportion remaining dependent on opiates (prescribed and illicit) at 12 months was higher in the heroin maintenance group (90% *v.* 70%). There were no differences between the groups for self-reported criminal activity, health or employment. This report led to greatly reduced enthusiasm for injectable opioid treatment. Another UK trial found no advantage between injectable methadone and oral methadone (Strang *et al*, 2000).

Injectable opioid treatment is claimed by some enthusiasts to engage users in treatment more effectively than oral alternatives. Opponents suggest that it perpetuates injecting behaviour and thereby postpones eventual abstinence from heroin and also, in effect, endorses injecting. The treatment is expensive and there is a risk of deep-vein thrombosis and infection. The prospect of being offered injectable opiates may also provide some users with a vested interest in poor adherence to methadone maintenance. Relatively few individuals are ever likely to receive the treatment, so the overall effects on crime will be small. Needle exchange programmes probably reduce health risks more than the prescription of injectables. The available evidence does not support the widespread adoption of injectable opioid treatment.

Psychosocial treatment (see also chapter 16)

Intensity of psychotherapy

Many studies have shown that the intensity and duration of involvement in drug misuse treatment programmes is one of the best predictors of outcome (National Consensus Development Panel, 1998). However, the 'more is better' idea is often based on uncontrolled follow-up studies, in which patient motivation and selection might be primarily responsible for the good outcome.

Kraft *et al* (1997) reported a trial of 100 opiate-addicted individuals, randomised to three psychosocial treatments of 6 months duration: minimum-contact methadone maintenance; methadone maintenance plus standard drug counselling three times weekly; and an enhanced programme of psychosocial treatment with daily counselling, family therapy and social work activity to improve job prospects, housing and address other social problems. However, many of the participants who were randomised to the enhanced programme actually attended only once each week, despite the offer of more-frequent sessions. All participants received 60–90 mg methadone per day. Abstinence from opiates and cocaine use at 1 year were 29%, 47% and 49% of participants in the minimum-contact, standard and enhanced groups respectively. Overall, the enhanced programme did not confer significant benefit over standard drug counselling, although it was better than minimum-contact methadone maintenance. A cost-effectiveness analysis confirmed this.

Narcotics Anonymous and its Twelve-Step Approach

Narcotics Anonymous provides support groups for problem drug users. These groups are widely available and are free to participants. Applying the disease model to substance misuse, they promote the Twelve-Step Approach. This involves recognition that addiction is a relapsing illness that requires complete abstinence (Box 1.2). Participants are required to acknowledge their addiction and the harm they are causing themselves and others. No randomised controlled trial has attempted to determine the effectiveness of Narcotics Anonymous or of 12-step approaches in opiate addiction. However, a study of 487 cocaine users, all of whom received group twelve-step drug counselling throughout the trial, involved randomisation to individual counselling (based on the Twelve-Step Approach), supportive–expressive psychotherapy or cognitive–behavioural therapy (CBT) with a 1-year follow-up (Crits-Christoph *et al*, 1999). One-third of the eligible cocaine users initially approached were recruited, of whom 28% completed the 6-month treatment programmes. Cocaine use was reduced from a mean of 10 days per month to only 3 days. However, 71% of the group receiving a combination of individual and group counselling were abstinent for at least 1 month, compared with 55–60% for combinations of group counselling with formal psychotherapy. The psychotherapy approaches were able to retain more participants in treatment (33% completed treatment *v.* 22% for drug counselling). Similarly, Wells *et al* (1994) report a controlled comparison of CBT-based relapse prevention *v.* 12-step approaches in out-patient treatment of 110 cocaine users. The two treatments were equally effective at 1 year, and the number of days of cocaine use halved. Overall, the evidence suggests that a 12-step approach is at least as effective as other structured psychotherapies.

Box 1.2 The Twelve Steps of Narcotics Anonymous

1 We admitted that we were powerless over our addiction, that our lives had become unmanageable.
2 We came to believe that a Power greater than ourselves could restore us to sanity.
3 We made a decision to turn our will and our lives over to the care of God as we understood Him.
4 We made a searching and fearless moral inventory of ourselves.
5 We admitted to God, to ourselves, and to another human being the exact nature of our wrongs.
6 We were entirely ready to have God remove all these defects of character.
7 We humbly asked Him to remove our shortcomings.
8 We made a list of all persons we had harmed, and became willing to make amends to them all.
9 We made direct amends to such people wherever possible, except when to do so would injure them or others.
10 We continued to take personal inventory and when we were wrong promptly admitted it.
11 We sought through prayer and meditation to improve our conscious contact with God as we understood Him, praying only for knowledge of His will for us and the power to carry that out.
12 Having had a spiritual awakening as a result of these steps, we tried to carry this message to addicts, and to practice these principles in all our affairs.

Relapse prevention and cognitive–behavioural therapy

Relapse prevention techniques using CBT are based on the work of Marlatt & Gordon (1985). The techniques assume that substance misuse is a means of coping with difficult situations, dysphoric mood and peer pressure. Treatment aims to help individuals recognise high-risk situations and either avoid or cope with them without drug use.

Irvin *et al* (1999) reported a meta-analysis of five randomised controlled trials of relapse prevention treatment for polydrug misuse. The overall effect was modest. For example, Carroll *et al* (1994) compared CBT-based treatment with routine clinical management over 1 year for cocaine addicts. They found that CBT was superior only for participants who were also depressed and for those with high levels of cocaine use. Wells *et al* (1994) found no difference between CBT-based relapse prevention and a 12-step approach in cocaine users (see above).

In one randomised controlled trial involving 64 amphetamine users, 2–4 CBT/motivational interviewing sessions were compared with provision of a self-help booklet. Participants typically attended half the sessions. Twenty-four (38%) of the treatment group abstained from amphetamine use, compared with 13 (21%) of the self-help group (Baker *et al*, 2001).

Overall, CBT approaches are better researched, but are probably no more effective than the other psychological methods used in addiction treatment.

Psychodynamic psychotherapy

There is a widespread opinion that psychodynamic psychotherapy is of low acceptability to drug misusers, as illustrated by a trial of interpersonal psychodynamic psychotherapy with 72 opiate addicts in methadone maintenance (Rounsaville *et al*, 1983). Weekly individual interpersonal therapy was compared with monthly 'low-contact' control treatment. Both treatments continued for 6 months. Only 5% of eligible clients agreed to attend psychotherapy and only 38% of these completed the interpersonal therapy programme. There were no significant differences in outcome between the two groups, although both made significant gains. Woody *et al* (1995) reported a similar randomised trial of supportive–expressive psychotherapy, in which the overall effect size was small (0.26). Other investigators have failed to find advantages for psychodynamic psychotherapy in substance misuse (Crits-Christoph *et al*, 1999).

Motivational interviewing/motivational enhancement therapy

Motivational interviewing is a technique described by Miller & Rollnick (2002). It is based on theories of cognitive dissonance and attempts to promote a favourable attitude towards change. Briefly, instructing addicts on the problems of dependency and the advantages of abstinence tends to provoke them to contradiction. This might reinforce continued dependence. Motivational interviewing encourages clients to give their own reasons for attempting to change their drug use (see chapters 16 and 17).

A systematic review identified five randomised trials of motivational interviewing in drug dependence, involving 800 participants (Dunn *et al*, 2001). Typical effect sizes were 0.5–0.6 (although confidence intervals were large). One randomised trial of 122 opiate addicts found that motivational interviewing compared with health education alone increased retention in methadone programmes at 6 months from 50% to 70% (Saunders *et al*, 1995). Booth *et al* (1998) reported a trial of 4000 intravenous drug users seeking HIV testing. Individuals were randomly assigned to either standard testing alone or testing plus three sessions of motivational counselling from a health educator. At 6-month follow-up, the latter group showed half the rate of drug injection (20% *v.* 45%) and were four times more likely to be abstinent (confirmed by urine analysis). They also had significantly lower arrest rates (14% *v.* 24%).

9

Community reinforcement, couple and family therapies

Reinforcement treatments typically involve clients' partners or families rewarding them for abstinence using agreed strategies. Stanton & Shadish (1997) performed a meta-analysis of 15 randomised controlled trials, involving 1571 opiate addicts, that compared couple/family therapy with individual counselling, peer-group therapy and family psychoeducation. Six of the trials involved adult clients. Family therapy methods had an effect size at 1 year that was 0.46 greater than that for non-family therapy. The drop-out rate was also lower in the family therapy group (~45% v. ~25%).

Community reinforcement using families and couples is feasible and shows some effectiveness, although it is often overlooked. Not all clients have family members or partners who are willing to be involved in substance misuse treatment. However, where they can be recruited as co-therapists, family members can be encouraged to provide agreed rewards to clients for abstinence. The nature of the reward needs to be negotiated in advance with the client and family member. Family members also provide a degree of surveillance over the clients and can provide supervision, support, advice or comment if clients begin using drugs again, feel tempted or put themselves in risk situations.

Therapeutic communities and residential rehabilitation units

These units typically require prolonged residence (often 12–18 months). Clients are closely involved in running the programmes, including selecting and discharging residents. Abstinence is usually a prerequisite. Several large studies suggest that therapeutic communities are beneficial, although completion rates for prolonged residential programmes are often below 20%.

Bale *et al* (1980) randomly assigned 585 male heroin addicts to methadone maintenance or therapeutic communities. The outcomes between the two groups were comparable. Roughly half of the participants who completed the programmes reported heroin use during the 12th (and final) month of the study. Unfortunately, only 18% of the participants randomised to the therapeutic communities actually began the 6-month residential programmes. Overall, only 10% of participants successfully engaged in either of the programmes to which they had been assigned.

The National Treatment Outcome Research study is a follow-up of 1075 clients (most of whom were addicted to heroin) attending UK drug treatment agencies (Gossop *et al*, 2003). At 5 years, 42% of those who were attending community methadone programmes at the start of the study were regularly using heroin, compared with 39% of those who were in residential programmes at intake (and were subsequently discharged). Although the study was not randomised, these results support North American research demonstrating that residential programmes are no more effective than community programmes, despite the greatly increased cost.

Other approaches

Drug treatment and testing orders were introduced in the UK under the Crime and Disorder Act 1998. Orders last from 6 months to 3 years. Under the relevant legislation, courts can require an offender to undergo treatment for drug misuse, subject to the offender's consent to such an order being made. Offenders are required to undergo testing for use of illicit substances and to 'submit' to treatment. If treatment is not satisfactory or clients reoffend, the court may sentence them again. Turnbull et al (2000) report the results of the pilot programmes, which involved 210 offenders. The percentage of opioid-positive urine tests (excluding methadone) fell from 42% to 13%. However, about half of the offenders were discharged from the orders for breach of terms. These results are disappointing, despite US reviews suggesting that coerced offenders do no worse than voluntary clients (Anglin & Hser, 1991). In the UK, a government report concluded that 'because of lack of investment in data and research, the nation is in no better position to evaluate the effectiveness of enforcement than it was 20 years ago' (National Research Council, 2002).

Needle exchanges have been widely adopted, their main purpose being to prevent transmission of HIV and hepatitis. Most surveys have concluded that they are effective in reducing needle sharing and blood-borne viruses and they encourage drug users to seek help. Needle exchange programmes do not appear to have caused an increase in injecting (Royal College of Psychiatrists, 2000: p. 161). An Australian study concluded that the cost-effectiveness of needle exchanges varied from Aus$50 to Aus$7000 per life-year saved. There are no randomised controlled trials of needle exchange schemes or drug treatment and testing orders.

Conclusion

What works in drug addiction? Methadone maintenance has been shown to be safe and very effective on a variety of measures, including preventing illicit drug use. Buprenorphine is probably equally effective, although it is more expensive in some countries. Reasonable evidence exists for the effectiveness of motivational interviewing. Few randomised controlled trials compare other psychosocial treatments and no or minimal contact. However, where evidence does exist, the effect size is often modest. Evidence for the effectiveness of detoxification is poor, even though this is one of the most widely used treatments. Residential treatments are not demonstrably more effective than community programmes.

References

Anglin, M. D. & Hser, Y. I. (1991) Criminal justice and the drug-abusing offender: policy issues of coerced treatment. *Behavioural Sciences and the Law*, **9**, 243–267.

Baker, A., Boggs, T. G. & Lewin, T. J. (2001) Randomised controlled trial of brief cognitive–behavioural interventions among regular users of amphetamine. *Addiction*, **96**, 1279–1287.

Bale, R. N., Stone, W. W. V., Kuldau, J. M., *et al* (1980) Therapeutic communities vs methadone maintenance. *Archives of General Psychiatry*, **37**, 179–193.

Barnett, P. G., Rodgers, J. H. & Bloch, D. A. (2001) A meta-analysis comparing buprenorphine to methadone for treatment of opiate dependence. *Addiction*, **96**, 683–690.

Bedenoch, J. (2002) A death following ultra-rapid opiate detoxification. *Addiction*, **97**, 475–477.

Booth, R. E., Kwiatkowski, C., Iguchi, M. Y., *et al* (1998) Facilitating treatment entry among out-of-treatment injection drug users. *Public Health Report*, **113** (suppl. 1), s116–s128.

Bruce, M. (2000) Managing amphetamine dependence. *Advances in Psychiatric Treatment*, **6**, 33–40.

Capelhorn, J. R. & Bell, J. (1991) Methadone dosage and retention of patients in maintenance treatment. *Medical Journal of Australia*, **154**, 195–199.

Carroll, K. M., Rounsaville, B. J. & Gordon, L. T. (1994) Psychotherapy and pharmacotherapy for ambulatory cocaine abusers. *Archives of General Psychiatry*, **51**, 989–997.

Crits-Christoph, P., Siquel, L., Blaine, J., *et al* (1999) Psychosocial treatments for cocaine dependence. *Archives of General Psychiatry*, **56**, 493–502.

de Lima, M. S., de Oliveria Soares, B. G., Reisser, A. A., *et al* (2002) Pharmacological treatment of cocaine dependence: a systematic review. *Addiction*, **97**, 931–949.

Department of Health (1999) *Drug Misuse and Dependence – Guidelines on Clinical Management*. TSO (The Stationery Office).

Dunn, C., Deroo, L. & Rivara, F. P. (2001) The use of brief interventions adapted from motivational interviewing across behavioural domains: a systematic review. *Addiction*, **96**, 1725–1742.

Fram, D. M., Marmo, J. & Holden, R. (1989) Naltrexone treatment – the problem of patient acceptance. *Journal of Substance Abuse Treatment*, **6**, 119–122.

Gossop, M., Marsden, J., Stewart, D., *et al* (2003) The national treatment outcome research study: 4–5 year follow-up results. *Addiction*, **98**, 291–303.

Gowing, L. R., Farrell, M., Ali, R. L., *et al* (2002) Alpha-2-adrenergic agonists in opioid withdrawal. *Addiction*, **97**, 49–58.

Hartnoll, R. L., Mitcheson, M. C., Battersby, A., *et al* (1980) Evaluation of heroin maintenance in controlled trial. *Archives of General Psychiatry*, **37**, 877–884.

Higgins, S. T., Budney, A. J. & Bickel, W. K. (1994) Incentives improve outcome in outpatient behavioural treatment of cocaine dependence. *Archives of General Psychiatry*, **51**, 568–576.

Irvin, J. E., Bowers, C. A., Dunn, M. E., *et al* (1999) Efficacy of relapse prevention: a meta-analytic review. *Journal of Consulting and Clinical Psychology*, **67**, 563–570.

Kakko, J., Svanborg, K. D., Kreek, M. J., *et al* (2003) 1-year retention and social function after buprenorphine-assisted relapse prevention treatment for heroin dependence in Sweden: a randomized, placebo-controlled trial. *Lancet*, **361**, 662–668.

Kirchmayer, U., Davloi, M., Vester, A. D., *et al* (2002) A systematic review of the efficacy of naltrexone maintenance treatment in opioid dependence. *Addiction*, **97**, 1241–1249.

Kleber, H. D., Riordan, C. E., Rounsaville, B., *et al* (1985) Clonidine in out-patient detoxification from methadone maintenance. *Archives of General Psychiatry*, **42**, 391–394.

Kraft, M. K., Rothbard, A. B. & Hadley, T. R. (1997) Are supplemental services provided during methadone maintenance really cost-effective? *American Journal of Psychiatry*, **154**, 1214–1219.

Marlatt, G. A., & Gordon, J. R. (1985) *Relapse Prevention*. Guilford Press.

McCarthy, J. J. & Borders, O. T. (1985) Limit setting on drug abuse in methadone maintenance patients. *American Journal of Psychiatry*, **142**, 1419–1423.

McLellan, A. I., Luborsky, L., Woody, G. E., *et al* (1980) An improved diagnostic instrument for substance abuse patients: the Addiction Severity Index. *Journal of Nervous and Mental Diseases*, **168**, 26–33.

Miller, W. R. & Rollnick, S. (2002) *Motivational Interviewing: Preparing People to Change Addictive Behaviour*. Guilford Press.

National Consensus Development Panel (1998) Effective medical treatment of opiate addiction. *JAMA*, **280**, 1936–1943.

National Research Council (2002) Executive summary of the National Research Council's report 'Informing America's policy on illegal drugs: what we don't know keeps hurting us'. *Addiction*, **97**, 647–652.

Newman, R. G. & Whitehill, W. B. (1979) Double-blind comparison of methadone and placebo maintenance treatment of narcotic addicts in Hong Kong. *Lancet*, **2**, 484–488.

O'Connor, P. G. & Kosten, T. R. (1998) Rapid and ultra-rapid opioid detoxification techniques. *JAMA*, **279**, 229–234.

Preston, K. L., Umbricht, A. & Epstein, D. H. (2000) Methadone dose increase and abstinence reinforcement for treatment of continued heroin use during methadone maintenance. *Archives of General Psychiatry*, **57**, 395–404.

Rounsaville, B. J., Glazer, W., Wilber, C. H., et al (1983) Short-term interpersonal psychotherapy in methadone-maintained opiate addicts. *Archives of General Psychiatry*, **40**, 629–636.

Royal College of Psychiatrists (2000) *Drugs: Dilemmas and Choices*. Gaskell.

Saunders, B., Wilkinson, C. & Phillips, M. (1995) The impact of a brief motivational intervention with opiate users attending a methadone programme. *Addiction*, **90**, 415–424.

Schottenfeld, R. S., Pakes, J. R. & Oliveto, A. (1997) Buprenorphine versus methadone maintenance treatment for concurrent opioid dependence and cocaine abuse. *Archives of General Psychiatry*, **54**, 713–720.

Simpson, D. D. & Friend, J. (1988) Legal status and long-term outcomes from addicts in the DARP follow-up project. In *Compulsory Treatment of Drug Abuse* (eds C. G. Leukefield & F. M. Tims), pp. 81–98 (National Institute of Drug Abuse Research Monographs, no. 86). US Department of Health and Human Services.

Simpson, D. D., Joe, G. W. & Rowan-Szal, G. A. (1997) Drug abuse treatment retention and process effects on follow-up outcomes. *Drug and Alcohol Dependence*, **47**, 227–235.

Stanton, M. D. & Shadish, W. R. (1997) Outcome, attrition and family-couples treatment for drug abuse: a meta-analysis and review of controlled, comparative studies. *Psychological Bulletin*, **122**, 170–191.

Stitzer, M. L., Iguchi, M. Y. & Flech, L. J. (1992) Contingent take-home incentive: effects on drug use on methadone maintenance patients. *Journal of Consulting and Clinical Psychology*, **60**, 927–934.

Strain, E. C., Bigelow, G. E., Liebson, I. A., et al (1999) Moderate- vs high-dose methadone: a randomised trial. *JAMA*, **281**, 1000–1005.

Strang, J., Marsden, M., Cummins, M., et al (2000) Randomised trial of supervised injectable versus oral methadone maintenance. *Addiction*, **95**, 1631–1645.

Turnbull, P. J., McSweeney, T., Webster, R., et al (2000) *Drug Treatment and Testing Orders: Final Evaluation Report* (Home Office Research Study 212). Home Office.

Ward, J., Hall, W. & Mattick, R. P. (1999) Role of maintenance treatment in opioid dependence. *Lancet*, **353**, 221–226.

Wells, E. A., Peterson, P. L. & Gainey, R. R. (1994) Outpatient treatment for cocaine abuse: a controlled comparison of relapse prevention and twelve-step approaches. *American Journal of Drug and Alcohol Abuse*, **20**, 1–17.

Woody, G. E., McLellan, A. T., Luborsky, L., et al (1995) Psychotherapy in community methadone programs. *American Journal of Psychiatry*, **152**, 1302–1308.

CHAPTER 2

The development of the drug treatment system in England

David Best, Sanju George and Ed Day

Summary   Addiction treatment in England has evolved gradually over a period of more than 100 years, as theoretical models of treatment have changed and public concerns about addiction have ebbed and flowed. However, the past 20 years have seen a greater level of public spending on reducing levels of drug addiction, and with this has come a greater level of scrutiny of treatment services. Central government targets have been set in relation to both attracting drug users into treatment and retaining them for set periods of time. This chapter outlines the historical developments in drug treatment provision, the current position in terms of both what is typically available and the underlying structures and systems, and suggests some indicators of whether a local treatment system is working effectively and delivering adequate outcomes.

Historical overview of policy developments and evolution of treatment services

We will begin by summarising key policy developments in England and the resulting addiction treatment services, with specific focus on the so-called 'British system' (Spear, 2005). Although this summary provides a chronological account of the evolution of Britain's drug policies (Box 2.1), it is recommended that it be read in conjunction with two key references: Strang & Gossop (2005a,b) and Spear (2002). Space precludes detailed descriptions of the socio-political context within which the various British drug policies have developed, although it is worth noting that dramatic and unplanned shifts in policy have often been the result of a combination of changing political ideals, social structures and medical ideologies, rather than the consequence of any better understanding of addiction.

The 18th and 19th centuries

Although the origins of the British system are often traced to the Rolleston Report of 1926 (Ministry of Health, 1926), Berridge (2005) describes three systems that existed in Britain in the 18th and 19th centuries: the lay or

---

Box 2.1 Chronology of the evolution of the British system

- The early British system
  - The lay/commercial system (18th and 19th centuries)
  - The pharmaceutical control system (Pharmacy Act 1868)
  - The medico-penal system (early 20th century)
- The new British system
  - The Rolleston Report (1926)
  - The First Brain Report (1961)
  - The Second Brain Report (1965)
- The harm reduction approach (1980s)
- The crime reduction approach (1990s)

---

commercial control system, the pharmaceutical control system and the medico-penal system. During the 18th and initial part of the 19th centuries, opium was freely available in pharmacies, grocers and other general stores. There was no regulation on its sale or purchase and, like alcohol, it was marketed just as any other product, i.e. subject to a lay or commercial control system. However, the Pharmacy Act of 1868 formalised a control system in which only pharmacies were allowed to stock and sell opium, although a doctor's prescription was still not required. This shift in policy came about not because of health concerns or the addictive properties of opium but because of an attempt by pharmacies to attain control of this lucrative business. The 20th century saw the emergence of the third British system – the medico-penal system, with greater cooperation between doctors and the Home Office ensuring that a doctor's prescription was required to buy opiates, and a greater degree of governmental regulation of the supply of drugs.

The Rolleston Report and the new British system

The term British system as we understand it today was first used by E. W. Adams, the secretary to the Departmental Committee on Morphine and Heroin Addiction (the Rolleston Committee) (Adams, 1937). The UK Department of Health set up the committee in 1924 to assess whether opiates could be prescribed to addicts for treatment purposes. The Rolleston Report (Ministry of Health, 1926) recommended heroin prescription under these circumstances as a valid treatment for managing withdrawal symptoms and helping addicts sustain a normal life. Although the Home Office was the overall regulatory body, the medical profession had considerable authority and autonomy in prescribing opiates for addicts. The new British system also enshrined the principle of close collaboration between the medical profession and the penal/legal system.

Until about the mid to late 1950s, the British system (of treating opiate addicts as patients rather than criminals, and legitimising the provision of substitute opiate treatment) was believed to have kept drug dependence in check. However, despite its strengths, it was not without critics, and has been interpreted as having a social-class bias, favouring 'professional addicts' (addicted doctors and nurses) and 'therapeutic addicts' (in whom addiction was induced as a consequence of medical treatment). It is also possible that the 'success' of the Rolleston Report was a result of, and not the cause of, the low prevalence of drug problems in the UK. Downes (1977: p. 89) summed up this dissatisfaction by describing the British system (which was neither a system nor strictly British) as 'little more than masterly inactivity in the face of what was an almost non-existent addiction problem'.

The 1960s and 1970s: the Brain Reports

From the end the Second World War until the 1960s, the number of identified opiate addicts in the UK had remained largely static and fairly small (typically 400–600). However, the 1960s saw a change in the sociocultural climate and an increase in heroin use by young people, such that by 1968 there were nearly 1300 known new non-therapeutic heroin addicts (Bewley, 2005). As the Rolleston Report and ensuing policy frameworks were not able to contain this 'heroin epidemic', the Ministry of Health established the Interdepartmental Committee on Drug Addiction, chaired by Sir Russell Brain. The Committee's initial remit was to examine the increasing prevalence of drug misuse and assess the need for policy change. Although the First Brain Report (Ministry of Health, 1961) made no recommendations for change, by 1964 the problem had worsened, prompting the Committee to reconvene. The resulting Second Brain Report (Ministry of Health, 1965) recommended the setting up of clinics to treat addicts, compulsory notification of addicts to the Home Office and the requirement that only doctors with a Home Office license would be permitted to prescribe heroin and cocaine.

The first drug treatment clinics were set up in 1967, mainly in London and often attached to district general hospitals (Ministry of Health, 1967). They were headed by consultant psychiatrists and included multidisciplinary teams, for the comprehensive assessment and treatment of addicts. Over the next two decades drug dependency units were opened by most regional health authorities across the UK. As the oral methadone maintenance approach gathered momentum and developed a robust evidence base in the USA, clinics providing this relatively new treatment started to appear in the UK. However, even in the early days such clinics offered a range of psychosocial interventions in addition to substitute medication, including the support of social workers, counselling and group therapy.

1980s: the harm reduction agenda

The introduction of the drug dependency units did not prevent widespread escalation in drug use or the increasing prevalence of intravenous administration of heroin and cocaine. When awareness of HIV and its causes first developed in 1985, public health experts began to take an interest in drug addicts and drug addiction. This resulted in the evolution of the 'harm reduction' movement and its associated interventions – needle and syringe exchange schemes, outreach working and easily accessible (so-called low-threshold) substitute prescribing. This represented the first of two significant paradigm shifts in the UK, from an individual health to a public health perspective. This translated into a shift in treatment goals from a primary focus on abstinence to a pragmatic approach emphasising the provision of services to reduce harm incurred by the user and accrued by the community, based on interventions targeting prevention of the dissemination of blood-borne viruses. In 1988 a report by the Advisory Council on the Misuse of Drugs entitled *AIDS and Drug Misuse* marked a major turning point in government policy towards harm reduction. The report stated that:

'the spread of HIV is a greater threat to individual and public health than drug misuse. Accordingly, we believe that services which aim to minimise HIV risk behaviour by all means should take precedence in development plans' (Advisory Council on the Misuse of Drugs, 1988: p. 75).

Although provision of clean injecting equipment was the core activity of the new needle exchange services, they also provided other harm minimisation measures such as advice on safe sex and safe injecting, general health advice and screening for blood-borne viruses. They also acted as a conduit into further, more structured treatment. By 1990 there were over 200 needle exchange schemes in the UK. Research evaluation has identified the great success of such harm minimisation measures in the UK, with lower rates of HIV infection seen here than in other parts of Europe (European Monitoring Centre for Drugs and Drug Addiction, 2006).

The 1980s also saw a massive expansion in substitute prescribing to opiate addicts, partly in response to increasing prevalence of use and the resulting harms. Such a development was also linked to an increased demand for evidence of the effectiveness of drug treatment, culminating in the report of the Task Force to Review Services for Drug Misusers (1996). The delivery of treatment services was also evolving. In 1982 the Advisory Council on the Misuse of Drugs called for the setting up of 'community drug teams' in each health authority. The purpose of these teams was to provide community-based treatment services for a much larger population of drug misusers, with less emphasis on hospital-based provision. Community drug teams have now been established in most regions of the UK to provide a range of interventions and to work in close collaboration with agencies such as criminal justice services, social services and local housing departments. Finally, the 1980s also saw the development of the 'district drug advisory committees', which could be considered the precursor of the current 'drug action teams'.

The 1990s: the crime reduction agenda

During the 1990s there was a second paradigm shift in the treatment of drug dependence, with the rationale for treatment moving from a public health agenda to a public safety agenda predicated on crime reduction. From the influential National Treatment Outcome Research Study (Gossop *et al*, 2001), a product of the Task Force review mentioned above, it had become evident that drug treatment was associated with marked reductions in involvement in acquisitive crime. The guiding mantra from the study adopted by policy makers was that for every £1 spent on treating drug users there is a saving in cost of £3 to society. In other words, tackling drug misuse was a mechanism by which seemingly intractable crime problems could be addressed.

This led to a raft of initiatives to expand access to treatment, particularly routes through the criminal justice system, targeting those who had never previously received treatment and those who had dropped out of contact with treatment services. This was part of a process of centralisation of drug treatment initially characterised by the introduction of a 'drugs czar' based in the Cabinet Office, in a team called the UK Anti-Drug Co-ordination Unit (UKADCU). This was superseded in 2001 by a more formal hierarchical structure involving three tiers. At the centre was the National Treatment Agency for Substance Misuse (NTA), linked to both the Department of Health and the Home Office, whose role was to oversee the implementation of the government's national strategy 'Tackling Drugs to Build a Better Britain' (Home Office, 1998). This was achieved through a regional structure involving teams based in the nine regional government offices in England, within which 149 local partnerships (called drug action teams and described later in this chapter) were responsible for managing the overall treatment budget and its links to target-setting.

This transition to a centralised interventionist policy was also associated with a shift in departmental ownership of drug policy and service funding within government, with the primacy of health being eroded and the Home Office coming to occupy a more prominent role in a system in which crime reduction had become the primary motivator for expanding drug treatment provision. Initially, this shift took the form of interventions mandated by the courts (in the form of drug treatment and testing orders – DTTOs), police custody initiatives (arrest referral schemes) and work in prisons (in the form of counselling, advice, referral, assessment and throughcare – CARAT – initiatives). However, increasingly the focus moved to bespoke interventions designed to address the needs of drug-using offenders. Preliminary evaluations (Turnbull *et al*, 2000; Finch *et al*, 2003) indicated that drug treatment and testing orders were a cost-effective, useful and patient-friendly means of treating drug misusers and protecting society, although Edmunds *et al* (1998) had shown equally positive outcomes for arrest referral schemes.

Intervention through the criminal justice service was formalised further by the introduction of the Drug Intervention Programme in 2003, effectively creating an umbrella agency to facilitate communication and integration between criminal justice (police, prisons, probation officers and courts) and treatment agencies. By joining up a variety of professional agencies, the aim of the Drug Intervention Programme was to make contact with drug-using offenders at the police station, in courts and through the prison system, and to direct them to treatment, using a range of incentives and mandates. Furthermore, attention was focused on the need for effective case management for drug-using offenders by linking them to the appropriate housing, employment, counselling and support services, and in doing so reducing both drug use and offending.

National strategies, local structures and target-setting

The increasingly complex drug treatment system has been coordinated through two successive national strategies: 'Tackling Drugs Together: A Strategy for England, 1995–1998' (Home Office, 1995) and 'Tackling Drugs to Build a Better Britain' (Home Office, 1998; Box 2.2). These documents were subsequently underpinned in 2001 by the launch of the above-mentioned three-tier hierarchical structure led nationally by the NTA. Much of the treatment provision described below is overseen by this structure.

Changing role of the GP within the British system

Although the role of the general practitioner (GP) appeared to have diminished with the development of specialised treatment centres for substance addiction, the GP has always been a critical part of the 'treatment system'. Thus, while the Second Brain Report (Ministry of Health, 1965) resulted in a diminution of the GP's role in treating addicts, this trend was reversed in the early 1980s in response to the increasing scale of the problem. In its 1982 report, the Advisory Council on the Misuse of Drugs stated that 'with strict safeguards there is a possible role for some doctors outside the specialist services to play a part in the treatment of problem drug takers' (p. 56). A further enhancement of this role came with the Council's first report on AIDS and drug misuse (Advisory Council on the Misuse of Drugs, 1988), which noted that 'the network of GPs offers an unrivalled system of health care provision with great opportunities for intervention with drug misusing patients' (Glanz, 2005).

This expansion of the GP role has gained further impetus in the past 10 years. The NHS Plan (Department of Health, 2000) saw the creation of the 'general practitioner with special interest' (GPwSI). It is intended that such

---

Box 2.2 Key elements of the 'Tackling Drugs to Build a Better Britain' strategy (1998–2008)

- Young people – to reduce drug misuse among young people
- Communities – to protect communities from drug-related crime
- Treatment – to provide drug misusers with biopsychosocial treatment
- Availability – to reduce the availability of drugs on the streets

---

Box 2.3 Definition of shared care

Shared care 'is the joint participation of specialists and GPs (and other agencies as appropriate) in the planned delivery of care for patients with a drug misuse problem, informed by an enhanced information exchange beyond routine discharge and referral letters. It may involve the day-to-day management by the GP of a patient's medical needs in relation to his or her drug misuse. Such arrangements would make explicit which clinician was responsible for different aspects of the patient's treatment and care. They may include prescribing substitute drugs in appropriate circumstances' (Department of Health, 1995).

---

individuals take referrals from fellow GPs, thus providing an intermediate level of expertise between the generalist and the specialist. To support this in the field of substance misuse, the Royal College of General Practitioners provides an accredited qualification for GPwSIs – the certificate in the management of drug misuse (http://www.rcgp.org.uk/substance_misuse/substance_misuse_home/substance_misuse_certificate.aspx). Similarly, the Department of Health (1999) recommended a 'shared care' framework (Box 2.3), based on close, collaborative working between primary (GPs) and secondary care (addiction specialists). This role has become particularly important in the Drug Intervention Programme initiative in which GPs, often employed on a part-time basis, provide both prescribing and essential medical services to offenders engaged in drug treatment. For further clarification on the potential roles of GPs, general psychiatrists and addiction psychiatrists see Royal College of Psychiatrists & Royal College of General Practitioners (2005).

Summary

The defining feature of the British system is its lack of rigid structure and tightly defined policies, and it is this that has given it the scope and flexibility to change shape and direction in response to changing circumstances. While commentators continue to debate the effectiveness of the British system, it has provided a flexible framework that has allowed shifts in policies and philosophies to be assimilated within a basic model of evidence-based clinical practice.

The current context and provision of drug treatment in England

The key starting point for describing the current drug treatment system is Models of Care for Treatment of Adult Drug Misusers (National Treatment Agency for Substance Misuse, 2002, 2006) (Box 2.4), the proxy national service framework for drug treatment provision for England.

Box 2.4 Key tenets of Models of Care, 2006

- Four-tiered commissioning model
- Local screening and assessment systems
- Care-planned and coordinated structured drug treatment
- Integrated care pathways

The Models of Care guidance requires commissioners within the 149 drug action team areas in England to provide services across four tiers:

- Tier 1   Generic agencies (such as the police and hospitals) that can screen problem substance misuse and refer to specialist agencies (normally Tier 3), including a wide range of professionals such as social workers, GPs, community pharmacists and teachers
- Tier 2   Open-access drug and alcohol treatment services, offering easy access to services (so-called low-threshold access) and providing harm reduction support and activities to drug users. These include advice, information and referral services, needle and syringe exchanges and outreach provision
- Tier 3   Structured community-based drug treatment services, including psychotherapeutic interventions such as structured counselling and opiate substitute maintenance programmes. These services have a higher threshold and require patients to sign a plan outlining treatment goals.
- Tier 4   Residential services for drug and alcohol misusers. Services are split into two distinct groups:
  - Tier 4a services are aimed at individuals with a high level of presenting need and they are provided in both specialist medically supervised (in-patient) settings and longer-term residential rehabilitation settings
  - Tier 4b services are highly specialised hospital services such as liver units and infectious disease units that drug and alcohol users may need to access on a residential basis.

See Box 2.5 for some examples of the four service tiers.

The underlying principle of the tiered system is that all drug action teams should have equality of access to all of the above provision (although the providers, particularly for residential services, will not necessarily be located within a particular team's regional boundaries). Models of Care specifies that treatment commissioning within each of the drug action team areas should be needs-led, and that strategic commissioning should ensure ease and speed of access to services that have been shown to be effective and are consistent with the expressed wishes and care-planned needs of service users.

Box 2.5   Examples of the four service tiers

Tier 1 – Housing, social services

Tier 2 – Harm reduction services, outreach services

Tier 3 – Community drug teams

Tier 4 – In-patient drug treatment (detoxification and rehabilitation) services

---

So how effectively has this package of treatment been delivered? The process for ensuring its delivery has been through a commissioning system in which regional NTA teams have worked with local partnerships (superseding drug action teams in many areas) through a detailed treatment planning process that attempts both to evaluate current provision and to plan future provision. This has undoubtedly been linked to a huge increase in treatment uptake. As shown in Fig. 2.1, the number of adults in England in contact with drug treatment services increased from around 80000 in 1998/99 to 153000 in 2004/05. This is in line with the Department of Health's Public Service Agreement target of doubling the numbers of problem drug users in contact with structured treatment services in the course of a year to 160000 by 2008. This target was based on an initial estimate of 280000 problem drug users (Frisher *et al*, 2004).

But what do people typically receive from the drug treatment system? There are two ways of examining this question: taking a cross-sectional

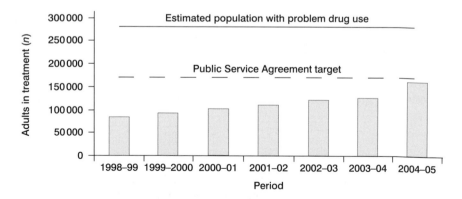

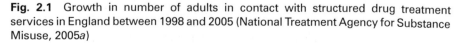

Fig. 2.1 Growth in number of adults in contact with structured drug treatment services in England between 1998 and 2005 (National Treatment Agency for Substance Misuse, 2005*a*)

approach or a longitudinal approach. A review of the effectiveness of local drug treatment systems attempted to map what is available in a local drug action team (or partnership) area (Prime Minister's Delivery Unit, 2005): Fig. 2.2 shows an example of such a systems model. The aim of the model is to describe the commissioning system within each drug action team area as the unit of analysis. Thus, clients should move through the system using the services they require within a 'treatment journey' (Audit Commission, 2004). One of the main concerns raised in the 2004 Audit Commission report was that services tended not to be integrated and so the kind of pathways demonstrated in Fig. 2.2 – where clients access different types of treatment as their recovery progresses – were often poorly conceptualised and integrated. The overall package of provision should include acute crisis intervention, stabilisation and maintenance provisions, detoxification options, longer-term recovery support (such as rehabilitation in both community and residential settings) and ongoing support in the local community.

Individuals will typically access drug treatment either through referral from a Tier 1 service (most commonly from their GP, but also from probation, housing, employment services and so on) or by self-referral, and will be assessed by a member of staff from one of the specialist treatment providers. Assuming that treatment needs are identified, a care plan will be agreed and an appropriate treatment package determined based on the severity and extent of the problem (such as urgent need for detoxification or safer injecting advice), additional complications (such as criminal justice, housing or mental health issues) and patient preference. Progression through the system should also be needs driven, with patient choice and problem severity determining whether the short- and medium-term goals of treatment are abstinence-oriented or focus on stabilising the individual and making gains in other areas such as relationships, accommodation, employment and health.

Although the model for services is now fairly clear, there is still great variability in treatment provision across England (Audit Commission, 2004). While it would be encouraging to assume that this results from the planning and commissioning of services to meet local needs, it is more likely to reflect historical practices and commissioner preferences (Best et al, 2005). Thus, the extent to which local treatment systems are led by specialist statutory healthcare providers (mental health or primary care trusts), non-statutory services or primary-care-based services varies enormously. Similarly, both the balance of service provision across the tiered system and the quality and consistency of pathways between them also vary according to commissioning factors and service delivery issues.

The Models of Care initiative should ensure that the appropriate package of pharmacotherapy, psychological / psychosocial support, case management and ancillary services is available to meet the needs of the full range of patients. Each system is also bound by commissioning arrangements that attempt to ensure equality of access to treatment (through waiting-time restrictions on providers) and guidance and targets on patient retention.

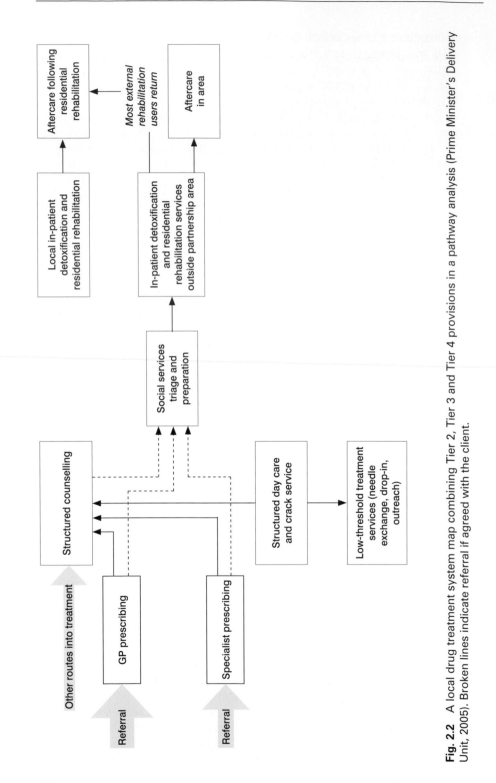

Fig. 2.2 A local drug treatment system map combining Tier 2, Tier 3 and Tier 4 provisions in a pathway analysis (Prime Minister's Delivery Unit, 2005). Broken lines indicate referral if agreed with the client.

Does the treatment system work?

The Audit Commission has produced two reviews of drug treatment services in the past 5 years. The first of these, on the commissioning and management of services (Audit Commission, 2002) was highly critical of the system, pointing to lengthy delays, limited treatment options and poor care management that resulted in high levels of treatment drop-out and failure. The authors also pointed out that individuals' needs were inadequately assessed and insufficiently addressed, and that drug treatment was generally delivered poorly and inconsistently. Although the later report, on reducing the local impact of drug misuse (Audit Commission, 2004), identified substantial improvements in this position, it still identified major problems. The report focused on assisting drug users through the treatment journey and suggested that services were still poorly coordinated, with interagency working often absent and unsatisfactory attempts to tailor services to the needs of users. In particular, reservations were expressed about the adequacy of aftercare provision and the availability of knowledge and evidence to support drug users in achieving and maintaining abstinence.

These concerns were the central target for the NTA's treatment effectiveness strategy, launched in 2005 (Box 2.6). The initiative focused on the concept of the addiction 'career' and the stages involved in treatment journeys, placing greater emphasis on linking services and requiring commissioners to focus on the coherence of the treatment system and the extent to which it involves service users in decision-making and treatment planning. In doing so, the NTA acknowledged that its emphasis on increasing numbers in treatment had to be supplemented by a new drive towards improved treatment quality, and that this would be the core task of the agency for the remainder of the current drug strategy (Tackling Drugs to Build a Better Britain, which runs until 2008).

Box 2.6 Key aims and targets of the NTA's treatment effectiveness strategy (2005–2008)

Aim I: Improving access to treatment
- Target: To give 85% of patients access to treatment within 3 weeks
- Target: To double numbers in treatment from 1998 levels by 2008

Aim II: Improving patient retention
- Target: To retain 62% of patients in treatment for at least 12 weeks

Aim III: Improving treatment delivery
- Target: To provide all patients with a formal, individualised care plan for treatment

---

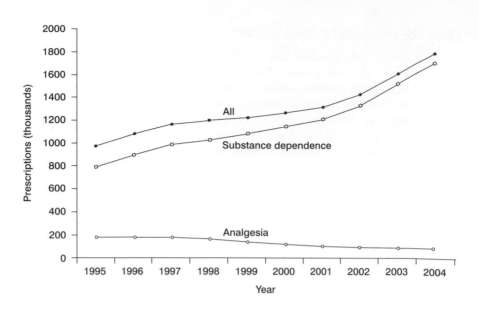

Fig. 2.3 Number of methadone prescriptions (000s) per year 1995–2004 (Department of Health, 2005). The number of prescriptions of methadone cough preparation remained unchanged, but was too low to show on this graph.

A further concern is that the system for the treatment of illicit drug use is dominated by substitute prescribing of opiates on a long-term maintenance basis, and so fails to meet the needs of non-opiate users (including users of stimulants such as crack cocaine and amphetamines) and those who wish to achieve abstinence.

As shown in Fig. 2.3, the total number of methadone prescriptions rose from fewer than 1 million in 1995 to 1.8 million in 2004, indicating the central role of methadone prescribing in current drug treatment. Such an increase has been underpinned by national guidelines on the clinical management of drug misuse and dependence (Department of Health, 1999), commonly referred to as the Orange Guidelines. However, when these guidelines are used as a benchmark of best practice in prescribing there is evidence of inconsistency across England, with considerable variation in dispensing practices and supervision processes (Best & Campbell, 2005).

Conclusion

The use of illicit substances is a complex problem in which multiple personal, environmental and societal factors come into play. The history of the development of treatment services mirrors this complexity, but current services are at their greatest ever level in terms of both quantity and sophistication. It is important to understand both the historical context of illicit drug use and the changing nature of the political response to this in order to comprehend the structure and function of contemporary treatment services.

References and further reading

Advisory Council on the Misuse of Drugs (1982) *Report on Treatment and Rehabilitation*. TSO (The Stationery Office).

Advisory Council on the Misuse of Drugs (1988) *AIDS and Drug Misuse, Part I*. TSO (The Stationery Office).

Adams, E.W. (1937) *Drug Addiction*. Oxford University Press.

Audit Commission (2002) *Changing Habits: The Commissioning and Management of Community Drug Treatment Services for Adults*. Audit Commission.

Audit Commission (2004) *Drug Misuse 2004: Reducing the Local Impact*. Audit Commission.

Berridge, V. (2005) The 'British System' and its history: myth and reality. In *Heroin Addiction and the British System. Vol. 1: Origins and Evolution* (2nd edn) (eds J. Strang & M. Gossop), pp. 7–17. Routledge.

Best, D. & Campbell, A. (2005) *Summary of the NTA's National Prescribing Audit*. National Treatment Agency for Substance Misuse.

Best, D., O'Grady, A. & Charalampous, I. (2005) *National Needs Assessment for Tier 4 Drugs Services in England*. National Treatment Agency for Substance Misuse.

Bewley, T. (2005) The drugs problem of the 1960s: a new type of problem. In *Heroin Addiction and the British System. Vol. 1: Origins and Evolution* (2nd edn) (eds. J. Strang & M. Gossop), pp. 43–52. Routledge.

Department of Health (1995) *Reviewing Shared Care Arrangements for Drug Misusers* (Executive Letter EL (95) 114). Department of Health.

Department of Health (1999) *Drug Misuse and Dependence: Guidelines on Clinical Management*. TSO (The Stationery Office).

Department of Health (2000) *The NHS Plan – A Plan for Investment, A Plan for Reform*. Department of Health.

Department of Health (2005) *Prescription Cost Analysis: England 2004*. Department of Health.

Downes, D. (1977) The drug addict as fold devil. In *Drugs and Politics* (ed. P. Rock). Transaction Books.

Edmunds, M., May, T., Hearnden, I., *et al* (1998) *Arrest Referral: Emerging Lessons from Research* (Drugs Prevention Initiative Paper no 23). Home Office.

European Monitoring Centre for Drugs and Drug Addiction (2006) *Annual Report 2006: The State of the Drugs Problem in Europe*. EMCDDA.

Finch, E., Brotchie, J., Williams, K., *et al* (2003) Sentenced to treatment: early experience of drug treatment and testing orders in England. *European Addiction Research*, **9**, 120–130.

Frisher, M., Heatlie, H. & Hickman, M. (2004) *Estimating the Prevalence of Problematic and Injecting Drug Use for Drug Action Team Areas in England: A Feasibility Study using the Multiple Indicator Method*. Home Office.

Glanz, A. (2005) The fall and rise of the general practitioner. In *Heroin Addiction and the British System. Vol. 2: Treatment Policy and Responses* (2nd edn) (eds J. Strang & M. Gossop), pp. 53–67. Routledge.

Gossop, M., Marsden, J., Stewart, D., *et al* (2001) Outcomes after methadone maintenance and methadone reduction treatments: two-year follow-up results from the National Treatment Outcome Research Study. *Drug and Alcohol Dependence*, **62**, 255–264.

Home Office (1995) *Tackling Drugs Together: A Strategy for England 1995–1998*. TSO (The Stationery Office).

Home Office (1998) *Tackling Drugs to Build a Better Britain: The Government's 10-year Strategy for Tackling Drugs Misuse*. (White Paper Cm 3945). TSO (The Stationery Office).

Home Office (2002) *Updated Drug Strategy 2002*. Home Office.

Ministry of Health (1926) *Rolleston Report: Departmental Committee on Morphine and Heroin Addiction*. TSO (The Stationery Office).

Ministry of Health (1961) *Drug Addiction. Report of the Interdepartmental Committee*. TSO (The Stationery Office).

Ministry of Health (1965) *Drug Addiction. Second Report of the Interdepartmental Committee*. TSO (The Stationery Office).

Ministry of Health (1967) *Treatment and Supervision of Heroin Addiction*. Health Circular 67/16. Ministry of Health.

National Treatment Agency for Substance Misuse (2002) *Models of Care for the Treatment of Adult Drug Misusers*. NTA.

National Treatment Agency for Substance Misuse (2005a) *National Needs Assessment for Tier 4 Services in England*. NTA.

National Treatment Agency for Substance Misuse (2005b) *Business Plan 2005/06: Towards Treatment Effectiveness*. http://www.nta.nhs.uk/publications/documents/nta_business_plan_2005_06.pdf. NTA.

National Treatment Agency for Substance Misuse (2006) *Models of Care for Treatment of Adult Drug Misusers: Update 2006*. NTA.

Prime Minister's Delivery Unit (2005) *Priority Review for Drug Treatment in England*. PMDU.

Royal College of Psychiatrists & Royal College of General Practitioners (2005) *Roles and Responsibilities of Doctors in the Provision of Treatment for Drug and Alcohol Misusers* (Council Report CR131). Royal College of Psychiatrists.

Spear, H. B. (2002) *Heroin Addiction: Care and Control: The British System (1916–1984)*. DrugScope.

Spear, B. (2005) The early years of Britain's drug situation in practice up to the 1960s. In *Heroin Addiction and the British System. Vol. 1: Origins and Evolution* (2nd edn) (eds. J. Strang & M. Gossop), pp. 17–42. Routledge.

Strang, J. & Gossop, M. (eds) (2005a) *Heroin Addiction and the British System. Vol. 1: Origins and Evolution* (2nd edn). Routledge.

Strang, J. & Gossop, M. (eds) (2005b) *Heroin Addiction and the British System. Vol 2: Treatment and Policy Responses* (2nd edn). Routledge.

Task Force to Review Services for Drug Misusers (1996) *Report of an Independent Review of Drug Treatment Services in England*. Department of Health.

Turnbull, P., McSweeney, T., Webster, R., *et al* (2000) *Drug Treatment and Testing Orders: Final Report*. Home Office.

United Kingdom Anti-Drugs Co-ordinator (2001) *Tackling Drugs to Build a Better Britain: United Kingdom Anti-drugs Co-ordinator's National Plan 2000/2001 (Second National Plan)*. Cabinet Office.

CHAPTER 3

Stimulant use still going strong

Nicholas Seivewright, Charles McMahon and Paul Egleston

Summary Amphetamines, cocaine and methylenedioxymethamphetamine (MDMA, 'ecstasy') are prominent on the UK drugs scene. Much cocaine is now in the form of 'crack', which produces particularly acute versions of well-known complications, including paranoid psychosis, mood disorders and cardiovascular problems. Ecstasy has additional hallucinogenic properties, and the slightly different range of psychiatric effects can be long-lasting. Assessment for stimulant misuse should include drug screening more than is currently common in general settings. Management comprises psychosocial (particularly behavioural counselling) and pharmacological approaches. A wide range of dopaminergic and other medications have been studied in cocaine misuse, and specialised substitute prescribing may be appropriate for heavy amphetamine injecting. There has been recent focus on problems of dual diagnosis, with particular strategies required to address stimulant misuse by people with severe mental illnesses.

In this chapter we revisit a subject that we reviewed almost a decade ago – the misuse of the most common illicit stimulant drugs (Seivewright & McMahon, 1996). In the drugs field, changes can certainly be expected in that length of time, particularly with substances linked to the so-called recreational drugs scene, where fashions and differences in usage come and go. Since the 1960s, when hallucinogens came into fashion, there has been prominence successively of barbiturates, pharmaceutical opioids and then smokable powdered heroin. In the decade leading up to our last review the widespread taking of methylenedioxymethamphetamine (MDMA, 'ecstasy') had emerged, and the long-established use of cocaine had increasingly transferred to its more potent 'crack' form. In 1996 we mainly considered four substances – amphetamine, powdered cocaine hydrochloride, crystalline 'crack' cocaine and MDMA – and since then all have remained highly prevalent on the drugs scene, with amphetamine and MDMA generally found in surveys to be the two most common drugs of misuse in the UK after cannabis.

Table 3.1 is an updated version of a table that appeared in our earlier review. It shows how the main stimulant drugs are used, approximate current street prices and their classification under the Misuse of Drugs Act 1971, which dictates the severity of penalties for supplying or possession.

Table 3.1 The main stimulant drugs of misuse

Drug	Description	Routes of administration	Current street price	Misuse of Drugs Act classification
Amphetamine	Usually light-coloured powder, low purity (roughly 10–20%). Also much stronger 'base', a moist paste, and some pharmaceutical preparations	Swallowed, snorted, intravenous	£10–15 per gram	B (A if prepared for injection)
Cocaine hydrochloride	White powder, moderate purity (up to 50%)	Snorted, intravenous	£40–60 per gram	A
Crack cocaine	Crystalline 'rocks'	Smoked, intravenous	£10–20 per 150 mg rock	A
MDMA	Various manufactured tablets, often with characteristic motifs	Swallowed	£5–10 per 100–120 mg	A

So what is different in assessing the problems caused by these drugs ten years on? Gratifyingly, there has been increasing recognition that people heavily injecting amphetamine require just as much attention as the opiate-dependent individuals who have typically predominated in drug services. Consequently, many agencies are devising protocols for stimulant users to run alongside their established methadone and other programmes. The most important psychosocial and pharmacological approaches, which we describe below, depend for their formal evidence base on studies conducted mostly on cocaine users and they have varying applicability to stimulants in general. The tendency for drugs agencies to solely deploy treatments for opiate dependence has been further challenged by the ongoing trends towards polydrug use, with additional cocaine use by by patients on opioid substitution programmes currently particularly problematic (Gossop *et al*, 2002). There has been no reversal, at least in the UK, of the rise in crack cocaine use, as distinct from intranasal use of the hydrochloride form. Particularly acute physical and psychological complications occur in crack users, who are often from marginalised social groups. The effects of MDMA are somewhat different in nature and there has been more progress in delineating the psychiatric problems that users of this drug can develop, as well as the medical complications, which can sometimes be fatal.

By way of overview, we would reiterate the relevance of stimulant misuse for the majority of psychiatrists, not just those working in substance misuse services. It is well known that, through their common action in enhancing central transmission of catecholamines, amphetamine and cocaine can produce psychoses resembling schizophrenia, which in acute circumstances are most likely to be treated in general psychiatric settings. Furthermore, as people with severe mental illness are predominantly managed in the community very large numbers take drugs, including stimulants. This creates additional problems, with such 'dual diagnosis' cases frequently requiring combined service provision and special attention to issues such as adherence to psychiatric medication regimens (Swofford *et al*, 2000; Weaver *et al*, 2003; also chapter 12, this volume). Careful assessment of the relative contributions of these drugs and of the underlying illness to observed clinical states is often necessary. Clinicians should be wary of the oversimplistic application of the term 'drug-induced psychosis' and be prepared to include drug misusers in systematic management schemes such as the UK's care programme approach (CPA) if their condition merits it. The need to 'mainstream' the care of people with dual diagnosis, with ready use of CPA and treatment within general mental health services wherever possible, has been formalised as policy in good practice guidelines from the Department of Health (2002).

Usage

Amphetamine

Most use of this drug is in the form of the relatively impure powder commonly known as 'speed' or 'whizz'. The majority of users take the drug orally, for instance by wrapping some in a cigarette paper and swallowing ('bombing'), or putting it in a drink. In the past decade there has been increased use of the 'base' preparation, which is moist to the touch and generally much more potent in its effects, including causing psychotic reactions. Methamphetamine ('ice') is a version used at high levels in southwest USA, Thailand, China and Japan, although not significantly in the UK at present. It can be made in home laboratories using relatively inexpensive ingredients, and its more pronounced effects on the central nervous system have led to major concern (National Institute on Drug Abuse, 2002). Confusingly some laboratory analyses label MDMA as methamphetamine. Pharmaceutical amphetamines are only rarely encountered in the street-drugs scene, although this may change if there is a significant increase in the very specialised area of substitute prescribing for some heavily injecting users (see below).

Cocaine

Cocaine hydrochloride is more expensive than other illicit drugs and use by snorting has sometimes been linked with executive lifestyles. This same powdered preparation has also long been injected by polydrug users. The crack form is generally more potent in terms of effects and withdrawal features. Rapid rises in blood levels, and hence a very quick high, occur after smoking crack in various kinds of pipe or container, but committed injectors use their preferred route.

MDMA (ecstasy)

Ecstasy was inextricably associated with the rise of the rave dance culture across Europe and elsewhere, and the links with 'clubbing' generally continue. Amphetamine and lysergic acid diethylamide (LSD) are frequently used in the same club scenes, and large numbers of individuals take these as part of perceived normalised socialising, with a mainly low likelihood of progression to dependent or injected drug use. Ecstasy tablets are made in illicit laboratories and may be stamped with various motifs, and users seek out their own favoured type. Periodically there have been additional concerns that totally unrelated substances such as the anaesthetic agent ketamine are being passed off as MDMA. The similar compounds 3,4-methylenedioxy-ethylamphetamine (MDEA) and 3,4-methylenedioxyamphetamine (MDA) are also sometimes encountered.

Surveys tend to show levels of usage of any stimulant drug in the UK as small, single-figure percentages of the general population, but in young people usage can rise to 5–10% or even more. There is an impression that the MDMA phenomenon is on the wane, and this was demonstrated in a survey of older school students by Plant & Miller (2000). They found that lifetime use by boys had decreased from 9% to 3% between 1995 and 1999, and by girls from 7% to 3%. The issue of sample selection in drug misuse research is crucial, as illustrated in one comprehensive comparison of MDMA use between a general population sample, regular users and 'purposive' samples of high-using and minority groups (Topp *et al*, 2004). Patterns of usage were well demonstrated in their study: notably, no individuals in any group were taking MDMA daily, and alcohol, cannabis and amphetamines were the most common additionally taken substances.

Clinical features

The clinical features of stimulant usage were described in our previous review (Seivewright & McMahon, 1996) and are generally well established. The main mechanism that produces the stimulant action and related effects comprises increased presynaptic release and inhibition of reuptake of catecholamines, with a direct action on dopaminergic terminals and effects in the common 'reward pathway'. The characteristic features, which we have classified into early, late and withdrawal effects, are indicated in Box 3.1.

The use of the term 'withdrawal' can be questioned by purists as the stimulants are not truly addictive, at least in the physical sense in which heroin, benzodiazepines and alcohol are. Nevertheless, there is a clear distinction between early effects, which are mainly the desired ones, the features that supervene, which are more adverse in nature and usually lead the individual to end the episode of usage, and finally the stage that users refer to as the come-down or crash. After the effects of stimulation, this withdrawal stage partly constitutes rebound (i.e. opposite) symptoms of oversleeping, overeating and depressed mood, but there may also be agitation,

Box 3.1   Effects of stimulant drugs

Early	Increased energy, elation, reduced appetite
Late	Overactivity, insomnia, confusion, paranoia
Withdrawal	Depression, irritability, agitation, craving, hyperphagia, sleep disturbance (hypersomnia, nightmares)

irritability and general distress, which commonly lead to other substance use in attempts at alleviation. Stimulant users often counteract withdrawal effects with alcohol, tranquillisers or cannabis, and heroin may also be used in this way and so lead to the development of opiate dependence. Cocaine and alcohol are also frequently used in a straightforward combination, with individuals presenting with combined dependence.

Cocaine is shorter-acting than amphetamine and each instance of use tends to be over more quickly, in sessions lasting perhaps a few hours. Many committed stimulant users, however, take their drug over 2–3 days, keeping awake during the nights and eating little. They readily use the term paranoia fairly accurately for the ideas of reference, other paranoid ideation and actual delusions that can develop after that length of time, usually recognising that they should stop the episode until they feel more normal again. This usually averts a fully developed paranoid psychosis, although this can, of course, occur especially after prolonged and heavy use of amphetamine or cocaine.

In addition to the general stimulant features, MDMA also has partly hallucinogenic, or 'psychedelic', effects resembling those of LSD. These include visual illusions, enhancement of sensory perceptions and states of altered consciousness, which along with a feeling of emotional closeness to others are basically the desired effects in typical usage. Common physical effects include tachycardia, dry mouth, dilated pupils, facial muscle stiffness and paraesthesia. Negative effects such as sickness, confusion, mood disturbances and ataxia are also experienced by many users (Handy *et al*, 1998).

Complications

The range of clinical features, including adverse and withdrawal effects, merge into more definite complications, a classification of which is given in Box 3.2. Some complications clearly relate to subgroups of users only, such as injectors or pregnant women; in the latter, stimulants appear to cause higher levels of obstetric complications than are expected from drug misuse in general.

Importantly, because of their primary effect on monoamines the stimulant drugs are relatively likely to produce vascular effects that can lead to myocardial

---

Box 3.2 Possible complications of stimulant misuse

Medical
- Cardiovascular: hypertension, arrhythmias, myocardial infarction, cerebrovascular accident
- Infective: abscesses, hepatitis, septicaemia, HIV
- Obstetric: reduced foetal growth, miscarriage, placental abruption, premature labour
- Other: hyperthermia, weight loss, dental problems, epilepsy

Psychiatric
- Anxiety
- Depression
- Aggressive behaviour
- Confusional state
- Paranoid psychosis

---

infarction and stroke. High proportions of young people who have died from these conditions in the USA have been found to be cocaine misusers.

Of the infective conditions, the one that has been recognised in the past decade to be of great significance is hepatitis C, which can lead to chronic liver impairment and is commonly found in up to 50%, and sometimes in over 90%, of drug injectors in different areas. Antiviral treatments can be used for the condition, although many units operate policies whereby injecting must have stopped before treatment is provided (Schaefer *et al*, 2004).

From the listed psychiatric effects it will already have become clear that stimulants frequently produce mood disturbances or confusion. The aggressive behaviour that can undoubtedly occur as a direct effect of drug intoxication needs to be distinguished from the more general antisocial personality features that are common in drug misusers (Bowden-Jones *et al*, 2004). Paranoid psychosis from amphetamine use has been recognised for decades, with even more acute similar syndromes increasingly occurring from crack cocaine. It seems that dopaminergic overactivity substantially accounts for this schizophrenia-like condition. There is now controversy as to the representativeness of the early reports of amphetamine psychosis, which described only a relatively short-lived condition that resolved if the drug was withdrawn (Curran *et al*, 2004). The exact relationships between transient psychotic symptoms, more persistent illness and the effects of substance misuse are not fully established, but in practice the misuse of stimulant drugs is highly likely to have a deleterious effect on any individual with a pre-existing psychotic condition. In stimulant psychoses tactile and visual hallucinations probably occur more frequently than in schizophrenia, and there may be hyperactivity and repetitive or compulsive behaviours. If the conditions do become chronic, for instance with ongoing drug use, there is less deterioration in terms of negative symptoms from the drug-related psychoses. One interesting study found higher levels of overt behavioural disturbance in individuals with substance use disorder and psychosis (dual diagnosis), but better preservation of social competence (Penk *et al*, 2000).

It was known when we last reviewed this subject that MDMA could produce a range of psychiatric after-effects such as anxiety states, depression, flashback experiences, persistent cognitive deficits and occasionally psychoses, and also that the drug could be fatal in isolated cases even after single usage. The literature on psychiatric sequelae continues to be mainly small case series, and the importance of other vulnerability factors and the confounding effects of additional substance use have been emphasised (Soar *et al*, 2001). Regarding severe physical consequences, it has become increasingly clear that as well as general stimulant adverse effects and other toxicity the most likely fatal syndrome from MDMA includes hyperthermia, rhabdomyolysis, renal failure and disseminated intravascular coagulation (Gowing *et al*, 2002). Dehydration is thought to contribute to this syndrome as well as the chemical itself, as MDMA is usually used in the context of prolonged dancing in hot crowded environments.

Management

Assessment

As in other areas of substance misuse, assessment is mainly through history, examination and relevant investigations. Details must be established of use of the drugs in question, bearing in mind that use of multiple substances is common. Additional assessments may be necessary for the various complications. It is important to establish a user's personal situation and the context in which they take drugs, as well as making a broad assessment of their motivation to change their behaviour.

The usage history should include amounts, frequency, routes of administration, duration of usage, relevant treatments received and significant drug-free periods. There are few specific physical signs of stimulant usage beyond dilated pupils and overactivity, although needle sites may be seen in injecting users. Physical examination can reveal medical complications, and drug screening often provides essential information, particularly when monitoring whether an individual with psychiatric complications is or is not abstaining from drugs. Managing a drug misuser without urine results is rather like treating a haematology patient without blood counts, and with the generally high levels of current drug use it would seem that there needs to be a greater awareness of testing in general psychiatric settings.

Table 3.2 summarises the main drug-screening methods and the period after a drug has been taken within which they are effective. Urine sampling is by far the most routine. The process is simple, using a plain bottle and either instant testing with a kit or laboratory analysis. Cooperation may be a problem in disturbed individuals, and the recent development of equipment

Table 3.2 Testing for misuse of stimulant drugs

Sample	Detection period	Remarks
Urine	1–3 days	Usual method; should be routine where drug use is possible. Laboratory testing or instant kits
Oral fluid	1–2 days	Specialised laboratory analysis of cheek cell fluid. Useful if there are compliance or authenticity problems with urine
Hair	Permanent	Specialised and relatively expensive. Examination of sections gives chronology of drug usage, e.g. for medico-legal cases

for easily obtaining cheek cell fluid samples provides a method that is often more acceptable. Hair testing is a specialised approach that has the advantage that most substances remain detectable for as long as the hair is present.

Harm reduction

Even with some recent developments in treatment the clinical management of stimulant misuse is not nearly as effective as that for opiate dependence, where treatments such as methadone and buprenorphine routinely enable substantial reductions in drug usage in the majority of individuals. Partly because there is no equivalent of these established and readily available substitution therapies, stimulant users are far less likely to present to medical services. However, stimulant users need harm reduction advice, which can be provided by community drug teams and specialised non-statutory services. Useful recommendations can be found in guidance issued to GPs by the Royal College of General Practitioners (2004). At the more informal end of the range of management approaches are drugs information, education about health risks, advice on safe practices and the provision of clean injecting equipment.

Psychosocial treatments

This term is applied to the more systematic counselling and behavioural approaches that are undertaken by nurses, psychologists or social workers in substance misuse or sometimes general psychiatry teams. Often there needs to be some focus on motivation to change, as this is not static and can be enhanced by well-established techniques of motivational interviewing, sometimes allied to other cognitive–behavioural strategies and coping skills training (Rohsenow *et al*, 2004). In a survey investigating treatments for cocaine use deployed in UK services, the overall category of counselling was by far the most common approach. Detailed follow-up of a subgroup of clients, mainly in residential rehabilitation units, showed good outcomes, with improvements in health and psychological adjustment (Seivewright *et al*, 2000). A large multicentre study of psychosocial treatments for cocaine dependence in the USA found that individual and group therapy based on treatment manuals compared favourably with some of the more specialised psychotherapeutic techniques (Crits-Cristoph *et al*, 1999).

Psychophysiological methods can be used by specialist practitioners, particularly for cocaine misuse, in which there is high arousal to drug-related cues that may be reduced through systematic exposure.

A very different behavioural approach has also been investigated, that of providing rewards such as retail vouchers for demonstrable abstinence from drugs during ongoing treatment. The latest in a series of studies using this 'community reinforcement therapy' with cocaine-dependent individuals from one centre in the USA demonstrates benefits in retention in treatment and social outcomes such as employment, and reduced drug and alcohol use (Higgins *et al*, 2003; see chapter 16). The idea of financially rewarding users to abstain is inevitably controversial, but the results have been impressive in comparison with other treatments.

A systematic programme comprising cognitive–behavioural therapy, family education, social support groups and individual counselling has also been found in a large multisite study to be beneficial for the treatment of methamphetamine dependence (Rawson *et al*, 2004), and such methods have broad relevance for managing stimulant misuse in the UK.

Pharmacological treatments

Both harm reduction and psychosocial treatments for stimulant users are extremely important, since there has been no major progress in demonstrating useful pharmacological treatments. As crack cocaine use escalated in many countries there was great pressure on researchers to find a medication as effective for that drug as methadone is for heroin dependence, but the nature of the dependent states is very different. Research efforts focused on dopaminergic drugs (including bromocriptine and amantadine), serotonergic reuptake inhibitors, other antidepressants, antipsychotics, mood-stabilising medications and even disulfiram, the last mainly to prevent cocaine misuse in individuals who only take the drug after alcohol. Although there have been positive results from uncontrolled studies, notably with desipramine and fluoxetine, the large meta-analyses (e.g. de Lima *et al*, 2002) now conclude that there is no strong evidence for any medication in cocaine dependence treatment. The most common direct usage in practice is of antidepressants to treat definite evidence of a depressive disorder, with other medications as indicated for psychiatric complications.

In UK drug services it is common for patients on methadone also to use cocaine (Gossop *et al*, 2002), and in such cases there is at least a theoretical advantage in changing the maintenance agent to buprenorphine, as this partial agonist leads to less in the way of combined subjective effects. The use of disulfiram for cocaine addiction has received a good deal of publicity, and it appears that as well as preventing individuals from taking cocaine after alcohol the medication may have a more specific effect on features of cocaine use (Carroll *et al*, 2004).

As we have noted, a substitution approach is not usually considered suitable in cocaine misuse, although there have been trials of both methyl-phenidate and dexamphetamine. It might indeed be assumed that the potentially destabilising and sometimes psychotic effects of stimulants would simply rule out such therapies, but some specialised units accommodate oral dexamphetamine prescribing for the heaviest and most problematic amphetamine users who otherwise inject the street preparation several times daily. Such prescribing is seen as based on harm reduction principles, and some reasonable results have been achieved (Grabowski *et al*, 2004). In practical terms many UK drug services operate a three-tier approach for amphetamine users, offering counselling alone for most cases, some use of symptomatic medications with individuals who find it particularly hard to overcome the period of withdrawal, and limited dexamphetamine prescribing in the most severe cases (Seivewright, 2000: pp. 128–132).

Some of the same management approaches may be relevant for MDMA users, but these individuals present relatively rarely to drug treatment services, typically seeing their drug-taking as 'recreational' despite the various adverse effects.

Although we have considered the treatment of stimulant misuse collectively, there are some important differences in emphasis between the substances, and these are summarised in Box 3.3.

Other

Complementary therapies are frequently deployed for stimulant users, particularly in non-clinical services, with acupuncture the most established method (Seivewright *et al*, 2000). There is little systematic evidence for effectiveness of the methods overall, or for the very different experimental approaches of enhancement of drug excretion and antibody formation from cocaine vaccination.

Treatments for psychiatric complications

As a basic principle, anxiety states, depression, paranoid psychosis, confusional states and other behavioural disturbances produced by stimulants should be managed in much the same way as such conditions of other aetiology (see chapters 14 and 15). The serotonergic antidepressants are sometimes favoured because they may reduce drug craving, although there is equal theoretical rationale for compounds such as desipramine, which act more on monoamines. A pragmatic consideration is the preferable avoidance of benzodiazepines in managing drug use, because of the potential for misuse. The issue of stimulant psychosis has received careful consideration in a review by Curran *et al* (2004), which addresses whether a kind of sensitisa-tion occurs to even limited drug exposure which might indicate ongoing

---

Box 3.3   Some distinctions within stimulant misuse management

Amphetamines
- Most cases minor, but heavy use merits systematic treatment
- General drug counselling is the mainstay, with limited evidence for anti-depressants in withdrawal
- Substitute prescribing sometimes undertaken in specialist services for daily injecting users

Cocaine
- Psychological and physical complications often acute, particularly with crack
- Very large number of medications trialled in studies but few positive results
- Specialised psychological treatments developed, e.g. cue exposure and behavioural reinforcement

MDMA
- Elective presentation for treatment is rare
- No special programmes available
- Likely area of involvement is advising on psychiatric after-effects

---

antipsychotic drug treatment. The examination of many studies suggests that this may sometimes be necessary despite the usual view that amphetamine psychosis is short-lived, and it is also concluded that stimulant misuse has the potential to worsen symptoms in individuals with severe mental illness even when they are adhering to antipsychotic drug regimens.

Issues of dual diagnosis

We have reiterated that individuals who misuse stimulants may become psychotic as a direct effect and that many people with illnesses such as schizophrenia additionally use various substances. The much-used term 'drug-induced psychosis' actually covers a range of phenomena, including the classic paranoid states, syndromes of a more organic nature with illusions and visual hallucinations produced by LSD or MDMA, briefer flashback experiences and/or worsening or alteration of pre-existing psychotic conditions (Poole & Brabbins, 1996). As the management of drug-induced states is basically along standard symptomatic lines, much of the recent specialised literature addresses the clinical approaches necessary for people with severe mental illness who develop substance misuse, given the implications that such dual diagnosis has for severity of psychiatric disturbance, adherence to treatments and overall prognosis (Seivewright et al, 2004).

Some units in the USA have developed ultraspecialised programmes solely for patients with dual diagnosis, often with high staffing levels and relatively small case-loads. The development of such centres in the UK seems unlikely, in light of the general policy preference to build on existing links between community mental health teams, substance misuse services and primary care, and to treat people with dual diagnosis in the mainstream as far as possible (see chapter 13). Nevertheless, clinical guidance from experienced units is very useful in identifying the principles often necessary in treating this group (Drake & Mueser, 2000). These include assertive outreach if adherence is a problem, close monitoring, integration between services and the ability to tackle very practical aspects such as finances and accommodation as well as deploying formal therapies.

A common difficulty in practice is that people with distressing psychiatric symptoms can subjectively feel that they gain relief from taking drugs, whether they be sedatives to subdue hallucinations or stimulants to counter lethargy, depression and negative symptoms. Consequently, careful advice on drug-related harms tailored to the requirements of this population needs to be provided. In general it can be expected that stimulant users presenting in psychiatric services who have not actually requested treatment for drug misuse will be suitable for motivational approaches in the first instance rather than the various forms of cognitive therapy.

A particularly comprehensive study of dual diagnosis in the UK (Weaver *et al*, 2003) included both a survey of all the individuals on the case-load of keyworkers in community mental health and substance misuse services in three cities on a given date, and thorough formalised assessments of a random subsample. Response rates were high and the research confirmed an impression that services currently mainly manage individuals with severe disorders, with 75% of the mental health interview sample having psychosis. Thirty-one per cent of that sample currently used illicit drugs (mainly stimulants, cannabis, tranquillisers and heroin), while of the interviewed drug misusers over 70% had significant additional psychiatric illness. A measure was included of risk factors that would indicate referral for CPA, and in general individuals with dual diagnosis had fewer contacts with reciprocal services than appeared necessary on clinical grounds.

Weaver *et al*'s study reinforces the need for more liaison and joint working, and it is to be hoped that education on the various manifestations of substance misuse problems and the management of relevant psychiatric conditions will help enable that.

References

Bowden-Jones, O., Iqbal, M. Z., Tyrer, P., *et al* (2004) Prevalence of personality disorder in alcohol and drug services and associated comorbidity. *Addiction*, **99**, 1306–1314.

Carroll, K. M., Fenton, L. R., Ball, S. A., *et al* (2004) Efficacy of disulfiram and cognitive behavior therapy in cocaine dependent outpatients: a randomized placebo-controlled trial. *Archives of General Psychiatry*, **61**, 264–272.

Crits-Cristoph, P., Siqueland, L., Blaine, J., *et al* (1999) Psychosocial treatments for cocaine dependence. *Archives of General Psychiatry*, **56**, 493–502.

Curran, C., Byrappa, N. & McBride, A. (2004) Stimulant psychosis: systematic review. *British Journal of Psychiatry*, **185**, 196–204.

de Lima, M. S., de Oliveira Soares, B. G., Reisser, A. A. P., *et al* (2002) Pharmacological treatment of cocaine dependence: a systematic review. *Addiction*, **97**, 931–949.

Department of Health (2002) *Mental Health Policy Implementation Guide: Dual Diagnosis Good Practice Guide.* TSO (The Stationery Office).

Drake, R. E. & Mueser, K. T. (2000) Psychosocial approaches to dual diagnosis. *Schizophrenia Bulletin*, **26**, 105–118.

Gossop, M., Marsden, J., Stewart, D., *et al* (2002) Changes in use of crack after drug misuse treatment: 4–5 year follow-up results from the National Treatment Outcome Research Study (NTORS). *Drug and Alcohol Dependence*, **66**, 21–28.

Gowing, L. R., Henry-Edwards, S. M. & Irvine, R. G. (2002) The health effects of ecstasy. *Drug and Alcohol Review*, **21**, 53–63.

Grabowski, J., Shearer, J., Merrill, J., *et al* (2004) Agonist-like, replacement pharmacotherapy for stimulant abuse and dependence. *Addictive Behaviours*, **29**, 1439–1464.

Handy, C., Pates, R. & Barrowcliff, A. (1998) Drug use in South Wales: who uses Ecstasy anyway? *Journal of Substance Misuse*, **3**, 82–88.

Higgins, S. T., Sigmon, S. C., Wong, C. J., *et al* (2003) Community reinforcement therapy for cocaine-dependent outpatients. *Archives of General Psychiatry*, **60**, 1043–1052.

National Institute on Drug Abuse (2002) *Methamphetamine Abuse and Addiction* (NIDA Research Report, NIH Publication no. 02-4210). National Institute on Drug Abuse.

Penk, W. E., Flannery, R. B. Jr, Irvin, E., *et al* (2000) Characteristics of substance-abusing persons with schizophrenia: the paradox of the dually diagnosed. *Journal of Addictive Diseases*, **19**, 23–30.

Plant, M. & Miller, P. (2000) Drug use has declined amongst teenagers in United Kingdom. *BMJ*, **320**, 1536–1537.

Poole, R. & Brabbins, C. (1996) Drug induced psychosis. *British Journal of Psychiatry*, **168**, 135–138.

Rawson, A. R., Marinelli-Casey, P., Anglin, M. D., *et al* (2004) A multi-site comparison of psychosocial approaches for the treatment of methamphetamine dependence. *Addiction*, **99**, 708–717.

Rohsenow, D. J., Monti, P. M., Martin, R. A., *et al* (2004) Motivational enhancement and coping skills training for cocaine abusers: effects on substance use outcomes. *Addiction*, **99**, 862–874.

Royal College of General Practitioners (2004) *Guidance for Working with Cocaine and Crack Users in Primary Care.* RCGP. http://www.smmgp.co.uk

Schaefer, M., Heinz, A. & Backmund, M. (2004) Treatment of chronic hepatitis C in patients with drug dependence: time to change the rules? *Addiction*, **99**, 1167–1175.

Seivewright, N. (2000) *Community Treatment of Drug Misuse: More Than Methadone.* Cambridge University Press.

Seivewright, N. & McMahon, C. (1996) Misuse of amphetamines and related drugs. *Advances in Psychiatric Treatment*, **2**, 211–218.

Seivewright, N., Donmall, M., Douglas, J., *et al* (2000) Cocaine misuse treatment in England. *International Journal of Drug Policy*, **11**, 203–215.

Seivewright, N., Iqbal, M. Z. & Bourne, H. (2004) Treating patients with comorbidities. In *Drug Treatment: What Works?* (eds P. Bean & T. Nemitz), pp. 123–141. Routledge.

Soar, K., Turner, J. J. D. & Parrott, A. C. (2001) Psychiatric disorders in Ecstasy (MDMA) users. A literature review focusing on personal predisposition and drug history. *Human Psychopharmacology*, **16**, 641–645.

Swofford, C. D., Scheller-Gilkey, G., Miller, A. H., *et al* (2000) Double jeopardy: schizophrenia and substance use. *American Journal of Drug and Alcohol Abuse*, **26**, 343–353.

Topp, L., Barker, B. & Degenhardt, L. (2004) The external validity of results derived from ecstasy users recruited using purposive sampling strategies. *Drug and Alcohol Dependence*, **73**, 33–40.

Weaver, T., Madden, P., Charles, V., *et al* (2003) Comorbidity of substance misuse and mental illness in community mental health and substance misuse services. *British Journal of Psychiatry*, **183**, 304–313.

41

CHAPTER 4

Adverse effects of khat: a review

Glenice Cox and Hagen Rampes

Summary *Catha edulis* (khat) is a plant grown in the countries around the Red Sea and on the eastern coast of Africa. Its leaves are chewed by the local people for their stimulant action. Its principal active constituents are cathinone and cathine, which have sympathomimetic actions. Migration of Africans from these countries has spread the habit of khat chewing to the West. Chewing khat has a number of important psychological and physical sequelae. 'Khat-related' psychosis is very similar to that seen following use of amphetamines.

Khat grows wild in countries bordering the Red Sea and along the east coast of Africa. The people of these countries have chewed khat for centuries. There are several names for the plant, depending on its origin: chat, qat, qaad, jaad, miraa, mairungi, cat and catha. In most of the Western literature, it is referred to as khat.

Khat is an evergreen shrub, which is cultivated as a bush or small tree. The leaves have an aromatic odour. The taste is astringent and slightly sweet. The plant is seedless and hardy, growing in a variety of climates and soils. Khat can be grown in droughts where other crops have failed and also at high altitudes. It is harvested throughout the year. Planting is staggered to obtain a continuous supply (Luqman & Danowski, 1976). Khat is mainly grown in Ethiopia, Kenya, Yemen, Somalia, Sudan, South Africa and Madagascar. It has also been found in Afghanistan and Turkestan. Previously, khat leaves were available only near to where they were grown. Recently, improved roads and air transport have allowed a much wider distribution. Khat is harvested in the early hours of the morning and sold in markets in late morning. It is presented as a bundle of twigs, stems and leaves, wrapped in banana leaves to preserve freshness (Fig. 4.1).

History of consumption and 'medical' use

Ethiopia is thought to be the country of origin of khat use. The chewing of khat leaves probably pre-dates the use of coffee. The earliest written record

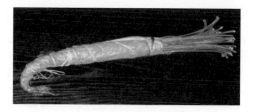

Fig. 4.1 Bundle of khat. The usual length of a bundle is 30–40 cm.

of the medical use of khat appears to be in the New Testament. Khat has been used to treat various ailments, including relieving the symptoms of depression. Some believe it to be a dietary requirement.

Legal aspects of use

In Kenya, Yemen, Uganda, Ethiopia and Madagascar prohibition has resulted in increased illegal importation. When prohibition was replaced in Somalia by import duty, khat chewing became a very common habit within a few years. In Saudi Arabia khat cultivation and consumption are forbidden and the ban is strictly enforced. However, khat circulates freely today in all of the above countries. In some countries, khat chewing is allowed, in others it is officially banned but there is no law enforcement (Elmi, 1983).

Obtaining khat in Western countries

In the UK, khat trade, possession and use are not illegal. Although cathinone and cathine, the major active constituents, are scheduled as class C drugs, khat itself is not a prohibited substance. An offence is committed only if cathinone or cathine are isolated from the plant. About 7 tonnes of khat pass through Heathrow airport each week, and smaller amounts are imported through other airports (Griffiths, 1998). Immigrants have spread the use of khat to the UK, Europe and the USA. Heathrow airport serves as a hub for the re-export of khat to other European countries and for its distribution to other locations in the UK (Goudie, 1987).

Ingestion of khat

The vast majority of those who ingest khat do so by chewing. Only a small number ingest it by making a drink from dried leaves, or, even more rarely, by smoking dried leaves. The chewer fills his or her mouth with leaves and stalks, and then chews slowly and intermittently to release the active components in the juice, which is then swallowed with saliva. The plant material is chewed into a ball, which is kept for a while in the cheek, causing a characteristic bulge (Nencini et al, 1986).

Behaviours associated with the ritual of khat chewing

Khat chewing usually takes place in groups in a social setting. Only a minority frequently chew alone. A session may last for several hours. During this time chewers drink copious amounts of non-alcoholic fluids such as cola, tea and cold water. In a khat chewing session, initially there is an atmosphere of cheerfulness, optimism and a general sense of well-being. After about 2 h, tension, emotional instability and irritability begin to appear, later leading to feelings of low mood and sluggishness. Chewers tend to leave the session feeling depleted.

Reasons for chewing khat

Chewing khat is both a social and a culture-based activity. It is said to enhance social interaction, playing a role in ceremonies such as weddings. In Yemen, Muslims are the most avid chewers. Some believe that chewing facilitates contact with Allah when praying. However, many Christians and Yemenite Jews in Israel also chew khat. Khat is a stimulant and it is used to improve performance, stay alert and to increase work capacity (Kalix, 1984). Workers on night shifts use it to stay awake and postpone fatigue. Students have chewed khat in an attempt to improve mental performance before examinations. Yemeni khat chewers believe that khat is beneficial for minor ailments such as headaches, colds, body pains, fevers, arthritis and also depression (Kennedy *et al*, 1983).

Epidemiology of khat use

Elmi (1983) studied khat chewers in the two main cities in Somalia: Mogadishu and Hargeisa. The results showed that traders and businessmen carried out business transactions during khat parties, whereas for the unemployed it was a way of overcoming feelings of frustration and boredom. Also in Somalia, Alem *et al* (1999) found that more men habitually chewed than women: 75% of men chewed khat regularly compared with only 7–10% of women. Kennedy *et al*'s (1983) Yemen studies had similar findings. Overall, it seems that khat is less appealing to women, although in Somalia chewing has recently become more popular among middle-class and educated women.

Use by immigrants in the UK and other Western countries

In the UK, the chewing of khat is largely confined to ethnic communities accustomed to its use, such as the Somali community (Gough & Cookson, 1984). Wherever Somalis reside, khat is available. Griffiths (1998) carried out a survey of 207 Somalis living in London: 78% of men and 76% of women had used khat and 6% were chewing on a daily basis; the average frequency of use was 3 days per week. Of those surveyed, 76% were using more khat in London than they had in Somalia; 20% had started chewing khat since coming to London. Participants felt that community use was greater in the UK than in Somalia. The explanation most commonly given was that, because of high unemployment, more free time was available for chewing. There was also a desire to maintain cultural identity by chewing khat.

Pharmacology of khat

Active constituents

Khat contains more than 40 alkaloids, glycosides, tannins, amino acids, vitamins and minerals (Halbach, 1972). Most of the effect of chewing khat is thought to come from two phenylalkylamines – cathinone and cathine – which are structurally related to amphetamine (Nencini *et al*, 1984). The presence of amphetamine and caffeine in khat has been excluded. A number of other constituents, including cathidine, eduline and ephedrine, have been identified, but it is unlikely that any of these, except tannin, play a role in khat's effects (Giannini *et al*, 1986).

Cathinone has been termed a 'natural amphetamine' (Fig. 4.2). It produces sympathomimetic and central nervous system stimulation analogous to the effects of amphetamine, hence its similar clinical effects. The difference in effect is due to slight pharmacodynamic variations between the stimulating substances, to other plant constituents (mainly tannins), and to differences in dosage and the mode of consumption.

Actions of cathinone and cathine

Cathinone is also named (–)-alpha-aminopropiophenone. It is considered to be the most active ingredient of khat. It has been isolated and synthesised and its effects have been shown to be similar to those of amphetamine, but with a lower potency. Cathinone is estimated to be 7–10 times more potent than cathine. It is difficult to synthesise, therefore it is unsuitable for marketing as a pure substance for drug misuse (Nencini *et al*, 1989).

Cathine is also named (+)-norpseudoephedrine and phenylpropanolamine. It had previously been isolated from the plant ephedra, which has effects similar to those of khat. Cathine has a milder psychostimulant action than cathinone and the effects last for only a short time, so the user must chew

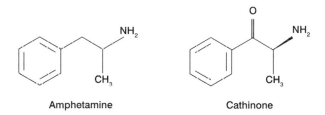

Amphetamine   Cathinone

Fig. 4.2 Chemical structures of amphetamine and cathinone.

leaves almost continuously. It plays only a minor role in the action of khat, but it is cathine that is responsible for the unwanted systemic effects. Normally, fresh leaves contain a higher proportion of the desirable cathinone, but on drying, cathinone breaks down into cathine. Therefore khat chewers prefer fresh leaves that contain a higher proportion of cathinone to cathine, so that they obtain a better stimulation with fewer systemic adverse effects.

Modes of action

The constituents of khat have been shown to exert their effects on two main neurochemical pathways: dopamine and noradrenaline. It has also been postulated that, like amphetamine, cathinone releases serotonin in the central nervous system. Both cathinone and amphetamine induce release of dopamine from central nervous system dopamine terminals and thus increase the activity of the dopaminergic pathways (Kalix & Braenden, 1985). Cathinone has a releasing effect on noradrenaline storage sites, which supports the conclusion that cathinone facilitates noradrenaline transmission. Drake (1988) also proposed that cathinone and cathine cause inhibition of noradrenaline uptake.

Pharmacokinetics

The euphoric effect appears shortly after the chewing begins, suggesting absorption from the oral mucosa. The effect of cathinone is greatest after 15–30 min. Metabolism of cathinone is rapid, occurring mainly during first passage through the liver. Only a small fraction (about 2%) appears unchanged in the urine. Most cathinone is metabolised to norephedrine and is excreted in this form. The rate of inactivation is about the same as the rate of absorption, which limits the cathinone blood levels attainable by chewing.

Cathine has a slower onset of action, with a serum half-life in humans of about 3 h. It is excreted unchanged in the urine within about 24 h. When taking khat, large amounts of non-alcoholic drinks are consumed. There is pharmacological synergism with drinks containing methylxanthines (e.g. tea and cola), which therefore enhance the effects of khat.

Addiction, tolerance and withdrawal

Cathinone is the dependence-producing constituent of khat leaves. It is a reinforcer and maintains very high rates of responding in animal experiments (Kalix & Khan, 1984). Debate exists as to whether khat, like amphetamines, can actually cause dependence. Some authors describe a psychological dependence rather than a physical one (Halbach, 1972). Tolerance to khat practically does not occur; if it does, the doses are increased only very slowly. This may be due to the intrinsic properties of khat or to the physical limits on the amount that can be consumed (Kalix, 1988).

There are conflicting opinions regarding the existence of a withdrawal syndrome. Physical withdrawal symptoms are documented, including lassitude, anergia, nightmares and slight trembling, which appear several days after ceasing to chew. Depressive disorder, sedation and hypotension are sometimes seen after withdrawal of khat. In one study only 0.6% of khat chewers continued to use it in order to prevent withdrawal symptoms (Alem *et al*, 1999).

Psychological sequelae of chewing khat

Chewers report their subjective experiences of khat use in a positive way when consuming small amounts. They describe a feeling of well-being, a sense of euphoria, excitement, increased energy levels, increased alertness, increased ability to concentrate, improvement in self-esteem and an increase in libido. Also experienced are an enhanced imaginative ability and capacity to associate ideas, an improvement in the ability to communicate and a subjective improvement in work performance. After chewing ceases, unpleasant after-effects tend to dominate the experience: insomnia, numbness, lack of concentration and low mood. Some chewers also experience unpleasant effects during the chewing process, describing anxiety, tension, restlessness and hypnagogic hallucinations.

Objectively, chewers can be seen to show a range of experiences, from minor reactions to the development of a psychotic illness. Minor reactions include over-talkativeness, overactivity, insomnia, anxiety, irritability, agitation and aggression.

Broadly, the main psychiatric manifestations linked to the use of khat are a short-lived schizophreniform psychotic illness, mania (Yousef *et al*, 1995) and, more rarely, depression (Pantelis *et al*, 1989). On occasions these presentations are associated with episodes of self-harm or harm to others. Owing to the mode of consumption, the dose of khat tends to be self-limiting, unlike amphetamines, which are available in a pure form for oral or parenteral administration. Therefore toxic psychosis as a result of excessive use is much less frequent with khat than with amphetamines.

Epidemiology and reporting of psychiatric complications

Most reports are of cases of psychosis and suggest a low incidence. The impression of low incidence may reflect the fact that in countries where it is most used, health facilities are lacking and people are managed at home by their family.

Dhadphale & Omolo (1988) studied psychiatric morbidity among khat users. They found that when khat was chewed in moderate quantities there was no excess morbidity, but when the amount chewed per day was greater than two bundles, morbidity was significantly increased. Other research

(Critchlow & Seifert, 1987; Alem & Shibre, 1997) confirms our clinical experience that adverse effects are dose-related. However, many researchers consider that khat precipitates a psychotic illness in those who are already predisposed.

Psychiatric care of these patients can be difficult, leading to less-than-optimal care. This is because individuals with the 'dual diagnosis' of khat misuse and a psychotic illness are often not recognised by substance misuse services. Furthermore, these services have had little experience with khat misuse in the UK. Khat users with psychosis therefore frequently present to general adult psychiatry services.

Psychoses

The literature outlining the characteristics of psychoses following the use of khat describes two main types: a paranoid or schizophreniform psychosis (similar to an amphetamine-like psychosis) and a manic psychosis.

Schizophreniform psychosis

Case histories typically describe a recent increase in khat use or heavy consumption. The patients typically present with paranoid delusions, fear, a hostile perception of the environment, auditory hallucinations (frequently of a persecutory or threatening type), ideas of reference, thought alienation and a tendency to isolate themselves, or alternatively displaying aggressive behaviour towards others. If khat consumption is ceased at this time, resolution of symptoms usually occurs within a short period (3–11 days), but there is a tendency for the psychosis to recur if khat chewing is restarted.

Manic psychosis

Several authors have described a manic-type psychosis. Giannini & Castellani (1982) reported the first case in the USA. The patient presented with hyper-activity, shouting, pressure of speech, grandiose delusions with flight of ideas and tangential thought processes, and a labile mood varying from euphoria to anger. The patient had used khat for the first time, chewing about 24 leaves (this is equivalent to a single dose of khat). Symptoms subsided spontaneously within about 8h of chewing. Drake (1988) also described a case of mania following prolonged chewing, with the patient 'running amok'.

Our own experience is of working in an adult mental health unit in Southall, west London. This area of London has a high number of Somali immigrants and refugees, a large proportion of whom are unemployed. Khat chewing in Somali cafes is a common pastime. Admissions to hospital due to khat-induced psychosis are not infrequent, usually associated with a recent increase in the amount consumed. Presentations are frequently similar to an amphetamine-like psychosis, with disturbed and violent behaviour. On occasions this requires compulsory hospital admission under the Mental Health Act 1983, often involving the use of Section 136 by the police.

Confusional states are rare; usually the paranoid reactions occur in clear consciousness. Kennedy *et al* (1983) stated that confusion and disorientation may occur as a transient phenomenon in the khat user, even without psychosis. Dhadphale & Omolo (1988) suggested that the people Kennedy *et al* studied were in fact exhibiting acute drug intoxication and were in a state of delirium. The level of sympathetic arousal is higher in acute khat intoxication than in heavy prolonged use, where some sympathetic tolerance occurs; this might be helpful in distinguishing between these situations (McLaren, 1987).

Depression

Several authors describe depression associated with chewing khat, but nearly all of these reports document that the depression arose on cessation of use. On occasions it was associated with self-harm and suicide. Such behaviour has also been reported following amphetamine use and cessation (Pantelis *et al*, 1989).

Self-harm, suicide and violence

Self-harm and suicide have been reported in the literature, although they are rare. Each has been documented during both chewing and the subsequent intoxication phase. One patient bit himself and repeatedly banged his head against the wall. Another took an overdose because of the distress caused by his paranoid symptoms. Suicide has been described by several authors in the context of a 'withdrawal state'.

Violent acts, including homicide, are also documented, usually in the context of paranoid or persecutory delusions. Alem & Shibre (1997) described a case where a patient murdered one of his wives and his daughter. He was acquitted of murder by the court, as he was deemed not responsible for his actions. Alem *et al* (1999) also reported a case of combined homicide and suicide after chewing increased amounts of khat.

Effects of long-term khat use

Intoxication with khat is self-limiting, but chronic consumption can lead to impairment of mental health, possibly contributing to personality disorders and 'mental deterioration' (Kalix & Braenden, 1985). Conversely, Dhadphale & Omolo (1988) reported no increased long-term psychiatric morbidity among khat chewers.

Physical sequelae

The physical effects of khat are well documented and can be described according to the physiological systems affected (Box 4.1).

Box 4.1 The physical adverse effects of khat

Cardiovascular system	Tachycardia, arrhythmias, palpitations, hypertension, vasoconstriction, ischaemia, infarction, pulmonary oedema, cerebral haemorrhage (Giannini *et al*, 1986). Exacerbation of pre-existing cardiac conditions
Respiratory system	Bronchitis, tachypnoea, dyspnoea, tuberculosis
Gastrointestinal system	Dry mouth, polydipsia, dental caries, periodontal disease, chronic gastritis, gastric ulcer, constipation (54% in one study, Elmi, 1983), paralytic ileus, anorexia, weight loss, increased risk of upper gastrointestinal malignancy
Hepatobiliary system	Cirrhosis
Genitourinary system	Spermatorrhoea, impotence, libido change, urinary retention (complicated by diuresis from increased fluid intake)
Obstetric effects	Low birth weight, stillbirths, impaired lactation
Metabolic and endocrine effects	Hyperthermia, perspiration, hyperglycaemia
Central nervous system	Dizziness, impaired concentration, insomnia, headaches, migraine, midriasis, conjunctival congestion, impaired motor coordination, fine tremor, stereotypical behaviour (Kalix, 1984)

Socio-economic effects

In communities where khat is used regularly it has a negative impact on health and socio-economic conditions.

Decreased productivity

Khat chewing leads to loss of work hours, decreased economic production, malnutrition and diversion of money in order to buy further khat. It is indirectly linked to absenteeism and unemployment, which may in turn result in a fall in overall national economic productivity. It is reported that habitual khat chewing has led to decreased productivity in Ethiopia, Somalia, Uganda and Kenya (Giannini *et al*, 1986). Others argue that moderate use improves performance and increases work output, owing to the stimulant and fatigue-postponing effects. Consequently, working hours and possibly productivity can decrease when khat is not used, because of anergia and reduced motivation.

Family and marital problems

Kalix & Khan (1984) estimated that in Djibouti about one-third of all wages were spent on khat. Many men secure their daily portion of khat at the expense of vital needs, indicating dependence. Family life is harmed because of neglect, dissipation of family income and inappropriate behaviour. Khat is quoted as a factor in one in two divorces in Djibouti. Acquisition of funds to pay for khat may lead to criminal behaviour and even prostitution (Elmi, 1983).

Economic perspectives of growing khat

The urban poor are the most negatively affected, but in rural areas scarce arable land and irrigation water are used for khat instead of for nutrient plants and the export crop, coffee. However, the economic benefit from selling and exporting khat is said to be high (Kalix, 1984).

Khat and cigarettes, alcohol and illicit drugs

A Home Office survey (Griffiths, 1998) noted that 60% of Somali khat chewers in London also smoked cigarettes; 75% of these were men, smoking 5–45 cigarettes per day. Only a minority used any other drugs and the most common was cannabis, used by 6% of the sample.

Heavy chewers use khat to stay awake, increase productivity or feel 'high'. They then need alcohol to rest, calm their nerves or sleep: alcohol is used to counteract the stimulating effect and sleeplessness caused by the khat. Omolo & Dhadphale (1987) investigated the use of alcohol with khat, and surveyed 100 general hospital out-patients in Kenya: 29 chewed khat, and of these, 20 also drank alcohol, 12 of them heavily. Khat has been linked to the misuse of other drugs. In Somalis living in London, high rates of concomitant heroin and cocaine use were found, but this was thought to be associated with the traditional availability of these drugs in their home country (Griffiths, 1998).

Interactions between khat and prescribed medication

Khat can interact with therapeutic drugs. Phenylpropanolamine, which can display synergism with khat, is widely available in over-the-counter cold and appetite-suppressant preparations and in prescription drugs. The use of monoamine oxidase inhibitors is to be avoided with khat users, as they are likely to precipitate a dangerous level of sympathetic stimulation, possibly leading to a hypertensive crisis. Reactions to surgical anaesthetics may be bizarre in chronic khat users and during the post-operative period patients may be agitated and overaroused.

Detection of khat

Urinalysis

In the UK, a commercially available biochemical test to detect khat constituents in the urine can now be used for confirmation of a suspected khat-induced state. Initially, a rapid screen by immunoassay detects amphetamine-related compounds. Then gas chromatography mass spectrometry is performed. This cannot detect cathinone directly, but a positive result indicates the presence of norephedrine, a cathinone metabolite. The test will give a positive result for up to about 48h after consumption of khat, although this is dependent on many factors, for example chronic consumption as opposed to a single episode of use, the quantity taken, the user's metabolism and dilution of urine following consumption of fluids. The test is highly sensitive, but not highly specific, and there are some cross-reactions with other metabolites (Lehmann et al, 1990). However, in the context of the clinical presentation together with the history of khat consumption, the urinalysis is a useful additional test. In many areas urine testing is not available, and an accurate history of (increased) khat consumption prior to the onset of clinical symptoms is equally important, if not more so.

Management of psychiatric problems related to khat use

There is a paucity of information in the literature regarding treatment of khat-induced psychiatric illnesses. Before the advent of antipsychotic drugs, and possibly currently in areas where access to modern health care is poor or not culturally acceptable, relatives and friends of patients managed the situation by locking them in their homes until the condition subsided, which may take several days. Physical restraint may sometimes be needed to ensure the safety of the patient and others.

Reports of pharmacological management

Many episodes of khat-induced psychosis resolve spontaneously within 1–2 days of cessation of use; sometimes symptoms subside within less than 24h. Most clinicians agree that, even when antipsychotics are given, the improvement is attributed to stopping the khat rather than taking antipsychotics. Occasionally, a psychotic episode may require longer periods of treatment (i.e. several weeks) with antipsychotics for full resolution.

Case reports of effective resolution of symptoms describe treatment with thioridazine at doses of 300–600 mg/day for 1 week, haloperidol (doses not specified) and, in one case, electroconvulsive therapy (Alem & Shibre, 1997). For several cases the duration of treatment with antipsychotics was not specified; however, reports of resolution of symptoms (dependent on cessation of khat use) were given as 'within 1 week'. Treatment with new or atypical antipsychotics has not yet been reported. Box 4.2 lists practice points for clinicians managing patients who misuse khat. The following fictional case report describes a common situation.

Fictional case report

A 22-year-old Somali male was admitted via the accident and emergency department. He had poor appetite, insomnia and grandiose delusions. He

---

Box 4.2 Practice points

- Enquire about use of khat in Somali or any other East African patients
- Khat use can be tested by urine sample on admission
- Interim use of benzodiazepine and antipsychotic medication is often necessary for symptom control
- Pure khat-induced psychosis resolves rapidly
- Mental and behavioural disorders due to the use of stimulants (khat) is often a comorbid diagnosis in such patients

---

had been talking and laughing to himself, and admitted to experiencing visual hallucinations in the form of scenes of people being tortured.

He admitted that he had chewed khat intermittently for about 6 years. His use of khat had increased for several weeks prior to admission.

On the ward he was verbally and physically aggressive. He was prescribed zuclopenthixol acetate. Oral regular antipsychotic medication was started with haloperidol and subsequently depot zuclopenthixol dihydrochloride 200 mg intramuscularly weekly. After initially responding with a decrease in his psychotic symptoms, he absconded from the ward. He returned later exhibiting bizarre behaviour and worsening of his mental state. His khat bundles were confiscated and disposed of. He admitted to chewing khat during the period of absence from the ward.

Continued regular depot medication led to a gradual decrease and disappearance of his psychotic symptoms over the next 4 weeks. He abstained from further use of khat (confirmed by negative urinalysis) and was discharged 8 weeks after admission.

References

Alem, A. & Shibre, T. (1997) Khat induced psychosis and its medico legal implication: a case report. *Ethiopian Medical Journal*, **35**, 137–141.

Alem, A., Kebede, D. & Kullgren, G. (1999) The prevalence and socio-demographic correlates of khat chewing in Butajira, Ethiopia. *Acta Psychiatrica Scandinavica Supplementum*, **100**, 84–91.

Critchlow, S. & Seifert, R. (1987) Khat-induced paranoid psychosis. *British Journal of Psychiatry*, **150**, 247–249.

Dhadphale, M. & Omolo, O. E. (1988) Psychiatric morbidity among khat chewers. *East African Medical Journal*, **65**, 355–359.

Drake, P. H. (1988) Khat-chewing in the Near East. *Lancet*, i, 532–533.

Elmi, A. S. (1983) The chewing of khat in Somalia. *Journal of Ethnopharmacology*, **8**, 163–176.

Giannini, A. J. & Castellani, S. (1982) A manic-like psychosis due to khat (*Catha edulis Forsk*). *Journal of Clinical Toxicology*, **19**, 455–459.

Giannini, A. J., Burge, H., Shaheen, J. M., *et al* (1986) Khat: another drug of abuse? *Journal of Psychoactive Drugs*, **18**, 155–158.

Goudie, A. J. (1987) Importing khat, legal but dangerous. *Lancet*, ii, 1340–1341.

Gough, S. P. & Cookson, I. B. (1984) Khat induced schizophreniform psychosis in UK. *Lancet*, i, 455.

Griffiths, P. (1998) *Qat Use in London: A Study of Khat Use among a Sample of Somalis Living in London* (Home Office Paper 26). TSO (The Stationery Office).

Halbach, H. (1972) Medical aspects of the chewing of khat leaves. *Bulletin of the World Health Organization*, **47**, 21–29.

Kalix, P. (1984) The pharmacology of khat. *General Pharmacology*, **15**, 179–187.

Kalix, P. (1988) Khat: a plant with amphetamine effects. *Journal of Substance Abuse and Treatment*, **5**, 163–169.

Kalix, P. & Braenden, O. (1985) Pharmacological aspects of the chewing of khat leaves. *Pharmacological Reviews*, **37**, 149–164.

Kalix, P. & Khan, I. (1984) Khat: an amphetamine-like plant material. *Bulletin of the World Health Organization*, **62**, 681–686.

Kennedy, J. G., Teague, J., Rokaw, W., *et al* (1983) A medical evaluation of the use of qat in North Yemen. *Social Science and Medicine*, **17**, 783–793.

Lehmann, T., Geisshüsler, S. & Brenneisen, R. (1990) Rapid TLC identification test for khat (*Catha edulis*). *Forensic Science International*, **45**, 47–51.

Luqman, W. & Danowski, T. S. (1976) The use of khat (*Catha edulis*) in Yemen: social and medical observations. *Annals of Internal Medicine*, **85**, 246–249.

McLaren, P. (1987) Khat psychosis. *British Journal of Psychiatry*, **150**, 712–713.

Nencini, P., Ahmed, A. M., Aminconi, G., *et al* (1984) Tolerance develops to sympathetic effects of khat in humans. *Pharmacology*, **28**, 150–154.

Nencini, P., Ahmed, A. M. & Elmi, A. S. (1986) Subjective effects of khat chewing in humans. *Drug and Alcohol Dependence*, **18**, 97–105.

Nencini, P., Grassi, M. C., Botan, A. A., *et al* (1989) Khat chewing spread to the Somali community in Rome. *Drug and Alcohol Dependence*, **23**, 255–258.

Omolo, O. E. & Dhadphale, M. (1987) Alcohol use among khat (*Catha*) chewers in Kenya. *British Journal of Addiction*, **82**, 97–99.

Pantelis, C., Hindler, C. G. & Taylor, J. C. (1989) Use and abuse of khat (*Catha edulis*): a review of the distribution, pharmacology, side effects and a description of psychosis attributed to khat chewing. *Pharmacological Medicine*, **19**, 657–668.

Yousef, G., Huq, Z. & Lambert, T. (1995) Khat chewing as a cause of psychosis. *British Journal of Hospital Medicine*, **54**, 322–326.

CHAPTER 5

What the clinician needs to know about magic mushrooms

Nicholas Seivewright and Olawale Lagundoye

Summary   Some species of mushrooms are classified as hallucinogenic drugs, although strictly speaking the phenomenology is usually in partial form, such as illusions. Some perceptual and associated mood disturbances can be highly distressing, and clinicians are more likely to encounter acute anxiety or confusional states than see mushroom users electively presenting at drug services. There are also short-term physical adverse effects, and severe poisoning may result if the 'wrong' type of mushroom is taken. Treatment of psychiatric complications is symptomatic, with no special approaches in this form of substance misuse.

'Magic mushrooms' refer to mushrooms that grow naturally and have hallucinogenic (sometimes called psychedelic) properties. Different species have been consumed in various cultures over the centuries, with use in ritual ceremonies in Mexico being particularly well known. In the UK at present the species most commonly used is *Psilocybe semilanceata*, also known as the liberty cap mushroom. This grows in many areas, particularly in dark places and after heavy rainfall, with fruition occurring from September to November. It is creamy-yellow or brown in colour, very small (5–15 mm across) with a thin fragile stalk. In the USA a closely related type is used.

The active chemical psilocybin is categorised in class A in the UK's Misuse of Drugs Act 1971, so in theory there can be severe penalties for offences. However, possession of the mushrooms in their natural state is not illegal; charges can be brought only if they have been prepared in some way for consumption (see below).

Usage

Psilocybe semilanceata mushrooms (to which the rest of this chapter refers) can be eaten raw, cooked or brewed into a liquid. They may also be dried, sometimes for keeping for later use, and the dried form can be put into cigarettes, a pipe or home-made capsules. There have apparently been rare instances of injecting the liquid form.

Because the mushrooms are small, about 10–100 are typically used at a time. Nearly all usage is personal or within small groups, and there is no significant illicit market. They are commonly used experimentally by young people: the 2006 British Crime Survey revealed that just under 1 in 10 people aged between 16 and 24 years admitted to having tried magic mushrooms (Home Office, 2006). Some experimenters become more regular users, and cases among older people often involve individuals with somewhat 'alternative' lifestyles. The most common other substances of misuse in mushroom users appear to be alcohol and cannabis. In general, mushrooms are consumed on their own.

In no sense can magic mushrooms be said to be truly addictive, with one particular measure finding them to be the least dependence-producing of all illicit substances (Gable, 1993). However, a degree of tolerance does occur, so that if they are consumed on two days running more will be required the second time to achieve the desired effects. This tolerance disappears within days, but effectively acts as a natural constraint against very frequent use.

Desired effects

It is well known that the effects of magic mushrooms broadly resemble those of lysergic acid diethylamide (LSD) (Leikin et al, 1989). The desired effects, which to some extent relate to the user's expectations, include a pleasant state of detachment and euphoria and then the hallucinatory experiences – more correctly, often illusions or pseudo-hallucinations, involving images, colours and sounds. In a report of cases seen in the early days of magic mushroom use in the UK (Peden et al, 1981), distortions of perception of faces received special comment. The phenomenon of synaesthesia, in which sensations cross between modalities (for instance, colours may appear to have a smell), has mainly been reported with LSD but may also occur with mushrooms. The overall experience is referred to as a 'trip', which starts within 20 min or so of ingestion and may last several hours, partly dependent on the amount taken and the route.

The effects of hallucinogenic drugs generally appear to be partly related to actions on the serotonergic transmission system, but the mechanisms relating to mushrooms in particular are not known.

Adverse effects

The possible adverse effects of magic mushrooms are summarised in Box 5.1.

Physical

If many mushrooms are taken, the user may experience nausea, vomiting, stomach pains and dizziness. There is general physiological arousal, with tachycardia more frequent than elevations in blood pressure (Peden et al,

---

Box 5.1   Adverse effects of magic mushrooms

- Nausea and vomiting
- Tachycardia
- Poisoning (if 'wrong' species taken)
- Accidents
- Anxiety, panic
- Acute confusion
- Psychotic reactions

1981). Pupils become enlarged but react to light. The main physical danger, however, occurs if similar-looking poisonous mushrooms such as the *Amanita* species in the UK are taken by mistake. Some species can be fatal, and in cases of accidental poisoning identification by a mycologist is recommended if the mushrooms are available. Individuals in states of mushroom-induced intoxication are also at risk of accidents of various kinds.

Psychological

Any hallucinogenic drug can produce a so-called 'bad trip' instead of the desired effects. In this there is anxiety and general mood disturbance, with the hallucinations and alterations in consciousness seeming alarming. This is more likely to occur in inexperienced users, or when dysphoria was present before taking the drug. Acute confusional states may develop, and the hallucinatory experiences can develop into a state that it is correct to term a psychotic disorder. Such states would be expected to subside completely in less than 24 h, but the clinical picture may be complicated if other drugs such as alcohol or cannabis have been used. The prototype of the hallucinogenic drugs in terms of effects and adverse effects is LSD, the psychiatric complications of which have been reviewed by Abraham & Aldridge (1993). It can be supposed that magic mushrooms produce modified forms of some of these typical effects, but it must be recognised that very little literature refers to mushrooms specifically.

Testing

Testing for psilocybin is not included in the routine urine (or hair) screening for drugs done by UK hospital laboratories. Special assays can be set up, but the short half-life of the chemical means that detection would be missed in some cases. Urine screening for the range of substances is, however, always clinically indicated where drug use is suspected, and clearly mushroom users may have used other substances. Also, it appears that sometimes non-hallucinogenic mushrooms are 'spiked' with drugs such as LSD.

Box 5.2 Possible ICD–10 diagnoses in use of magic mushrooms

F16.0   Acute intoxication

F16.1   Harmful use

F16.5   Psychotic disorder

Classification of disorders

The ICD–10 (World Health Organization, 1992) specifies mental and behavioural disorders that can occur due to any psychoactive substance use, which may be applied to hallucinogens as one of the nine categories of drugs (there is also a coding for disorders due to multiple drug use). Box 5.2 shows the diagnoses that could possibly be made in relation to magic mushrooms.

Management

As seen currently in the UK, the use of magic mushrooms is either experimental in nature or represents a lifestyle feature. Users would hardly ever view themselves as having a problem with the drug, with the possible exception of some of its acute effects. It is therefore virtually unheard of for users to present to drug services asking for help with cutting down or stopping, although such advice could be given if necessary. In practice, the relevant management is of complications such as toxicity or confusional or brief psychotic states, and is largely supportive, with symptomatic treatment as necessary. There are no features of mushroom use that would lead to selection of specific treatments within such management.

Conclusion

The main clinical messages regarding magic mushrooms are indicated in Box 5.3.

Whenever psychiatrists encounter cases of drug misuse, consideration must be given to possible additional diagnoses. The strongest overall association is with personality disorder (Grant *et al*, 2004), with studies indicating that about one-half of drug misusers have this diagnosis, usually the antisocial category. However, many studies are of opiate misusers in treatment settings, and it is reasonable to assume a lower rate in users of the more 'recreational' drugs, although such use may still be an indicator of personal problems of various kinds.

Box 5.3 Main learning points

- Magic mushrooms are not addictive, but produce physiological effects and sometimes significant psychiatric complications
- Although 'recreational', the use of magic mushrooms may be one indicator of conduct or personality disorder
- Urine testing cannot usually detect the psilocybin constituent of mushrooms, but should be done to screen for other drugs
- Management of complications is symptomatic, with no specific approaches indicated

---

Clinicians will rarely be called upon to advise users regarding their magic mushroom use, but knowledge is necessary of the possible direct psychiatric complications and the occasional need for management.

References

Abraham, H. D. & Aldridge, A. M. (1993) Adverse consequences of lysergic acid diethylamide. *Addiction*, **88**, 1327–1334.

Gable, R. S. (1993) Toward a comparative overview of dependence potential and acute toxicity of psychoactive substances used non-medically. *Journal of Drug and Alcohol Abuse*, **19**, 263–281.

Grant, B. F., Stinson, F. S., *et al* (2004) Co-occurrence of 12-month alcohol- and drug-use disorders and personality disorders in the US. Results from the National Epidemiological Survey of Alcohol and Related Conditions. *Archives of General Psychiatry*, **61**, 361–368.

Home Office (2006) *Drug Misuse Declared: Findings from the 2005/2006 British Crime Survey*. Home Office.

Leikin, J. B., Krantz, A. J., Zell-Kanter, M., *et al* (1989) Clinical features and management of intoxication due to hallucinogenic drugs. *Medical Toxicology and Adverse Drug Experience*, **4**, 324–350.

Peden, N. R., Bisset, A. F., Macaulay, K. E. C., *et al* (1981) Clinical toxicology of 'magic mushrooms' ingestion. *Postgraduate Medical Journal*, **57**, 543–545.

World Health Organization (1992) *The ICD–10 Classification of Mental and Behavioural Disorders. Clinical Descriptions and Diagnostic Guidelines*. WHO.

CHAPTER 6

What works in alcohol use disorders?

Jason Luty

Summary Treatment of alcohol use disorders typically involves a combination of pharmacotherapy and psychosocial interventions. About one-quarter of people with alcohol dependence ('alcoholics') who seek treatment remain abstinent for over 1 year. Research has consistently shown that less intensive, community treatment (particularly brief interventions) is just as effective as intense, residential treatment. Many psychosocial treatments are probably equally effective. Techniques for medically assisted detoxification are widespread and effective. More recent evidence provides some support for the use of drugs such as acamprosate to prevent relapse in the medium to long term.

There has been much recent debate and criticism of UK alcohol policy (Drummond, 2004; Hall, 2005). Over the past 20 years, per capita alcohol consumption in Britain has increased by 31%, leading to large increases in the prevalence of alcoholic cirrhosis, alcohol-related violence and heavy alcohol use. Alcohol misuse causes at least 22 000 premature deaths each year and costs the taxpayer an estimated £20 billion (Prime Minister's Strategy Unit, 2003). The key features of alcohol dependence and harmful use are listed in Box 6.1. About 5% of the UK population are dependent on alcohol (Farrell *et al*, 2001) and 8 million Britons drink more than recommended levels.

In their review of seven multicentre studies in the USA and Europe, involving over 8000 treatment-seeking individuals, Miller *et al* (2001) found that overall mortality at 1-year follow-up was about 1.5%. Clients reported an 87% reduction in alcohol consumption, with abstinence on 80% of days. Overall, 24% were abstinent for the entire year, and a similar proportion resumed controlled, problem-free drinking. These results were validated using confidants (often the client's spouse). Most relapses occurred within the first 3 months. These results are supported by other studies, including a more recent review of alcohol treatment from the Scottish Executive (Ludbrook *et al*, 2005). By contrast, Vaillant (1983) estimated that 2–3% of alcohol-dependent individuals in the USA abstain spontaneously each year in the community.

Box 6.1 Alcohol dependence and harmful use

Key features[1] of ICD–10 dependence include:

- Compulsion to drink
- Problems in controlling drinking
- Physiological withdrawal symptoms
- Escalating consumption, owing to tolerance
- Preoccupation with alcohol, to the exclusion of other pursuits
- Increasing time lost to hangovers
- Disregard of evidence that excessive drinking is harmful
- Harmful alcohol use
- Harmful use is diagnosed if there is evidence that alcohol is damaging an individual's mental or physical health, but criteria for dependence are not met

1. Full diagnostic criteria appear in ICD–10 (World Health Organization, 1992: pp. 75–76).

Unfortunately there are many uncertainties in the evidence base for treatment of alcohol use disorders – not least of which is the cost-effectiveness of therapy. Many in-patient and residential alcohol services in the UK were downsized following the famous trials by Edwards (see below). Controversies also remain concerning the benefits of disulfiram and controlled drinking.

Ideally, trials of alcohol treatment should follow more than 70% of participants for 1 year and confirm alcohol consumption using relatives or other confidants. Clients should be breathalysed at follow-up interviews. Appropriate outcome measures include time to first drink, time to relapse (more than five standard drinks in one day), biochemical markers (especially γ-glutamyl transferase and carbohydrate-deficient transferase) and functional outcome scales such as the Alcohol Problems Questionnaire. A number of the published trials fail to meet these ideals. Another common problem is an unusually high rate of adherence to medication regimens (often exceeding 70%) or conclusions based on very small samples.

Home *v.* in-patient detoxification

Detoxification is a treatment designed to control both the medical and psychological complications that may occur temporarily after a period of heavy and sustained alcohol use. Clinical procedures for managing detoxification are well described in chapter 7. These usually involve chlordiazepoxide at diminishing doses over 7–10 days, with parenteral thiamine supplementation. Ideally the dose of medication should be titrated against withdrawal symptoms. The mean cell volume has been identified as the best predictor of withdrawal complications such as hallucinations or fits. These occur in 5–10% of patients and would indicate in-patient detoxification (Metcalf *et al*, 1995). Unfortunately a history of previous alcohol withdrawal seizures has little predictive value.

In the 1960s in-patient psychotherapy over several weeks was the preferred method of therapy for alcohol dependence. However, published reports have consistently failed to find any difference in outcome between long and short in-patient detoxification programmes (Miller & Hester, 1986). For example Foster *et al* (2000) report a study of 64 alcohol-dependent patients admitted for either 7 or 28 days. About 60% relapsed (drank more than the recommended weekly intake) over the 3-month follow-up period.

Edwards & Guthrie (1967) reported a classic trial of 40 alcohol-dependent men who were randomly assigned to in-patient or 'intensive' out-patient treatment. Treatment duration for both groups was 7–9 weeks. Participants were followed up each month for 1 year. Social worker support and medication were used to provide assistance where necessary, for example by encouraging return to work. There was no significant difference in outcome between the groups when assessed by independent raters.

Edwards & Guthrie's influential paper encouraged the development of home detoxification procedures that have become the preferred method of treatment for most people dependent on alcohol. Clients can usually complete home detoxification in 5–9 days. In ideal circumstances they are visited twice daily for the first 3 days and medication is supervised by a relative. Clients are breathalysed and medication withheld if they have consumed significant amounts of alcohol.

Hayashida *et al* (1989) reported a randomised trial of in-patient (77) and out-patient (87) detoxification using oxazepam with daily clinic visits. In-patient detoxification was significantly shorter than out-patient detoxification (6.5 *v*. 9.2 days). Fewer out-patients completed the procedure (72 *v*. 95%). There were no serious medical complications in either group. Both groups had improved at 6 months, with no significant differences; nearly half the participants were completely abstinent. In-patient detoxification cost 9–20 times more than out-patient detoxification. Hayashida *et al* noted that the Veterans Administration Medical Center in Philadelphia had reported the out-patient detoxification of more than 6000 individuals with no serious adverse consequences. Many of these people had no supportive friends or relatives. Home detoxification can also be conducted by a nurse or general practitioner without recourse to a specialist. Other trials have shown no difference in outcome between in-patient and home detoxification (Irvin *et al*, 1999).

Treatment intensity

Research has consistently shown that less intensive treatments are as effective as the more intensive options (Chick *et al*, 1988). For example, Edwards *et al* (1977) reported another classic trial of 100 alcohol-dependent men randomised to a treatment group or an advice-only group. The treatment group received a 12-month programme involving introduction to Alcoholics Anonymous (AA), calcium cyanamide, drugs to cover withdrawal, regular contact with a psychiatrist, advice on abstinence strategies and interpersonal problems, and regular support for the patient's wife from a social worker. If out-patient management failed, participants were offered in-patient detoxification for around 6 weeks. Participants in the advice-only group were offered just a sympathetic explanation that the responsibility for improvement lay with them and they were advised to abstain from alcohol completely. There was no difference between the two groups on outcome measures, including alcohol consumption. For example, 50–60% of each group still had significant drinking problems at 12 months.

These results have been confirmed in other populations. For example, Chapman & Huygens (1988) reported a study of 113 alcohol-dependent men in New Zealand randomised to a single confrontational interview or a 12-week programme involving 6 weeks' in-patient treatment. There was no difference between groups, with about one-third of participants abstinent after 18 months.

In the USA, Project MATCH (see below) showed very similar outcomes between the three forms of psychotherapy under study (Project MATCH Research Group, 1997). The four-session motivational enhancement therapy was just as effective as the 12-session treatments (twelve-step facilitation therapy or cognitive–behavioural therapy). Furthermore UKATT, the UK Alcohol Treatment Trial (2005), which is also discussed below, found that three-session motivational enhancement therapy was 48% cheaper but equally as effective as an eight-session social behaviour/network therapy.

Brief interventions

Brief interventions are short, focused discussions (often of less than 15 min) that can reduce alcohol consumption in some individuals with hazardous drinking (Wallace *et al*, 1988; Fleming *et al*, 1997). Brief interventions are designed to promote awareness of the negative effects of drinking and to motivate change. Most share a set of common components such as feedback about the adverse effects of alcohol, comparison of the individual's consumption with drinking norms and discussion of the adverse effects of drinking. They are often based on motivational interviewing (see below).

Many reviews have shown the effectiveness of brief interventions (e.g. Wilk *et al*, 1997; Hall, 2005). Moyer *et al* (2002) report a meta-analysis of 34 controlled trials comparing brief interventions (fewer than five sessions) offered to treatment-seeking and non-treatment-seeking people with alcohol misuse. Brief interventions were shown to be moderately effective in the non-treatment-seeking groups, especially for those with less severe alcohol problems (effect sizes of 0.14–0.67 were reported). However, this analysis found no similar evidence for people from the treatment-seeking populations. Other reviewers estimated that brief interventions reduce alcohol consumption by around 24% compared with control conditions (Effective Health Care Team, 1993). Many of these trials included people with severe alcohol problems.

A UK trial involving 909 men and women with excessive alcohol consumption randomly assigned to brief interventions or usual care showed that mean alcohol consumption in men was reduced by 18 drinks per week compared with 8 for the control group (Wallace *et al*, 1988). Project TrEAT (Trial for Early Alcohol Treatment) involved 723 people with problem drinking randomly assigned to brief interventions or no treatment. At 12 months the mean number of drinks per week had fallen from 19 at baseline to 11 in the intervention group and to 15.5 in controls (Fleming *et al*, 1997).

The great debate: abstinence *v.* controlled drinking

The controversial idea that some people recovering from alcohol dependence ('recovering alcoholics') can resume drinking was suggested by Davis (1962). This followed a study at London's Maudsley Hospital of 93 alcohol-dependent individuals, of whom seven had become 'normal' drinkers. The goal of controlled (moderate or non-problem) drinking usually includes some limit on alcohol consumption (e.g. 4 units per day) provided that drinking does not lead to signs of dependence, intoxication or social, legal or health problems. This runs contrary to the abstinence-based philosophy of Alcoholics Anonymous.

Controlled drinking may be an option for young, socially stable drinkers with short, less severe drinking histories (e.g. alcohol consumption of less than 4 units per day and normal liver function tests). An individual's belief that controlled drinking is an achievable goal is also a good prognostic factor. Most authors agree that controlled drinking should not be recommended for people with heavy dependence or those with protracted alcohol problems (Rosenberg, 1993). Controlled drinking is an attractive option for public health strategies aimed at non-dependent problem drinking.

The majority of studies of controlled drinking involve very different treatment interventions, as well as different goals. Hence it has been difficult to distinguish the effect of the advice (controlled drinking or abstinence) from other aspects of treatment. However, Sanchez-Craig *et al* (1984) reported one of the few randomised controlled trials. A sample of 70 people with early-stage problem drinking received six sessions of weekly cognitive–behavioural therapy and were randomised to groups with either a controlled drinking or an abstinence goal. There was no difference in outcomes at 2 years. In both groups at 6 months, drinking had been reduced from 51 to 13 drinks per week and 40–50% of participants had relapsed. These results were similar to those of a randomised controlled study by Foy *et al* (1984). Whereas the debate between controlled drinking and abstinence is unresolved, the trials indicate that clients themselves decide which of these goals to follow and that they are often uninfluenced by the agenda set by the therapist.

Alcoholics Anonymous

Alcoholics Anonymous is a worldwide organisation that has provided mutual aid for alcoholics for over 60 years. It uses the twelve-step approach (see Box 1.2, p. 8), and involves the recognition that alcoholism is a relapsing illness that requires complete abstinence. Clients are required to acknowledge their alcoholism and also the harm they are causing themselves and others. New participants are encouraged to attend '90 meetings in 90 days'. Participants may engage the support of a sponsor who is an AA member who has been sober for at least 1 year. Overall, around half of new AA participants continue for at least 3 months, and about two-thirds of all members have been sober for over 1 year (Chappel, 1997).

Alcoholics Anonymous groups are widely available, inexpensive and popular, but it has been difficult to demonstrate their effectiveness. Randomised controlled trials have not found AA groups or the twelve-step approach to be superior to alternative treatments (Nowinski et al, 1992; McCrady et al, 1996), but the evidence suggests that the twelve-step approach is at least as effective as most structured psychotherapies. A meta-analysis by Tonigan et al (1996) of 74 studies demonstrated a modest improvement in overall drinking patterns in AA members. However, participants are often involved in other forms of treatment, and studies are typically small and rarely randomised.

Project MATCH

Project MATCH (Matching Alcohol Treatments to Client Heterogeneity) was a multicentre US trial involving two groups of participants (Project MATCH Research Group, 1997). One group, of 774 individuals (the after-care group), was recruited from patients receiving care after in-patient treatment for alcoholism. The other, of 952 individuals (the out-patient-only group), was recruited from people about to receive out-patient treatment for alcoholism. Participants in each group were randomly assigned to three forms of manualised psychotherapy: four sessions of motivational enhancement therapy, 12 sessions of twelve-step facilitation or 12 sessions of cognitive–behavioural therapy. There was no control group. Stringent efforts were made to ensure that the treatment manuals were followed, including tape-recording each consultation. Follow-up was at 1 and 3 years. Rigorous entry criteria were applied, which led to high treatment adherence but might also have resulted in a degree of favourable patient selection. Participants receiving each of the three treatments showed significant improvements, although there was no significant difference between the three treatment modalities. At 1 year, 35% of the after-care clients (who had undergone in-patient detoxification) had remained completely abstinent, compared with 20% of the out-patient-only sample. Project MATCH was hugely expensive and is the largest trial of any form of psychotherapy in history.

UKATT

The United Kingdom Alcohol Treatment Trial (UKATT) involved 742 people seeking treatment for alcoholism at seven sites around the UK. Participants were randomised to social behaviour and network therapy or to motivational enhancement therapy, with follow-up at 3 and 12 months. Both groups reported similar, substantial reductions in alcohol consumption and alcohol-related problems, better mental health and improved quality of life based on a variety of measures (UK Alcohol Treatment Trial, 2005). For example the number of days abstinent from alcohol increased from 30% at baseline to 46% at 1 year, whereas average alcohol consumption per drinking day fell from 27 units to 19. Much like Project MATCH, only 23% of the 3241 treatment-seeking clients ultimately completed the trial. This may have produced a degree of favourable patient selection.

Psychological therapies (see chapters 16 and 17)

Motivational enhancement therapy

Motivational enhancement therapy is based on the process of motivational interviewing, and has been largely developed by William Miller (Miller & Rollnick, 2000, see also chapter 17). The technique, based on theories of cognitive dissonance, attempts to promote a favourable attitude to change. Instructing people on the error of their ways tends to provoke resistance to change. In motivational interviewing, clients themselves draw up a list of problems caused by their behaviour and give reasons why they should alter it. Box 6.2 gives the FRAMES formulation that encompasses the principles of motivational interviewing.

Box 6.2 Principles of motivational interviewing: the FRAMES formulation

- F   Provide Feedback on behaviour
- R   Reinforce the patient's Responsibility for changing behaviour
- A   State your Advice about changing behaviour
- M   Discuss a Menu of options to change behaviour
- E   Express Empathy for the patient
- S   Support the patient's Self-efficacy

After Miller & Rollnick (2000)

Project MATCH showed motivational enhancement therapy to be effective, although only four sessions were used, compared with 12 sessions of the other treatments. Motivational interviewing is an ideal brief therapy for patients with problem drinking in primary care.

Motivational enhancement therapy in UKATT comprised three sessions, each of 50 min, over 8–12 weeks. It combined counselling in the motivational style with objective feedback. Significant others were generally excluded from the sessions, in contrast to Project MATCH.

Twelve-step facilitation

Twelve-step facilitation is a form of structured intervention to enhance engagement with AA (Nowinski *et al*, 1992). In Project MATCH it was delivered individually rather than at conventional AA groups. However, the objectives included encouraging participants to become members of AA groups and to accept the AA philosophy.

Cognitive–behavioural therapy

Cognitive–behavioural therapy (cognitive–behavioural coping skills) for alcoholism assumes that alcoholism is a maladaptive habit rather than a purely physiological response to alcohol. Drinking becomes a means of coping with difficult situations, unpleasant moods and peer pressure. Consequently, coping skills are taught to deal with these high-risk situations (Carroll & Schottenfeld, 1997).

Cognitive–behavioural therapy involves several techniques, many of which have been studied in isolation. The terminology is confusing and varied. In general, cognitive–behavioural therapy for alcoholism includes techniques such as relapse prevention, behavioural marital therapy, social skills training and community reinforcement approaches. Many of these techniques are subsumed under the heading of behavioural skills training. Exhaustive reviews (Finney & Monahan, 1996; Miller & Wilbourne, 2002) identified variations of these techniques as some of the most effective treatments for alcoholism.

Many forms of relapse prevention treatment are based on cognitive–behavioural therapy. Irvin *et al* (1999) reported a meta-analysis that included ten randomised controlled trials of relapse prevention treatment in alcoholism. The overall effect size was 0.37, conventionally regarded as medium to large. Follow-up periods ranged from 6 months to 1 year. Significantly, there was a greater effect on psychosocial function than on drinking behaviour.

Social skills training

Social skills training is a component of cognitive–behavioural therapy. The method assumes that a larger repertoire of coping skills will reduce the stress of high-risk situations and provide alternatives to alcohol use. Techniques involve assertiveness training, modelling and role-playing of skills such as refusal of alcohol and dealing with interpersonal problems.

At least 25 controlled trials of social skills training have been published. One of these was a randomised trial of eight weekly 90-min sessions of social skills training or group discussion (Ericksen *et al*, 1986). Over 1 year clients in the social skills training group drank one-third less than those in the discussion group, had twice as many sober days (77 *v*. 32%) and remained abstinent for six times as long after discharge.

The community reinforcement approach

The community reinforcement approach (CRA) was developed in North America (Sisson & Azrin, 1986) and is a form of behavioural marital and family therapy. According to the original programme, a friend or family member, usually the spouse, uses the provision or removal of agreed reinforcers to reward periods of sobriety and punish drinking. Reinforcers include access to radio, television, newspapers, telephone and driving licence. The spouse may also be shown how to identify and take advantage of moments when the drinker is most motivated to enter treatment, reinforce attendance at relapse prevention groups (usually AA) and supervise disulfiram. The prescribing of disulfiram, early access to a counsellor in the event of relapse and the involvement of neighbours and friends were introduced to enhance the programme's effectiveness. These programmes typically require 30 h of the client's time.

Many of the randomised studies by enthusiasts of the community reinforcement approach report more than 90% abstinent days compared with 10–45% for individual counselling (Edwards & Steinglass, 1995). Dramatic reductions in alcohol consumption were observed even while the spouse was undergoing training before the partner began treatment. UKATT provides some information on the use of a variation of community reinforcement and cognitive–behavioural therapy in the UK, although it is impossible to determine the effectiveness of each component. The effectiveness of the community reinforcement approach itself has not been confirmed in the UK.

Social behaviour and network therapy

Social behaviour and network therapy (SBNT) is based on the principle that people with serious drinking problems need to develop a social network that supports change. It uses techniques adapted from cognitive–behavioural therapy and the community reinforcement approach to help clients build these networks. The therapy was developed for UKATT, where it involved eight 50-min sessions over 8–12 weeks (Copello *et al*, 2002).

Contingency management

Contingency management is particularly useful when there is no significant other to provide forms of community reinforcement. The four principal components of contingency management are shown in Box 6.3.

Box 6.3   Principal components of contingency management

- The clinician arranges the environment such that alcohol use is readily detectable
- Reinforcers are arranged to reward abstinence
- Incentives are withheld following alcohol use
- Reinforcement from alternative sources (employment, family or social) is increased to compete with that from alcohol

---

Petry *et al* (2000) described a North American study of a contingency management technique whereby abstinence (a negative breathalyser test) or the completion of various steps towards treatment goals earned participants the right to draw vouchers from a bowl and win prizes ranging from $1 to $100 in value (from a $1 meal voucher to a hand-held television). No negative consequences resulted from self-reported alcohol use. Forty-two alcohol-dependent people were randomised to receive standard treatment plus contingency management or standard treatment alone. Standard treatment involved attending 5 days per week for 5 h each day for the first 4 weeks, with follow-up sessions ranging from 1 to 3 per week for a further 4 weeks. After 8 weeks each participant in the contingency management group had earned an average of $200 worth of prizes. Eighty-four per cent of the contingency management group completed the treatment course compared with 22% of the controls. Furthermore, 69% were abstinent compared with 39% of controls.

Although contingency management is an effective addition to many forms of treatment, it creates an ethical controversy by 'paying' alcoholics not to drink. Furthermore, there is a tendency to relapse when the reinforcing regime is ended. This may explain the reluctance of many services to introduce contingency management.

Cue exposure

When someone who has been dependent on alcohol encounters cues previously paired with drinking, such as a bottle or the smell of alcohol, they may experience responses such as craving and withdrawal-like symptoms which can motivate them to drink. Cue exposure involves repeated exposure to such stimuli in an attempt to extinguish the cravings and other undesirable responses. Although results for this approach have been variable, there is now some evidence of the benefit of cue exposure from the Mesa Grande project (Drummond & Glautier, 1994; Miller *et al*, 2001; Ludbrook *et al*, 2005). In one trial, 100 alcohol-dependent individuals were randomised to ten sessions of cue exposure plus coping skills training or to a meditation and relaxation control condition (Rohsenow *et al*, 2001). At 12-month follow-up individuals in the experimental group who had lapsed reported fewer heavy drinking days (12%) than those in the meditation and relaxation group (25%). They also made greater utilisation of coping skills techniques.

Therapeutic communities and residential rehabilitation

Therapeutic communities typically require prolonged residence (often 12–18 months) and clients are closely involved in their running, including selecting and discharging residents. Abstinence is usually a prerequisite. Despite the long tradition of this approach and its continued popularity, very little critical research has been performed into its effectiveness. Although therapeutic communities are extremely expensive, of the 361 controlled studies of in-patient treatment for alcohol dependence, involving 72 000 clients, reviewed by Miller & Wilbourne (2002) only one involved treatment in a therapeutic community. This showed no benefit over the control treatment.

Most studies of therapeutic communities are conducted without control groups, and the lack of randomisation probably leads to selection bias in favour of more motivated patients. One such, reported by Van de Velde *et al* (1998), involved 881 participants, three-quarters of whom had alcohol dependence, residing in a Dutch therapeutic community providing a 1-year programme. Forty-five per cent of the participants remained in the therapeutic community for at least 5 months. At 2.5 years the proportion drinking heavily (more than 4 units per day) had fallen from 77% to 20%. Almost half of those who had been dependent on alcohol were abstinent after 4.5 years.

Drug treatments

Disulfiram

Disulfiram prevents the breakdown of alcohol by acetaldehyde dehydrogenase. This leads to accumulation of acetaldehyde, causing headache, flushing, palpitations, nausea and vomiting. Disulfiram was extremely popular in the 1950s and 1960s and was hailed as a 'cure' for alcoholism. This enthusiasm has waned with the results of more recent trials. Hughes & Cook (1997) reviewed 24 outcome studies for oral disulfiram and 14 for disulfiram implants from 1967 to 1995. Most studies were flawed and reported no significant benefits for disulfiram. There was no good evidence in favour of disulfiram implants. In the largest trial 605 men were randomly assigned to three groups, including oral disulfiram compared with placebo over 1 year. There was no overall difference in drinking outcome (Fuller *et al*, 1986). For example, the proportion continuously abstinent was 19% in the disulfiram group compared with 16% in the control group. However, disulfiram did lead to a reduction in the number of drinking days (49 *v.* 86). Only 20% of participants had acceptable adherence with the medication regimens.

Chick *et al* (1992) report one placebo-controlled trial involving 126 alcohol-dependent individuals randomised to receive supervised disulfiram or placebo (although participants were not masked to treatment). Over the 6-month follow-up period, the average increase in the number of abstinent days was 100 for the disulfiram group and 69 for the placebo group. Alcohol use was reduced by 70–80% in the disulfiram group compared with 50% in placebo group. Fifty-five per cent of participants adhered to the protocol. Although this trial was really a composite of disulfiram and community reinforcement, it is nevertheless one of the few convincing trials to show significant benefits of disulfiram.

Disulfiram causes potentially fatal acute hepatotoxicity in about 1 in 25 000 patients. This has led several authors to recommend either frequent (every 2 weeks) liver function tests or avoidance of disulfiram in those with abnormal liver function (Fuller & Gordis, 2004).

Naltrexone

Naltrexone is an orally active opiate receptor antagonist that is thought to reduce the pleasurable effects of drinking. At least 10 controlled trials, involving 1500 participants, have been published (Kiefer *et al*, 2003). Two early randomised controlled trials compared naltrexone with placebo in people with alcohol dependence (O'Malley *et al*, 1995). Overall, 54% of participants remained abstinent at 12 weeks in the naltrexone group compared with 31% in the placebo group. However, the difference became less dramatic after 6 months (O'Malley *et al*, 1996).

Chick *et al* (2000*a*) reported a double-blind randomised controlled trial involving 169 individuals assigned to naltrexone or placebo after medical detoxification. Fewer than half completed the 12-week trial. Intention-to-treat analysis revealed no significant difference in drinking outcomes between the groups (complete abstinence occurred in about 20%). However, the quantity of alcohol consumed and the number of non-abstinent days were halved in the 70 participants in the naltrexone group who took 80% of the tablets given to them.

Volpicelli *et al* (1997) reported a study of 97 alcohol-dependent individuals randomised to naltrexone or placebo. The relapse rate at 12 weeks was 53% in controls and 35% in participants receiving naltrexone. The proportion of drinking days was 11% in controls and 6% in those receiving naltrexone. However, adherence to treatment was exceptionally good, with 73% reporting that they had taken over 90% of the prescribed tablets.

Overall these studies report a medium to large effect size of 0.3–0.6 (Kiefer *et al*, 2003). By comparison, the largest double-blind randomised controlled trial of naltrexone involved 627 participants. At 1 year there was no difference between groups (Krystal *et al*, 2001). For example, the proportion of drinking days was 15–19% in the two groups receiving naltrexone and

18% in the placebo group, while the mean time to relapse was 72 days in those receiving naltrexone and 62 days in those taking the placebo. (Relapse is conventionally defined as consuming more than five standard drinks on 1 day.) Adherence to the medication regimen was 44% over the year.

Although recent meta-analyses indicate that naltrexone may be as effective as acamprosate, naltrexone does not have a licence for treatment of alcohol dependence in the UK. Furthermore, research has shown less evidence of efficacy in European trials than in the USA (Soyka & Chick, 2003).

Acamprosate

Early studies suggested that acamprosate (an analogue of the inhibitory neurotransmitter γ-aminobutyric acid) approximately doubled the chances of achieving continuous abstinence following detoxification and increased the number of abstinent days by 30–40% (e.g. Sass *et al*, 1996). At least 14 controlled trials, involving 4000 participants, have been published (Kiefer *et al*, 2003). However, Chick *et al* (2000*b*) reported the largest single study of acamprosate: the United Kingdom Multicentre Acamprosate Study. This involved 581 individuals (one-third of whom were episodic drinkers, the rest dependent) randomly assigned to acamprosate or placebo under double-blind conditions. Overall adherence to treatment was poor (35%) and there was no significant difference in drinking outcomes between groups at 6 months. The mean total number of abstinent days was 77 in the acamprosate group compared with 81 in the placebo group, and complete abstinence was achieved by 12% and 11% respectively. Since this time, several other trials have reported more encouraging results, to the extent that the number needed to treat for acamprosate has been estimated at 8 (Soyka & Chick, 2003). Another review, based on data from Belgium and Germany, has calculated that acamprosate prescription may result in a healthcare cost saving of £600 per patient (Ludbrook *et al*, 2005).

Kiefer *et al* (2003) reported a randomised double-blind placebo-controlled study of 160 alcohol-dependent in-patients receiving naltrexone, acamprosate, a combination of naltrexone and acamprosate, or placebo. The relapse rate was about 50% in the placebo group and 30% for those receiving active medication. The relapse rate in the combination group was 25%. However, 80% adhered to the medication protocol and 90% attended follow-up appointments. Although 782 in-patients were informed about the study, only 160 chose to take part. These facts suggest a bias in favour of more highly motivated patients.

Conclusion

Research has consistently shown that less intensive, community-based treatment for alcoholism is just as effective as prolonged in-patient care. Large trials such as Project MATCH and UKATT show no significant difference between the various forms of psychosocial treatment. The dramatic improvements suggested by early trials of pharmacotherapy in relapse prevention have seldom been supported by later studies. There remains concern about trials of relatively expensive drugs (such as acamprosate and naltrexone) that report unusually high treatment adherence rates. Nevertheless more recent evidence provides some encouragement for the use of these agents. It is salient to note that some of the most effective means of reducing alcohol consumption, such as increasing taxation and restricting access, are being abandoned by governments 'bent on deregulation' (Hall, 2005). Government policy is likely to be influenced by the facts that the alcohol industry generates over £13 billion each year for the UK exchequer and employs well over 1.4 million people (Raistrick, 2005).

References

Carroll, K. M. & Schottenfeld, T. (1997) Nonpharmacologic approaches to substance abuse treatment. *Medical Clinics of North America*, **81**, 927–944.

Chapman, P. L. H. & Huygens, I. (1988) An evaluation of three treatment programmes for alcoholism an experimental study with 6- and 8-month follow-ups. *British Journal of Addiction*, **83**, 67–81.

Chappel, N. (1997) Addiction psychiatry and long-term recovery in 12-step programs. In *The Principles and Practice of Addictions in Psychiatry* (ed. N. S. Miller). W. B. Saunders.

Chick, J., Ritson, B., Connaughton, J., *et al* (1988) Advice versus extended treatment for alcoholism: a controlled study. *British Journal of Addiction*, **83**, 159–170.

Chick, J., Gough, K., Falkowski, W., *et al* (1992) Disulfiram treatment of alcoholism. *British Journal of Psychiatry*, **161**, 84–89.

Chick, J., Howlett, H., Morgan, M. Y., *et al* (2000a) A multicentre, randomised, double-blind, placebo-controlled trial of naltrexone in the treatment of alcohol dependence or abuse. *Alcohol and Alcoholism*, **35**, 587–593.

Chick, J., Howlett, H., Morgan, M. Y., *et al* (2000b) The United Kingdom Multicentre Acamprosate Study. *Alcohol and Alcoholism*, **35**, 176–187.

Copello, A., Orford, J., Hodgson, R., *et al* (2002) Social behaviour and network therapy. *Addictive Behaviors*, **27**, 345–366.

Davis, D. L. (1962) Normal drinking in recovered alcohol addicts. *Quarterly Journal of Studies on Alcohol*, **23**, 94–104.

Drummond, D. C. (2004) An alcohol strategy for England: the good, the bad and the ugly. *Alcohol and Alcoholism*, **39**, 377–379.

Drummond, D. C. & Glautier, S. (1994) A controlled trial of cue exposure treatment in alcohol dependence. *Journal of Consulting and Clinical Psychology*, **41**, 809–817.

Edwards, G. & Guthrie, S. (1967) A controlled trial of in-patient and out-patient treatment of alcohol dependence. *Lancet*, **i**, 555–559.

Edwards, G., Orford, J., Egert, S., *et al* (1977) Alcoholism: a controlled trial of "treatment" and "advice". *Journal of Studies on Alcohol*, **38**, 1004–1031.

Edwards, M. E. & Steinglass, P. (1995) Family therapy treatment outcomes for alcoholism. *Journal of Marital and Family Therapy*, **21**, 475–509.

Effective Health Care Team (1993) Brief interventions and alcohol use. *Effective Health Care Bulletin*, **7**. Royal Society of Medicine Press.

Ericksen, L., Bjornstad, S. & Gotestam, K. G. (1986) Social skills training in groups for alcoholics. *Addictive Behaviours*, **11**, 309–329.

Farrell, M., Howes, S., Bebbington, P., *et al* (2001) Nicotine, alcohol and drug dependence and psychiatric comorbidity. Results of a national household survey. *British Journal of Psychiatry*, **179**, 432–437.

Finney, L. & Monahan, G. (1996) The cost-effectiveness of treatment for alcoholism. *Journal of Studies on Alcohol*, **57**, 229–243.

Fleming, M. F., Barry, K. L., Manwell, L. B., *et al* (1997) Brief physician advice for problem drinkers. A randomised controlled trial in community-based primary care practices. *JAMA*, **277**, 1039–1045.

Foster, J. H., Marshall, E. J. & Peters, T. J. (2000) Outcome after in-patient detoxification for alcohol dependence. *Alcohol and Alcoholism*, **35**, 580–586.

Foy, D. W., Nunn, L. B. & Rychtarick, R. G. (1984) Broad-spectrum behavioural treatment for chronic alcoholics. *Journal of Consulting and Clinical Psychology*, **52**, 218–230.

Fuller, R. K. & Gordis, E. (2004) Does disulfiram have a role in alcoholism treatment today? *Addiction*, **99**, 21–24.

Fuller, R. K., Branchey, L., Brightwell, D. R., *et al* (1986) Disulfiram treatment of alcoholism. *JAMA*, **256**, 1449–1455.

Hall, W. (2005) British drinking: a suitable case for treatment? *BMJ*, **331**, 527–528.

Hayashida, M., Alterman, A., McLellan, A. T., *et al* (1989) Comparative effectiveness and cost of in-patient and out-patient detoxification of patients with mild to moderate alcohol withdrawal syndrome. *New England Journal of Medicine*, **320**, 358–365.

Hughes, J. C. & Cook, C. C. H. (1997) The efficacy of disulfiram: a review of outcome studies. *Addiction*, **92**, 381–395.

Irvin, J. E., Bowers, C. A., Dunn, M. E., *et al* (1999) Efficacy of relapse prevention: a meta-analytic review. *Journal of Consulting and Clinical Psychology*, **67**, 563–570.

Kiefer, F., Jahn, H., Tarnaske, T., *et al* (2003) Comparison and combining naltrexone and acamprosate in relapse prevention of alcoholism. *Archives of General Psychiatry*, **60**, 92–99.

Krystal, J. H., Joyce, J. A., Krol, W. F., *et al* (2001) Naltrexone in the treatment of alcohol dependence. *New England Journal of Medicine*, **345**, 1734–1739.

Ludbrook, A., Godfrey, C., Wyness, L., *et al* (2005) *Effective and Cost-Effective Measures to Reduce Alcohol Misuse in Scotland*. Scottish Executive.

McCrady, B. S., Epstein, E. E. & Hirsch, L. S. (1996) Issues in the implementation of a randomised clinical trial that includes Alcoholics Anonymous. *Journal of Studies on Alcohol*, **57**, 604–612.

Metcalf, P., Sobers, M. & Dewey, M. (1995). The Windsor Clinic Alcohol Withdrawal Assessment. *Alcohol and Alcoholism*, **30**, 367–372.

Miller, W. & Hester, R. (1986) Inpatient alcoholism treatment. *American Psychologist*, **41**, 361–366.

Miller, W. R. & Rollnick, S. (2000) *Motivational Interviewing* (2nd edn). Guilford Press.

Miller, W. R. & Wilbourne, P. L. (2002) Mesa Grande: a methodological analysis of clinical trials of treatment for alcohol use disorders. *Addiction*, **97**, 265–277.

Miller, W., Walters, S. T. & Bennett, M. E. (2001) How effective is alcoholism treatment in the United States? *Journal of Studies on Alcohol*, **62**, 211–220.

Moyer, A., Finney, J. W., Swearingen, C. E., *et al* (2002) Brief interventions for alcohol problems. A meta-analytic review of controlled investigations in treatment-seeking and non-treatment-seeking populations. *Addiction*, **97**, 279–292.

Nowinski, J., Baker, S. & Carroll, K. M. (1992) *Twelve-Step Facilitation Therapy Manual*. National Institute on Alcohol Abuse and Alcoholism.

O'Malley, S. S., Croop, R. S., Wroblewski, J. M., *et al* (1995) Naltrexone in treatment of alcohol dependence: a combined analysis of two trials. *Psychiatric Annals*, **25**, 681–688.

O'Malley, S. S., Jaffe, A. J., Chang, C., *et al* (1996) Six month follow-up of naltrexone and psychotherapy for alcohol dependence. *Archives of General Psychiatry*, **53**, 217–224.

Petry, N. M., Martin, B., Conney, J. L., *et al* (2000) Contingency management for alcoholism. *Journal of Consulting and Clinical Psychology*, **68**, 250–257.

Prime Minister's Strategy Unit (2003) *Strategy Unit Alcohol Harm Reduction Project: Interim Analytical Report*. Cabinet Office. http://www.number10.gov.uk/files/pdf/SU%20interim_report2.pdf

Project MATCH Research Group (1997) Matching Alcohol Treatments to Client Heterogeneity: posttreatment drinking outcomes. *Journal of Studies on Alcoholism*, **58**, 7–29.

Raistrick, D. (2005) The United Kingdom: alcohol today. *Addiction*, **100**, 1212–1214.

Rohsenow, D. J., Monti, P. M., Rubonis, A. V., *et al* (2001) Cue exposure with coping skills training for alcohol dependence. *Addiction*, **96**, 1161–1174.

Rosenberg, H. (1993) Prediction of controlled drinking by alcoholics and problem drinkers. *Psychological Bulletin*, **113**, 129–139.

Sanchez-Craig, M., Annis, H. M., Bornet, A. R., *et al* (1984) Random assignment to abstinence and controlled drinking. *Journal of Consulting and Clinical Psychology*, **52**, 390–403.

Sass, H., Soyka, M., Mann, K., *et al* (1996) Relapse prevention by acamprosate. *Archives of General Psychiatry*, **53**, 673–680.

Shaw, G. K. (1978) Alcohol and the nervous system. *Clinics in Endocrinology and Metabolism*, **7**, 385–404.

Sisson, R. W. & Azrin, N. H. (1986) Family member involvement to initiate and promote treatment of problem drinkers. *Journal of Behaviour Therapy and Experimental Psychiatry*, **17**, 15–21.

Soyka, M. & Chick, J. (2003) Use of acamprosate and opioid antagonists in the treatment of alcohol dependence. *American Journal of Addictions*, **12** (suppl. 1), S69–S80.

Tonigan, J. S., Toscova, R. & Miller, W. R. (1996) Meta-analysis of the literature on Alcoholics Anonymous. *Journal of Studies on Alcohol*, **57**, 65–72.

UK Alcohol Treatment Trial (2005) Effectiveness of treatment for alcohol problems: findings of the randomised UK alcohol treatment trial (UKATT). *BMJ*, **331**, 541–547.

Vaillant, G. E. (1983) *The Natural History of Alcoholism*. Harvard University Press.

Van de Velde, J. C., Schaap, G. E. & Land, H. (1998) Follow-up at a Dutch addiction hospital and effectiveness of therapeutic community treatment. *Substance Use and Misuse*, **33**, 1611–1627.

Volpicelli, J. R., Rhines, K. C., Rhines, J. S., *et al* (1997) Naltrexone and alcohol dependence. Role of subject compliance. *Archives of General Psychiatry*, **54**, 737–742.

Wallace, P., Cutler, S. & Haines, A. (1988) Randomised controlled trial of general practitioner intervention in patients with excessive alcohol consumption. *BMJ*, **297**, 663–668.

Wilk, A. I., Jensen, N. M. & Havigan, T. C. (1997) Meta-analysis of randomised control trial addressing brief interventions in heavy alcohol drinkers. *Journal of General Internal Medicine*, **12**, 274–283.

World Health Organization (1992) *The ICD–10 Classification of Mental and Behavioural Disorders. Clinical Descriptions and Diagnostic Guidelines*. WHO.

CHAPTER 7

Management of alcohol detoxification

Duncan Raistrick

Summary   In many respects detoxification is a stand-alone medical procedure. None the less, the key to successful detoxification is preparation and a clear understanding of how the detoxification procedure fits in with the overall care plan. Detoxification is often straightforward, but clinicians need to be aware of potential risks and monitor accordingly. The problem for the clinician is predicting the severity of the withdrawal syndrome and anticipating the individual's response to medication when there are complicating factors such as other medication and mental or physical health problems. Depending on the level of risk, detoxification can be undertaken in a variety of settings, ranging from in-patient monitoring to self-directed home detoxification. Chlordiazepoxide or diazepam remain the first-line pharmacotherapies.

The majority of people with an alcohol dependence problem that is uncomplicated by serious mental illness or social chaos receive treatment in the community. There is strong evidence supporting the move towards briefer and community-based treatments, although intensive and in-patient treatments are needed for people with more complicated problems (Raistrick *et al*, 2006). It follows that the traditional sequencing of care, which might be characterised as having four phases – assessing and engaging service users, detoxification, specific therapy and aftercare – is less tidy than it used to be. Detoxification is seen much more as a stand-alone procedure that should be undertaken when the service user is ready, rather than as a prerequisite of starting treatment. Of course, there are also instances where detoxification may be required as an expedient, for example during an unplanned admission to hospital, or where regular high levels of intoxication are a barrier to effective intervention. Equally, where the focus of treatment is on mental illness rather than alcohol dependence, then detoxification may well be viewed as a necessary first step.

Given the high proportion of people who have a combined problem of mental illness and alcohol dependence, it is inevitable that general psychiatrists will need to be skilled in the management of detoxification, but whether they should also have skills specific to substance misuse treatments is more contentious. Service users, their friends and relatives and sometimes also doctors become so desperate when faced with a catalogue of alcohol-related harms that they seek a solution in detoxification; in itself, this may provide respite and be a caring intervention, but it cannot be expected to have an enduring effect on drinking behaviour. Detoxification should not take place in isolation. Rather it should be integrated with a suitable psychosocial therapy or, where mental illness is judged the primary problem, with the usual treatment for the mental illness. The particular purpose of detoxification is to minimise the severity of withdrawal symptoms that occur when alcohol consumption is abruptly stopped or markedly reduced, and thereby to achieve an alcohol-free state with maximum safety and minimum discomfort to the service user. *Models of Care for Alcohol Misusers* (Department of Health, 2006) sets detoxification within the framework of an integrated treatment system.

Alcohol withdrawal

Anyone may develop a tolerance to the effects of alcohol within a matter of days or weeks provided that they take a sufficiently high and regular dose. However, the manifestation of withdrawal typically occurs some way into a drinking career and is considered a marker of severe dependence. Descriptions of withdrawal symptomatology, including alcoholic delirium, can be found throughout historical texts. The scientific demonstration of alcohol tolerance and withdrawal, based on both observational and laboratory studies, is relatively recent and followed on from the classic study by Isbell *et al* (1955). Another classic study (Gross, 1977) concluded that the severity of the alcohol withdrawal syndrome relates to the abruptness of stopping drinking, modified by the contribution of residual effects of previous drinking. Gross's description of withdrawal has changed little in the intervening years and is now thought of as comprising three symptom clusters.

1   A tremulous state occurs within a few hours of stopping or markedly reducing alcohol intake and symptoms may include tremor, sweating, restlessness, anxiety, depression, fleeting hallucinations, nausea and vomiting, insomnia and nightmares.
2   Seizures may occur without antecedent tremulousness and are usually of the grand mal variety. Partial (focal) seizures are usually due to trauma.
3   Alcoholic delirium is often preceded by seizures and most commonly occurs days after stopping or reducing drinking. Seizures and alcoholic delirium occur in less than 5% of problem drinkers.

Tremulousness and seizures seem to exist along a continuum of severity, whereas delirium, once triggered, runs a more independent course. Many of the symptoms that commonly occur in alcohol withdrawal are also found in mental illnesses, stress disorders and intoxication with a variety

Box 7.1 The 10 most common and the 10 most specific symptoms of alcohol withdrawal (adapted from Hershon, 1977)

Most common symptoms
- Depression
- Anxiety
- Irritability
- Tiredness
- Craving
- Restlessness
- Insomnia
- Confusion
- Sweating
- Weakness

Most specific symptoms
- Whole body shaking
- Hand or finger shaking
- Facial tremulousness
- Cannot face the day
- Panic
- Guilt
- Nausea
- Visual hallucinations
- Weakness
- Depression

of psychoactive drugs (Box 7.1). Negative mood states are highly likely to provoke drinking, which in turn is likely to relieve the symptoms: this holds true not only for people experiencing withdrawal, but also during periods of total abstinence from alcohol. In other words, negative mood states are a powerful relapse precipitant.

These characteristics of alcohol withdrawal are well known. For the majority of service users, there are no complications from withdrawal and there comes to be an expectation that all detoxification is risk-free. The danger is that clinicians may not exercise sufficient vigilance when monitoring withdrawal and may find themselves dealing with avoidable problems or, at worst, a fatality. It is the timing of withdrawal symptomatology that is particularly unpredictable – the tremulous state typically peaks within 6–24 h of stopping or reducing alcohol consumption. Illusionary or transient hallucinatory phenomena superimposed on the tremulous state, but occurring within a similar time scale, should alert clinicians to a more severe withdrawal and the need to review medication. The peak incidence of seizures occurs at about 36 h and of delirium at about 72 h after drinking has ceased or reduced, although both of these phenomena may occur while a person is still drinking. Probably the most important determinant of severity of withdrawal is the rate of fall in blood alcohol level, which in turn is a function of peak blood alcohol level. The clinician is often unable to get a full history and so observation is all-important.

Preparation for detoxification

The presence of withdrawal symptoms is sometimes seen to be the essence of addiction or at least of physical dependence. This preoccupation with withdrawal, which is often also associated with an emphasis on its pharmacological treatment, is unhelpful and distracting. In psychological terms, detoxification reduces the severity of withdrawal and thereby eliminates the negative reinforcement of relief drinking. In practice, a broad spectrum of drinking cues are diminished as the process of detoxification progresses. Neuroadaptation, that is, tolerance and withdrawal, is a function of recent alcohol intake that correlates highly with alcohol dependence but is theoretically distinct. Placing undue emphasis on substance-specific withdrawal fails to recognise the variety of cues and cue complexes that act as sources of reinforcement and contribute to building dependence, fails to take account of the transferability of dependence from one substance to another, and fails to take account of persistent dependence in people who have achieved long periods of abstinence. All of these have practical implications for future treatment plans.

The key to a successful, planned detoxification is preparation. The first job of therapy is to bring the individual to a point of readiness to change their drinking behaviour. In terms of the popular 'stages of change' model (DiClemente & Prochaska, 1998) this means at least reaching the determination stage. At this stage, individuals are sufficiently well motivated to make a sustained effort to change. In other words, they have reached a good-quality decision to change rather than opting for detoxification because they feel physically unwell, are under pressure from family or work, or simply feel the need for a temporary break from drinking. Motivation is not necessarily something that individuals either have or do not have. Practitioners can help to build motivation by consistently using motivational dialogue (Raistrick & Tober, 2007). Once the therapist is certain that the individual has reached the determination stage there is, ideally, a second step, which involves more detailed and more practical preparation work.

This work is probably best handled with the assistance of a leaflet or workbook that the individual can take away as homework. Allen et al (2005) found that individuals are likely to have fears about where the detoxification will happen, the severity of the withdrawal, the medication and life without alcohol. They will have difficulty reaching the action stage until these fears are dealt with. The key feature of the action stage is having a positive outcome expectancy or, more simply, the individual needs to believe that life is going to be better after detoxification. Individuals often assume that this will be the case, but have not really thought through the implications of not drinking, which will often mean not seeing friends or drinking mates and having unfilled time. Not doing something is inherently unrewarding and it is crucial that positive alternatives to drinking are planned.

It follows that individuals need to be given accurate information about what to expect during detoxification. Information-giving is likely to reduce the severity of the withdrawal and increase adherence to medication (Phillips et al, 1986). As part of information-giving, it is often useful to map out a timetable for the week in which detoxification will take place and for the following week. Filling out such a timetable in some detail is a convenient

or who need social support in order to stay away from alcohol. The essential therapeutic skill is the ability rapidly to form a working alliance with the service user while having confidence to refer to Tier 2 when necessary. Some sophistication can be added by the use of the increasingly popular 'feel good' therapies such as acupuncture, massage or homoeopathy.

Tier 2 – Open-access services

This tier is suitable for people with a moderate severity of withdrawal, but who none the less require some pharmacological treatment. It may be that the medical and nursing input available is quite limited and from staff who do not have specific addiction training. In these circumstances, it is sometimes useful to have a fixed-dose prescribing regimen in place (Table 7.1). Primary care, medical and psychiatric out-patient clinics and some voluntary sector agencies provide services at this tier.

Tier 3 – Specialist community-based services

This is for people with moderate to severe withdrawal problems, many of whom can be treated successfully by specialist staff working in the community or in a day facility. This tier requires medical and nursing staff who are trained and experienced in the management of addiction problems and who can handle complicated prescribing regimes. It is possible to care for service users who are hallucinating and who have a history of seizures provided that control of the withdrawal syndrome is rapidly achieved. This tier is likely to be part of a larger consultant-led service.

Tier 4 – Specialist residential services

This is for people with the most severe withdrawal, which usually includes delirium and often includes seizures or other medical complications associated

Table 7.1 Fixed-protocol chlordiazepoxide for severe withdrawal

	Dose, mg				
	Morning	Midday	Evening	Night-time	Total daily
Day 1	30	30	30	30	120
Day 2	30	20	20	30	100
Day 3	20	20	20	20	80
Day 4	20	10	10	20	60
Day 5	10	10	10	10	40
Day 6	10	10	0	10	30
Day 7	10	0	0	10	20

with severe withdrawal, such as hypertension, Wernicke's encephalopathy, hepatic failure, subdural haematoma, hypoglycaemia, electrolyte imbalance (especially magnesium deficiency) and polydrug use. People with a severity of withdrawal requiring Tier 4 services should be regarded as a medical emergency requiring care from an experienced medical team.

Pharmacotherapy for withdrawal

Alcohol enhances the inhibitory effects of the neurotransmitter gamma-aminobutyric acid (GABA) and diminishes the activity of the excitatory N-methyl-D-aspartate (NMDA) receptors. Pharmacotherapy of withdrawal is therefore based on depressant drugs that enhance GABA. In turn, GABA influences other transmitter systems that are thought to contribute to the alcohol withdrawal syndrome (Nutt, 1999) – dopaminergic induction of psychotic symptoms, NMDA excitability that reduces the seizure threshold, and glutamate overdrive of noradrenergic sympathetic activity.

Regardless of what medication is chosen there are three delivery regimens to consider:

- fixed-dose regimen
- front-loading regimen
- symptom-triggered regimen.

The first is the simplest method and requires little staff expertise; indeed, it can be managed by sensible family and friends. The second method, described by Day *et al* (2004), involves assessing the severity of withdrawal at the start of detoxification and then every 90 min. If the severity rating is above a predetermined 'trigger' score, then 20 g diazepam is given until two successive ratings fall below the trigger score. The third method is most demanding of competent staff and aims to tailor dose to severity of symptoms. In general the more sophisticated the delivery method the less medication is used and the more rapid the recovery.

When medication is used to treat uncomplicated alcohol withdrawal, chlordiazepoxide is recognised as the gold standard (Williams & McBride, 1998; Lingford-Hughes *et al*, 2004); diazepam has been used as if equivalent to chlordiazepoxide, although theoretically it has greater dependence-forming potential because it is more rapidly absorbed. The efficacy of chlordiazepoxide is similar to that of other benzodiazepines but it has the advantages of having a low dependence-forming potential and unique metabolites that can be detected on urinary toxicology screening. This may be helpful where polydrug use is an issue. Often, doses of chlordiazepoxide of 100–200 mg daily are required. Where there are prodromal signs of delirium, a loading dose of 100 mg chlordiazepoxide can be effective in aborting progression to delirium. The different pharmacological properties of other benzodiazepines determine their therapeutic place: for example, oxazepam can be useful where there is liver insufficiency, and lorazepam, which is well absorbed intramuscularly, is useful to achieve a loading dose rapidly.

> **Box 7.5** Common adjunctive medication
>
> - Hypertension: beta-blockers
> - Seizures: carbamazepine
> - Hallucinations: haloperidol
> - Poor nutrition: thiamine and magnesium

There is evidence that chlormethiazole is superior to benzodiazepines at preventing alcoholic delirium; however, this drug has a high dependence-forming potential, a risk of fatal respiratory depression if taken with alcohol and can quickly accumulate to toxic levels if there is liver damage. The evidence points to using chlormethiazole on an in-patient basis only and as a second-line medication.

Carbamazepine has been used where there is a history of withdrawal seizures and it is a rational alternative to chlordiazepoxide (Williams & McBride, 1998). Carbamazepine is thought to diminish the kindling process that causes successive episodes of seizure activity to lower the threshold for future seizures. Medicated withdrawal has the disadvantage of prolonging abnormal brain activity to a degree that may trigger further drinking, so detoxification should always move to relapse prevention as soon as possible.

As the severity of withdrawal increases, so does the likelihood of additional medical conditions. The rule of thumb is to treat these according to standard therapy (Box 7.5). For example, where paranoid thoughts are a feature of withdrawal, olanzapine might be the treatment of choice. Different considerations apply when assessing nutritional status. People who misuse alcohol are at particular risk of Wernicke's encephalopathy, because they have low levels of stored thiamine and because the metabolism of alcohol requires significant amounts of thiamine. Where there is any suggestion of dietary neglect or in any case where there is a high withdrawal score, there is strong evidence in favour of giving multivitamin supplements delivering at least 300 mg thiamine daily and magnesium (Cook & Thomson, 1997).

Audit of practice

Most people receiving treatment for alcohol dependence at some time enter a detoxification programme. Achieving successful detoxification is an important part of the overall treatment plan. Failure in detoxification is likely to engender a sense of hopelessness among both service users and staff. Significant resources are used for detoxification. For all these reasons, it is important that an effective audit system is in place. Audit should be a routine part of practice in specialist units, but is more difficult to organise in general psychiatry or primary care settings.

On the face of it, detoxification has a clearly defined endpoint – being alcohol-free – and is therefore easy to evaluate. Certainly, it is important to know how many people successfully become alcohol-free, but equally it is important to know the quality of the detoxification delivered. There is a further problem in that most clinicians see completion of detoxification, that is reaching an alcohol-free state, to be an unsatisfactory endpoint. Although not strictly part of detoxification, it is certainly part of the overall programme to see that effective steps have been taken to prevent relapse in the immediate post-detoxification period. Exactly what these steps might be varies from one service to another but might, for example, include prescribing disulfiram and ensuring attendance at an aftercare appointment. Box 7.6 summarises the audit measures used by the Leeds Addiction Unit. A follow-up at 1 month post-detoxification has been judged to allow enough time to check that the detoxification team has succeeded in starting aftercare plans, but not enough time for undue contamination by factors beyond the control of the detoxification programme.

Conclusion

Detoxification is not usually a technically difficult procedure. Whether detoxification is an expedient, or part of a planned care programme, it is always an opportunity to help people change their drinking behaviour. There is a persuasive argument in favour of selecting chlordiazepoxide as the first-line pharmacotherapy for most alcohol withdrawal problems. Other benzodiazepines have equal efficacy and may be preferred by clinicians, but their pharmacokinetics are generally less suitable than those of chlordiazepoxide. It may be necessary to prescribe high doses in order to achieve rapid containment of the withdrawal syndrome.

What has changed in recent years is the pattern and range of alcohol treatment services. There has been a broadening of the base of treatment both in terms of the settings in which it commonly occurs and also the variety of staff now involved in therapy. This all means that integrating detoxification into an overall care plan becomes more difficult. Wherever practical, detoxification followed by a 3–4 week period of abstinence from psychoactive drugs should precede making any definitive diagnosis or commencing treatment for mental illness.

References

Allan, C. A., Smith, I. & Mellin, M. (2002) Changes in psychological symptoms during ambulant detoxification. *Alcohol and Alcoholism*, 37, 241–244.

Allen, J., Copello. A. & Orford, J. (2005) Fear during alcohol detoxification: views from the clients' perspective. *Journal of Health Psychology*, 10, 503–510.

Alwyn, T., John, B., Hodgson, R. J., et al (2004) The addition of a psychological intervention to a home detoxification programme. *Alcohol and Alcoholism*, 39, 536–541.

Box 7.6 Alcohol detoxification audit schedule

The following items appear on the Leeds Addiction Unit's audit of detoxification

Pre-detoxification
- Age
- Gender
- LDQ score
- CORE–OM score
- Drinking history:
  - units of alcohol
  - duration of drinking
- Other substance misuse
- Medication
- Urine toxicology screen
- Illnesses
- Detoxification preparation
- Substance use (ICD code)
- Individual's stage of change
- Setting in which detoxification is to take place

Day 1 to final day of detoxification
- Windsor Clinic rating scale
- Pulse and blood pressure
- Medication
- Side-effects

Final day of detoxification
- Adverse events
- Duration of detoxification (days)
- Dropped out or completed
- Disulfiram prescribed?
- Date of next appointment with keyworker

1 month after detoxification
- Current drinking (units of alcohol)
- Medication
- LDQ score
- CORE–OM score
- Therapist contact
- Psychiatric diagnosis (ICD code)
- Substance use (ICD code)
- Treatment satisfaction questionnaire

LDQ, Leeds Dependence Questionnaire (Raistrick *et al*,1994); CORE–OM (Evans *et al*, 2002)

Cook, C. H. & Thomson, A. D. (1997) B-complex vitamins in the prophylaxis and treatment of Wernicke–Korsakoff syndrome. *British Journal of Hospital Medicine*, **57**, 461–465.

Day, E., Patel, J. & Georgiou, G. (2004) Evaluation of a symptom-triggered front-loading detoxification technique for alcohol dependence: a pilot study. *Psychiatric Bulletin*, **28**, 407–410.

Department of Health (2006) *Models of Care for Alcohol Misusers (MoCAM)*. Department of Health.

DiClemente, C. C. & Prochaska, J. O. (1998) Towards a comprehensive, transtheoretical model of change: stages of change and addictive behaviors. In *Treating Addictive Behaviors* (2nd edn) (eds W. R. Miller & N. Heather), pp. 3–24. Plenum.

Driessen, M., Arolt, V., John, U., *et al* (1996) Psychiatric comorbidity in hospitalised alcoholics after detoxification treatment. *European Addiction Research*, **2**, 17–23.

Evans, C., Connell, J., Barkham, M., *et al* (2002) Towards a standardised brief outcome measure: psychometric properties and utility of the CORE–OM. *British Journal of Psychiatry*, **180**, 51–60.

Gross, M. M. (1977) Psychobiological contributions to the alcohol dependence syndrome: a selective review of recent research. In *Alcohol Related Disabilities* (eds G. Edwards, M. M. Gross, M. Keller, *et al*), pp. 107–131 (WHO Offset Publication No. 32). World Health Organization.

Gross , M. M., Rosenblatt, S. M., Chartoff, S., *et al* (1971) Evaluation of acute alcoholic psychoses and related states. *Quarterly Journal of Studies on Alcohol*, **32**, 611–619.

Hershon, H. I. (1977) Alcohol withdrawal symptoms and drinking behavior. *Journal of Studies on Alcohol*, **38**, 953–971.

Isbell, H., Fraser, H. F., Wikler, A., *et al* (1955) An experimental study of the etiology of 'rum fits' and delirium tremens. *Quarterly Journal on Studies of Alcohol*, **16**, 1–33.

Johnston, A. L., Thevos, A. K., Randall, C. L., *et al* (1991) Increased severity of alcohol withdrawal in in-patient alcoholics with a co-existing anxiety diagnosis. *British Journal of Addiction*, **86**, 719–725.

Lingford-Hughes, A., Welch, S. & Nutt, D. (2004) Evidence based guidelines for the pharmacological management of substance misuse, addiction, and co-morbidity: recommendations from the British Association for Psychopharmacology. *Journal of Psychopharmacology*, **18**, 293–335.

Metcalfe, P., Sobers, M. & Dewey, M. (1995) The Windsor Clinical Alcohol Withdrawal Assessment Scale (WCAWAS): investigation of factors associated with complicated withdrawals. *Alcohol and Alcoholism*, **30**, 367–372.

Moos, R., Moos, B. S. & Timko, C. (2006) Gender, treatment and self-help in remission from alcohol use disorders. *Clinical Medicine and Research*, **4**, 163–174.

Mortimer, R. & Edwards, J. G. (1994) Detoxification in a community-based alcohol recovery unit and psychiatric department of a general hospital. A comparative study. *Psychiatric Bulletin*, **18**, 218–220.

Nutt, D. (1999) Alcohol and the brain. Pharmacological insights for psychiatrists. *British Journal of Psychiatry*, **175**, 114–119.

Phillips, G. T., Gossop, M. & Bradley, B. (1986) The influence of psychological factors on the opiate withdrawal syndrome. *British Journal of Psychiatry*, **149**, 235–238.

Raistrick, D. & Tober, G. (2007) Motivational Dialogue 2 – special treatment situations. In *Motivational Dialogue: Preparing Addiction Professionals for Motivational Interviewing Practice* (eds G. Tober & D. Raistrick), pp. 212–228. Routledge.

Raistrick, D., Bradshaw, J., Tober, G., *et al* (1994) Development of the Leeds Dependence Questionnaire. *Addiction*, **89**, 563–572.

Raistrick, D., Heather, N. & Godfrey, C. (2006) *Review of the Effectiveness of Treatment for Alcohol Problems*. National Treatment Agency for Substance Misuse.

SCAN Inpatient Treatment Working Party (2006) *Inpatient Treatment of Drug and Alcohol Misusers in the National Health Service*. Specialist Clinical Addiction Network (SCAN).

Soyka, M. & Horak, M. (2004) Outpatient alcohol detoxification: implementation efficacy and outcome effectiveness of a model project. *European Addiction Research*, **10**, 180–187

Williams, D. & McBride, A. J. (1998) The drug treatment of alcohol withdrawal symptoms: a systematic review. *Alcohol and Alcoholism*, **33**, 103–115.

CHAPTER 8

Nicotine addiction and smoking cessation treatments

Jason Luty

Summary   Tobacco smoking is the biggest public health problem in Western society and the biggest cause of preventable deaths. It persists primarily because of the highly addictive properties of nicotine, although many of the health problems arise from the inhalation of other chemicals. Techniques such as nicotine administration and group therapy have been developed to help people stop smoking. Although cessation rates with these are modest (perhaps 17% above the rates in control groups), they are eminently cost-effective, owing to the immense health problems produced by tobacco.

It is estimated that 29% of adults in the UK smoke tobacco (Office for National Statistics, 2000). Each year smoking kills 120 000 people (13 deaths per hour), making it the single most common preventable cause of death in Britain (Callum, 1998). Around half of all smokers will die prematurely because of their addiction (Peto *et al*, 1994). Their overall life expectancy is, on average, 8 years less than for non-smokers (Callum, 1998). About a decade ago it was estimated that smoking cost the National Health Service (NHS) £1500 million per year, with around 1000 admissions every day for smoking-related illnesses (Parrott *et al*, 1998). At the same time, the UK treasury earned £8 billion in tax on tobacco sold in the UK alone, in addition to the enormous revenue from overseas markets.

Smoking is a major risk factor for at least 20 diseases, including coronary and peripheral vascular disease, chronic bronchitis and at least 80% of lung cancers (Callum, 1998). Blood coagulates in smokers more easily than in non-smokers, fibrinogen levels are higher and platelets are more likely to aggregate. These effects all contribute to thromboembolic diseases. Although nicotine itself is not carcinogenic, tobacco smoke contains over 200 other compounds that are potential carcinogens and smoking itself is the greatest single risk factor for lung cancer. Cigarette smoking significantly contributes to several other nasopharyngeal and upper gastrointestinal carcinomas (Benowitz, 1988).

Is nicotine addictive?

A 1988 US Surgeon General's report stated that nicotine is as addictive as drugs such as heroin and cocaine (Stolerman & Jarvis, 1995). This represents the culmination of a gradual political shift from viewing smoking as a bad habit to seeing it as a behavioural form of habituation and, ultimately, a formal addiction (Box 8.1). The ICD–10 criteria for addiction clearly regard the nicotine in tobacco smoke as addictive (World Health Organization, 1992). These criteria include compulsive use, tolerance, development of withdrawal symptoms and tendency to relapse after stopping. Furthermore, nicotine in tobacco smoke activates brain reward areas in a way comparable to that of other addictive drugs.

Less than 4% of smokers smoke less frequently than daily. The majority smoke at least 10 cigarettes per day and most light a cigarette within half an hour of waking. The persistent nature of nicotine use is shown by the fact that 48% of smokers in a UK study had been unable to abstain from smoking for any period in excess of 1 week in the previous 5 years (Russell, 1986). In the same study, craving was reported in 47% of smokers following attempts to stop. Stolerman & Jarvis (1995) report that over 50% of smokers said they wished to give up but only 13% thought they were likely to succeed. Only about 2% of smokers quit per year without professional advice or help. Furthermore, less than 20% of those embarking on an intensive treatment aimed at abstinence succeed for more than 1 year. To put these facts into perspective, 40% of smokers who have had a heart attack return to smoking while still in hospital, and 50% of smokers who have undergone surgery for lung cancer resume the habit. These facts clearly indicate a compulsion (an irresistible urge) to smoke.

Numerous studies also show a clear withdrawal syndrome in humans (Benowitz, 1988). The symptoms include irritability, poor concentration, anxiety, restlessness, increased hunger, depressed mood and craving for tobacco (Hughes, 1992). Symptoms develop within 12h and can persist for 3 weeks, although appetite is increased for over 10 weeks (Benowitz,

---

Box 8.1 Addictive properties of nicotine in tobacco smoke

- Compulsive use and craving
- Tolerance (especially to adverse effects)
- Withdrawal syndrome
- Tendency to relapse after cessation
- Use to relieve withdrawal symptoms
- Persistent use despite evidence of harm

1988). These symptoms also occur to some degree after withdrawal of nicotine replacement therapy (NRT) or smokeless tobacco. This suggests that symptoms represent a physiological withdrawal from nicotine rather than a behavioural response to the process of smoking cigarettes.

A large number of studies have shown that tolerance to nicotine develops, particularly to its adverse effects such as nausea (Swedberg *et al*, 1990). Tolerance is reported in humans within days of starting to smoke.

Finally, the relapse rate among smokers who quit is comparable to rates in heroin addicts and alcoholics (Hughes, 1992).

Pharmacology of nicotine in tobacco smoke

Nicotine is a tertiary amine whose levorotatory isomer produces the majority of its physiological effects. This is the predominant isomer present in tobacco smoke. Nicotine is a weak base and can readily cross cell membrane and the blood–brain barrier at physiological pH. It is an agonist at the nicotinic acetylcholine receptors of the autonomic ganglia, adrenal medulla and neuromuscular junction and nicotinic receptors in the brain (Benowitz, 1988). Nicotine causes an acute increase in blood pressure and heart rate, although rapid tolerance to these effects develops. Nicotine also increases circulating catecholamine levels. It causes a reduction in body weight of 4–5 kg. These effects occur at the plasma nicotine concentrations to which smokers are exposed.

In the UK, a typical smoker consumes 14–17 cigarettes per day (Stolerman & Jarvis, 1995). Each cigarette provides around 1 mg of nicotine. An average smoker inhales 10–80 mg of nicotine per day to maintain a plasma concentration of 10–50 ng/ml. Nicotine is distilled from the tobacco burning on tar droplets that are inhaled and deposited in small airways and alveoli. This allows even more rapid absorption through the lungs than occurs with intravenous administration. Smoking a single cigarette produces peak increments of plasma nicotine concentrations of 5–30 ng/ml within minutes. Hence, cigarettes are excellently designed methods of rapidly administering and adjusting plasma nicotine concentrations. Smokers appear to be able to regulate the plasma concentration of nicotine on a puff-by-puff basis depending on the type of tobacco and rate and depth of puffing. Unfortunately, so-called low-tar cigarettes appear to deliver a dose of nicotine similar to that of other cigarettes because smokers inhale more deeply when smoking them (Benowitz, 1988).

Nicotine has a half-life of 2 h and is eliminated by direct renal excretion and metabolism to cotinine and nicotine-*N*-oxide. Nicotine therefore accumulates during the early part of the day and is almost completely eliminated overnight. Hence, the majority of smokers are beginning to suffer withdrawal symptoms on waking. (Incidentally, cotinine in urine or saliva is commonly used to monitor adherence to smoking cessation programmes.)

Box 8.2 General measures to encourage smoking cessation: the four As

- Ask about smoking at least once each year
- Advise smokers to stop and refer to specialist services if possible
- Assist smokers to stop (e.g. by referral to a specialist clinic and by providing nicotine replacement therapy or bupropion)
- Arrange follow-up if appropriate

Laboratory studies in rats, monkeys, dogs and humans clearly show the rewarding effects of nicotine (Goldberg et al, 1981). Animal studies also suggest that its effects more closely resemble the effects of stimulants (amphetamine and cocaine) than of other addictive drugs (sedatives or opiates). In humans who smoke, nicotine has been shown to improve attention, learning, reaction times, problem-solving and behavioural arousal (Henningfield, 1984). However, this appears to be primarily due to relief from withdrawal states. Nicotine administration in dependent animals produces release of dopamine in the nucleus accumbens, which is part of the putative reward pathway that is activated by most addictive drugs, including alcohol, opiates and stimulants (Stolerman & Jarvis, 1995).

Smoking cessation

The UK government has made smoking cessation one of its top 13 priorities. The Royal College of Physicians published smoking cessation guidelines (Raw et al, 1998) that were subsequently updated (West et al, 2000).

General measures to encourage and assist smoking cessation are the mainstay of NHS smoking cessation treatment (Box 8.2). General practitioners (GPs) and all health professionals are asked to give brief opportunistic advice to all smokers. Those who express any interest in stopping should then be referred to specialist services (West et al, 2000). General practitioners should aim to advise all smokers to stop, and record having done so, at least once a year. Primary care teams should also ensure that their records are kept up to date concerning the smoking status of their patients.

Assistance to stop smoking is best provided by a specialist smoking cessation clinic or full-time dedicated health professional. General practitioners should reinforce this advice or provide such assistance in the absence of a dedicated service. It takes around 5 min to give basic advice such as that shown in Box 8.3.

Specialist smoking cessation services are intended both to treat all smokers who wish to quit and to train other professionals to provide brief

---

Box 8.3 Advice to help people stop smoking

- Choose a 'quit' day
- Use nicotine replacement therapy (it is safer than continued exposure to the nicotine in cigarettes) or bupropion
- Review what may have caused past relapses
- Enlist the help of family and friends

---

interventions. West *et al*'s (2000) guidelines indicate that specialist services should be set up in each health authority (typically serving 500000 people by providing a throughput of around 1500 clients per year). It is preferable to provide either a central smoking cessation clinic or, in rural areas, arrange for a peripatetic service to visit local clinics over a wider locality. Specialist clinics and other support services should be staffed by individuals specially trained and employed for the purpose rather than attempting to fit the job in with other duties. They may come from a variety of professional groups, including nurses and pharmacists.

Smoking cessation clinics usually work with groups of clients, although individual treatment is also used. The format of smoking cessation programmes varies, but common features are shown in Box 8.4. A group meeting held in the 1- or 2-week gap prior to the quit date enables clients to start bupropion or obtain nicotine replacement therapy in advance of the quit date. The first week proper is introductory and smokers are expected to stop smoking completely after this session. Nicotine replacement products are distributed and discussed. All tobacco, cigarettes, lighters and other smoking-related items are disposed of before or during this session. Subsequent sessions concentrate on the group discussion of members' problems with quitting and on encouraging each other. This group-centred motivational approach may work better than didactic teaching by therapists, although this has yet to be confirmed in controlled trials. Groups typically work well with 15–25 participants and two therapists (Hajek *et al*, 1985). At the start

---

Box 8.4 Common features of smoking cessation programmes

- First group is held 1–2 weeks prior to quit date
- Groups meet for 1-hour weekly sessions over 6 weeks
- Groups include 15–25 participants
- Instruction is given on nicotine replacement therapy and use of bupropion
- Group members encourage and support each other in their attempt to quit

---

of each meeting, expired carbon monoxide is measured using commercial hand-held devices, to test for abstinence. At the end of the course, occasional follow-up sessions are usually offered.

Bupropion

Bupropion is an atypical antidepressant that inhibits neuronal reuptake of both dopamine and noradrenaline (Asher *et al*, 1995). It is unclear whether its anti-smoking action is related to its antidepressant activity. However, some research shows that bupropion is equally effective in smokers both with and without depression (Hughes *et al*, 1999). It has been licensed in the USA as an antidepressant since 1989, where anecdotal reports suggested that it might help patients to stop smoking. A slow-release preparation was licensed in the UK in 2000 for use in smoking cessation. This has been found to be at least as effective as nicotine replacement therapy in placebo-controlled double-blind studies involving 1500 smokers (Jorenby *et al*, 1999).

Treatment with bupropion should begin while the patient is still smoking, typically within 2 weeks of the proposed quit date. A 7- to 12-week course of bupropion is recommended. Side-effects are generally mild and typical of antidepressants (dry mouth, headache and insomnia). There is also a small risk of inducing seizures (1 in 1000) (Rosentien *et al*, 1993). Bupropion treatment currently costs about £80 for a 2-month course.

Many centres now suggest using both bupropion and nicotine replacement therapy.

Varenicline was released in the UK in 2006 to assist smoking cessation. It has been approved by the National Institute for Health and Clinical Excellence. This drug acts as a partial agonist of nicotinic receptors – it blocks the effect of nicotine from tobacco smoke, although it does have some stimulant effect at nicotinic receptors in the brain itself. The main side-effects are nausea, abnormal dreams and headaches. Varenicline is unusual in that the manufacturers (Pfizer) recommend starting at a low dose 1–2 weeks before quitting smoking (see manufacturer's data sheet).

Nicotine replacement therapy

All health professionals should know that nicotine replacement therapy is now available on the NHS. It is recommended that smokers use nicotine replacement therapy for up to 3 months after quitting. Box 8.5 summarises the forms in which it can be provided. Six such formulations are available in the UK both on prescription and as over-the-counter medications (Anonymous, 1999).

Nicotine chewing-gum releases nicotine over 30 min, and it enters the bloodstream through the oral mucosa. Chewing-gum is available in 2 and 4 mg formulations, and no more than 15 pieces should be chewed each day. It may be more effective for heavier smokers (i.e. more than 20 cigarettes a day) to use the 4 mg formulations. Nicotine microtabs provide sublingual release

---

Box 8.5 Forms of nicotine replacement therapy

- Chewing-gum
- Transdermal patches
- Inhalators
- Nasal sprays
- Sublingual microtabs
- Lozenges

---

of nicotine. These are also available in 2 and 4 mg formulations. Up to 80 mg can be taken daily. Sugar-free mint lozenges are also available, containing 1 mg of nicotine. Up to 25 lozenges can be used each day. Transdermal nicotine patches release nicotine for 16–24 h. They can be placed anywhere on the body, although it is sensible to vary the site each day and also to apply the patches to areas of skin where they are less likely to be rubbed off. Patches are usually applied or changed first thing in the morning. Nicotine inhalators contain a cartridge that releases nicotine vapour when the individual sucks on the device. The nicotine is absorbed through the oropharyngeal mucosa rather than the lungs. Up to 12 cartridges can be used each day, although 6 are usually sufficient. All of these nicotine replacement formulations produce a peak blood nicotine concentration after 20–30 min. Nicotine nasal sprays are used in each nostril, which gives rapid absorption through the nasal lining. With nasal sprays, blood nicotine concentration reaches a peak after 10–15 min, and they can be used every 30 min.

None of the nicotine replacement formulations produces a peak nicotine concentration as rapidly as that following smoking. Although replacement therapy can partially prevent withdrawal symptoms, none of the currently available products (perhaps with the exception of the nasal spray) gives sufficiently rapid absorption to have an acute effect that is subjectively rewarding (Hughes *et al*, 1994). This may partly explain the relatively high failure rates of nicotine replacement therapy in smoking cessation. Nicotine replacement therapy approximately doubles cessation rates; the proportion of clients who remain abstinent at 6 months is raised from 11% following brief advice from clinicians to 18% with the addition of nicotine replacement therapy, regardless of the setting (Anonymous, 1999).

The manufacturers of several nicotine replacement products also provide telephone counselling services and advice regarding various other psychosocial supports. However, the uptake rates for these helplines is very low and their value is therefore uncertain (Lando *et al*, 1997). Nevertheless, many randomised controlled trials have shown that psychosocial support significantly enhances quit rates when compared with nicotine replacement therapy alone (see Effectiveness of treatment, below).

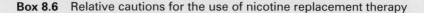

> **Box 8.6**   Relative cautions for the use of nicotine replacement therapy
>
> - Cardiovascular disease
> - Gastritis
> - Peptic ulcer disease
> - Systemic hypertension
> - Diabetes mellitus
> - Hyperthyroidism
> - Phaeochromocytoma
> - Renal or hepatic insufficiency
>
> Note: nicotine replacement therapy presents a lesser hazard than smoking

Nicotine replacement therapy in people with medical problems

Every hospital should have a dedicated specialist counsellor to advise hospital patients who smoke and wish to quit. Nicotine replacement products have not been shown to increase rates of heart disease and hypertension or to exacerbate other cardiovascular disorders (Benowitz, 1998). Nevertheless, there has been some concern expressed about the routine use of nicotine replacement therapy by people who have medical problems such as those listed in Box 8.6. However, several data sheets for nicotine replacement products clearly state that:

'Although nicotine's cardiovascular effects may be deleterious to patients with a history of coronary artery disease, [nicotine replacement therapy] presents a lesser hazard than smoking, which introduces carbon monoxide as an additional toxic factor' (Association of the British Pharmaceutical Industry, 2000).

Smoking introduces over 200 additional compounds into the body, many of which are atherogenic, thrombogenic and carcinogenic (Benowitz, 1998). Furthermore, the blood levels of nicotine produced by nicotine replacement formulations are typically lower than those produced by smoking (Oates & Wood, 1988).

These facts indicate that it is certainly in a patient's best interest to use nicotine replacement therapy to stop smoking, even in the presence of certain medical conditions, assuming that they cannot quit without it. There have been at least five cases in the USA where smokers on nicotine replacement therapy suffered serious cardiac events. However, in each instance, case investigation by the US Food and Drug Administration determined that nicotine replacement therapy was not responsible (Benowitz & Gourlay, 1997). The most recent smoking cessation guidelines for health professionals state that:

'NRT [nicotine replacement therapy] can be recommended for use in patients with cardiovascular disease but only with the agreement of the patient's physician if the disease is acute or poorly controlled' (West *et al*, 2000).

Nicotine replacement therapy and dependence

Early trials suggested that up to one-third of smokers who quit use nicotine replacement therapy for 1 year. However, this figure is probably much too high and, in practice, very few smokers who quit use nicotine replacement therapy for longer than the time suggested on the product label. Nevertheless, abrupt cessation of nicotine replacement therapy can produce nicotine withdrawal symptoms (Hughes, 1989). These facts have raised worries that nicotine replacement therapy is itself addictive. However, the Association of the British Pharmaceutical Industry advises that nicotine replacement therapy rarely leads to dependence, and if it does the dependence is less harmful and easier to break than smoking dependence (Association of the British Pharmaceutical Industry, 2000).

Smoking cessation in pregnancy

Specialist counsellors should be available to advise pregnant smokers who wish to quit. The safety of nicotine replacement therapy and bupropion have not been established in pregnancy. As with most other medications, manufacturers are reluctant to licence the use of these products in pregnancy (see chapter 19). Smoking exposes the foetus to much higher peak levels of nicotine than nicotine replacement therapy does and also introduces many other potential teratogens such as carbon monoxide. Current recommendations are to give "firm and clear advice to stop smoking throughout pregnancy, and give assistance when it is required" (Parrott *et al*, 1998). Unfortunately, there is no clear advice regarding whether pharmacotherapy should be used or not to help pregnant women quit. However, current guidelines do state that use of nicotine replacement therapy in pregnancy may benefit the foetus and the mother if it leads to smoking cessation (West *et al*, 2000).

Effectiveness of treatment

At least 80 randomised controlled trials have studied smoking cessation therapies using nicotine replacement therapy, and many other trials have analysed the effects of alternative forms of psychosocial treatments. Expert committees, including the Cochrane Tobacco Addiction Review Group in the UK and its US equivalent, the Agency for Health Care Policy Research, have concluded that treatment for smoking cessation is effective. Overall, smoking cessation treatments in the UK cost under £1000 per life-year saved. Even the most intensive smoking cessation treatment, involving specialist clinics, nicotine replacement therapy and behavioural advice, costs about £873 per life-year saved. By comparison, the median cost to the NHS of life-saving treatment and interventions for continuing smokers is around £17 000 per life-year saved (Parrott *et al*, 1998).

Brief advice from GPs increases abstinence rates at 6 months by 1–3% above control levels. This advice should be given to all smokers every year, whether or not they wish to quit. It has been estimated that 40% of smokers make some attempt to quit in response to advice from a GP. Overall, this would take up 20–40 hours of GP time each year (about 8 hours of GP time would be required per ex-smoker created). This translates to a cost of £174 per life-year saved (Parrott *et al*, 1998).

Specialist smoking cessation clinics can increase long-term (1-year) quit rates by 17% above control levels by combining behavioural and pharmacological techniques in those who are motivated to attend (West *et al*, 2000). Controlled trials suggest that intense psychosocial treatments are more effective than low-intensity support (such as routine care by a GP). However, nicotine replacement therapy and bupropion approximately doubled cessation rates in placebo-controlled trials in several different treatment settings, regardless of the form of nicotine replacement therapy and the nature, if any, of additional psychosocial measures (Anonymous, 1999).

References

Anonymous (1999) Nicotine replacement to aid smoking cessation. *Drug and Therapeutics Bulletin*, **37**, 52–54.

Association of the British Pharmaceutical Industry (2000) *ABPI Data Sheet Compendium 1999/2000*. ABPI.

Asher, J. A., Coles, J. O. & Colin, J.-N. (1995) Bupropion: a review of its antidepressant activity. *Journal of Clinical Psychiatry*, **56**, 395–401.

Benowitz, N. L. (1988) Pharmacologic aspects of cigarette smoking and nicotine addiction. *New England Journal of Medicine*, **319**, 1318–1330.

Benowitz, N. L. (1998) *Nicotine Safety and Toxicity*. Oxford University Press.

Benowitz, N. L. & Gourlay, S. G. G. (1997) Cardiovascular toxicity of nicotine: implications for nicotine replacement therapy. *Journal of the American College of Cardiology*, **29**, 1422–1431.

Callum, C. (1998) *The Smoking Epidemic*. Health Education Authority.

Goldberg, S. R., Spealman, R. D., & Goldberg, D. M. (1981) Persistent behaviour at high rates maintained by intravenous self-administration of nicotine. *Science*, **214**, 573–575.

Hajek, P., Belcher, M. & Stapleton, J. (1985) Enhancing the impact of groups. *British Journal of Clinical Psychology*, **24**, 289–294.

Henningfield, J. E. (1984) Behavioural pharmacology of cigarette smoking. In *Advances in Behavioural Pharmacology* (eds T. Thompson, P. B. Dews & J. E. Barrett), pp. 131–210. Academic Press.

Hughes, J. R. (1989) Dependence potential and abuse liability of nicotine replacement therapies. *Biomedical Pharmacotherapy*, **43**, 11–17.

Hughes, J. R. (1992) Tobacco withdrawal in self-quitters. *Journal of Consulting Clinical Psychology*, **60**, 689–697.

Hughes, J. R., Higgins, S. T. & Bickel, W. K. (1994) Nicotine withdrawal versus other drug withdrawal syndromes. *Addiction*, **89**, 1461–1470.

Hughes, J. R., Goldstein, M. G., Hurt, R. D., *et al* (1999) Recent advances in pharmacotherapy of smoking. *JAMA*, **281**, 72–76.

Jorenby, D. E., Leischow, S. J. & Mides, M. A. (1999) A controlled trial of sustained-release bupropion, a nicotine patch, or both for smoking cessation. *New England Journal of Medicine*, **340**, 685–691.

Lando, H. A., Rolnick, S., Klevan, D., *et al* (1997) Telephone support as an adjunct to transdermal nicotine in smoking cessation. *American Journal of Public Health*, **87**, 1670–1674.

Oates, J. A. & Wood, A. J. J. (1988) Pharmacologic aspects of cigarette smoking and nicotine addiction. *New England Journal of Medicine*, **319**, 1318–1330.

Office for National Statistics (2000) *Results from the 1999 General Household Survey*. TSO (The Stationery Office).

Parrott, S., Godfrey, C., Raw, M., *et al* (1998) Guidance for commissioners on the cost effectiveness of smoking cessation interventions. *Thorax*, **53** (suppl. 5), S2–S37.

Peto, R., Lopez, A. D. & Boreham, J. (1994) *Mortality from Smoking in Developed Countries, 1950–2000*. Oxford University Press.

Raw, M., McNeill, A. & West, R. (1998) Smoking cessation guidelines for health professionals – a guide to effective smoking cessation interventions for the health care system. *Thorax*, **53** (suppl. 5), S1–S18.

Rosentien, D. L., Nelson, C. & Jacobs, S. C. (1993) Seizures associated with anti-depressants. *Journal of Clinical Psychiatry*, **54**, 289–296.

Russell, M. A. H. (1986) Conceptual framework for nicotine substitution. In *The Pharmacologic Treatment of Tobacco Dependence* (ed. J. K. Ockene), pp. 90–107. Harvard University Press.

Stolerman, I. P. & Jarvis, M. J. (1995) The scientific case that nicotine is addictive. *Psychopharmacology*, **117**, 2–10.

Swedberg, M. D. B., Henningfield, J. E. & Goldberg, S. R. (1990) Nicotine dependency: animal studies. In *Nicotine Psychopharmacology: Molecular, Cellular and Behavioural Aspects* (eds S. Wonnacott, M. A. H. Russell & I. P. Stolerman), pp. 38–76. Oxford Science Publications.

West, R., McNeill, A. & Raw, M. (2000) Smoking cessation guidelines for health professionals. *Thorax*, **55**, 987–999.

World Health Organization (1992) *The ICD–10 Classification of Mental and Behavioural Disorders*. WHO.

CHAPTER 9

Pathological gambling: an overview of assessment and treatment

Sanju George and Vijaya Murali

Summary   Pathological gambling has received scant attention in the psychiatric literature. It has a prevalence rate of about 1% in most countries, and with the deregulation of gambling in the UK the prevalence is set to rise here. Pathological gambling can adversely affect the individual, family and society, and also carries high rates of psychiatric comorbidity. Early identification and appropriate treatment can limit the long-term adverse consequences and improve outcome. This chapter reviews assessment techniques and tools, and treatment strategies.

Gambling is a common, socially acceptable and legal leisure activity in most cultures across the world. It involves wagering something of value (usually money) on a game or event whose outcome is unpredictable and determined by chance (Ladouceur *et al*, 2002). The various types of gambling activities commonly available in the UK are the national lottery, scratch cards, internet gambling, casino games, sports betting, bingo, slot machines and private betting. Results from the most recent British Gambling Prevalence Survey indicate that nearly three-quarters of the adult population had gambled in the previous year and that over half had gambled in the previous week (Sproston *et al*, 2000). For the large majority, gambling is a recreational activity with no adverse consequences. However, for a significant minority it progresses to pathological gambling, defined in DSM–IV as 'a persistent and recurrent maladaptive gambling behaviour that disrupts personal, family or vocational pursuits' (American Psychiatric Association, 1994).

The wide array of choices available to the modern-day gambler, combined with the deregulation of gambling in the UK, is likely to result in an increase in the number of pathological gamblers and gambling-related problems (Griffiths, 2004). As it is an important public health issue, associated with high rates of psychiatric comorbidity and wide-ranging personal, family and societal problems, it is crucial that mental health professionals become familiar with this disorder, its assessment and treatment.

Epidemiology

Pathological gambling typically begins in early adolescence in males (later in females) and runs a chronic, progressive course, punctuated by periods of abstinence and relapses. Although gambling is currently more common among men, the prevalence among women is on the increase. Women are usually older than men when they take up gambling, but once started they develop gambling-related problems more rapidly. In a meta-analysis of 119 prevalence studies, Shaffer *et al* (1999) found the lifetime and past-year prevalence rates of pathological gambling in adults to be 1.6% and 1.14% respectively (adolescents had rates of 5.77% and 3.88%). The British Gambling Prevalence Survey (Sproston *et al*, 2000) estimated the prevalence of problem gambling in British adults to be 0.8%, and this is likely to increase in the coming years. It is important to note that the prevalence of pathological gambling in psychiatric patients ranges from 6 to 12%.

Adolescents are more vulnerable than adults to gambling and gambling-related problems. Although gambling is illegal for people under 18 years old, surveys have found that nearly three-quarters of adolescents had gambled in the previous year and that rates of problem and pathological gambling in adolescents were nearly twice those in adults. Gambling in this group is strongly associated with alcohol and drug misuse and with depression, and there is some evidence linking early onset of gambling to more severe later gambling and more negative consequences. Other at-risk populations include minority ethnic groups, those from lower socio-economic groups, and those with mental health or substance misuse problems.

Adverse consequences

Pathological gambling adversely affects the individual, the family and society. It can negatively influence the gambler's physical and mental health. Gamblers have been noted to report high rates of various psychosomatic disorders and psychiatric problems such as affective, anxiety, substance misuse and personality disorders. Excessive gambling can have a significant impact on the individual's financial situation, often resulting in large debts, poverty and even bankruptcy. To fund their gambling, some resort to criminal activities, ranging from theft and prostitution to violent crime, with obvious legal consequences. Gambling can also adversely affect the gambler's interpersonal relationships and can result in relationship problems, neglect of the family, domestic violence and child abuse (Jacobs *et al*, 1989). Children of pathological gamblers have been found to be at increased risk of behavioural problems, depression and substance misuse (Raylu & Oei, 2001). Costs of gambling borne by society include the cost of the crimes committed by gamblers and the various health and social care costs.

Psychiatric comorbidity

Research has consistently noted the very high rates of Axis I and Axis II comorbidity in pathological gamblers. Cunningham-Williams *et al* (1998) found that people with problem or pathological gambling were many times more likely than the general population to report major psychiatric disorders: major depression, antisocial personality disorder, phobias and current or past history of alcohol misuse. Depression is probably the most common psychiatric disorder comorbid with pathological gambling. Prevalence figures quoted range from 50% to 75% (Becona *et al*, 1996). Two theories have been put forward to explain the relationship between gambling and depression. One is that gambling-related losses and other adverse consequences result in depression. The second is that gambling is an activity engaged in to alleviate a depressed state – it is used as an 'antidepressant'.

Suicidal ideation, suicide attempts and completed suicides are much more common in pathological gamblers than in the general population. The rate of suicidal ideation in pathological gamblers has been estimated to range from 20% to 80% and that of suicide attempts from 4% to 40%. Severe gambling, large debts, coexisting psychiatric disorders and substance use have all been associated with an increased suicide risk.

Black & Moyer (1998), in a study of 30 pathological gamblers, found that 64% had a lifetime diagnosis of substance misuse. In a retrospective chart review of 113 pathological gamblers, Kausch (2003) noted that 66.4% had a lifetime diagnosis of substance misuse or dependence. Other disorders commonly comorbid with pathological gambling are personality disorders, impulse-control disorders, anxiety disorders and attention-deficit hyperactivity disorder. For an excellent overview of psychiatric comorbidity in pathological gamblers see Crockford & El-Guebaly (1998).

The assessment

A good assessment will help the clinician to formulate a comprehensive and effective treatment plan. The key areas to be explored are summarised in Box 9.1. Many gamblers feel ashamed and embarrassed to reveal the true extent of their problems. Hence, the clinician needs to be sensitive and tactful in exploring the individual's gambling behaviour. Sometimes, it might even be appropriate to obtain collateral information from the patient's partner, spouse or friends (with consent from the patient). It is good to ask the patient to describe in his or her own words the initiation, development and progression of the gambling behaviour in a chronological sequence. The key DSM–IV diagnostic criteria for pathological gambling include preoccupation with gambling, tolerance (the need to wager increasing amounts to achieve excitement), inability to control or stop gambling and 'chasing' one's losses, all of which adversely affect the individual's interpersonal, social and occupational functioning. Features

---

Box 9.1 Summary of key aspects of assessment of the pathological gambler

- Full psychiatric history, including history of presenting complaints, and psychiatric, family, treatment, past and personal histories
- Detailed assessment of gambling behaviour:
  - initiation
  - progression
  - current frequency (days per week or hours per day)
  - current severity (money spent on gambling proportionate to income)
  - types of games played
  - maintaining factors
  - features of dependence
- Consequences: financial, interpersonal, vocational, social and legal
- Reasons for consultation, motivation to change and expectations of treatment
- Assessment of suicide risk
- Assessment of Axis I and II comorbidity, including substance use disorders
- Comprehensive mental state examination

---

of tolerance, craving, withdrawal symptoms and other diagnostic criteria, if present, will readily confirm the diagnosis, but this forms only part of the assessment.

As maintaining factors can often inform specific interventions, it is important to ask individuals why they gamble. Most commonly reported maintaining factors include negative mood state, boredom and the need to overcome financial problems.

Previous attempts to cut back or quit gambling and treatments tried should inform the clinician in planning the current treatment type and setting. A sensitive exploration of the individual's financial situation (personal and family income and financial stability) and financial problems (gambling debts, bankruptcy) will guide the clinician in suggesting feasible and realistic solutions. The clinician must evaluate the impact of gambling on work (being late, absences, job losses, etc.) and interpersonal and marital life (strained relationships, neglect of family, domestic violence, etc.).

An understanding of a gambler's reasons for consultation will provide indicators of motivation to engage in treatment. A useful question to ask is 'Why are you seeking treatment now?' Individuals should also be specifically asked about their expectations of treatment, in terms of its type, duration and setting.

Despite the high rates of psychiatric comorbidity in pathological gamblers, they often go unrecognised and untreated. A detailed psychiatric history and mental state examination should establish whether there is comorbidity. Gamblers should also be asked about their use/misuse of psychoactive

> **Box 9.2**   Commonly used screening, assessment and diagnostic instruments
>
> - DSM–IV diagnostic criteria: 312.31 (American Psychiatric Association, 1994)
> - ICD–10 diagnostic criteria: F63.0 (World Health Organization, 1992)
> - The South Oaks Gambling Screen (SOGS; Lesieur & Blume, 1987)
> - The Lie/Bet Questionnaire (Johnson et al, 1997)
> - Gamblers Anonymous's Twenty Questions (GA–20; Gamblers Anonymous, 2005)

substances and, even more important, their use of alcohol and drugs during gambling sessions.

Assessment of suicide risk (past attempts at self-harm and ongoing suicidal thoughts and plans) forms a crucial part of the overall assessment.

Assessment instruments

In addition to the clinical interview, several structured instruments have been developed for the screening, diagnosis and assessment of the severity of pathological gambling. The most commonly used of these are listed in Box 9.2. More recently, many tools have been developed that attempt to assess gambling-related attitudes, beliefs, cognitions and urges. These are useful in formulating specific treatments and in monitoring response to treatment.

The clinician has a wide range of instruments to choose from, and the choice should be informed by the individual patient, the purpose of assessment and the instrument's psychometric properties. It may also be reasonable to use a combination of instruments to capture the complex, multidimensional aspects of gambling.

Aetiology

A detailed discussion of the various aetiological models of pathological gambling is beyond the scope of this chapter. Various theories have been postulated: psychoanalytic (unconscious desire to lose, unresolved Oedipal conflicts), learning theories (monetary gain and excitement acting as positive reinforcers), cognitive theories (cognitive distortions such as magnification of one's gambling skills, superstitious beliefs, interpretive biases) and neurotransmitter theories (serotonin, noradrenaline and dopamine dysfunction). To date, no single model fully explains the complex and heterogeneous nature of pathological gambling. The currently preferred approach to its aetiological understanding is eclectic, viewing pathological gambling as the result of a complex interaction between psychological, behavioural, cognitive and biological variables.

Pharmacological interventions

Selective serotonin reuptake inhibitors

Conceptualising pathological gambling as either an impulse-control disorder or an obsessive–compulsive-spectrum disorder implicates the serotonergic system in its aetiology. There is also considerable neurobiological evidence to support serotonin (5-HT) system dysfunction in pathological gambling. Hence, fluvoxamine, citalopram, paroxetine, sertraline and fluvoxetine have all been tried with some success in treatment trials for pathological gamblers.

Hollander *et al* (2000), in a double-blind placebo-controlled study of the use of fluvoxamine (mean dose 195 mg/day) with 15 pathological gamblers, noted significant improvements in the treatment group. However, this study had a small sample size (5 of the 15 dropped out) and was of relatively short duration (16 weeks). However, Blanco *et al* (2002), in a larger and longer study (32 gamblers, 6 months), failed to demonstrate any significant superiority of fluvoxamine over placebo. They also noted a high placebo response rate (59%). In a study of 53 pathological gamblers, Kim *et al* (2002) noted paroxetine to be superior to placebo.

An open-label trial of citalopram with 15 pathological gamblers found considerable improvements on various gambling measures in 87% of participants (Zimmerman *et al*, 2002). The therapeutic gains usually occurred in the first few weeks of treatment and were sustained at 12 weeks; they were also found to be independent of the drug's antidepressant effects.

Sertraline was no better than placebo in the treatment of pathological gambling in a double-blind, placebo-controlled study of 60 individuals (Saiz-Ruiz *et al*, 2005).

Naltrexone

Naltrexone, a μ-opioid receptor antagonist, is effective in the treatment of a range of impulsive behaviours/disorders such as kleptomania, self-injury and borderline personality disorder. It is also useful in reducing high-urge and craving states in people dependent on alcohol and heroin. Naltrexone's predominant mechanism of action is via the modulation of the mesolimbic dopamine pathway involved in reward and reinforcement. Hence, it is postulated that naltrexone could be used to reduce the rewarding and reinforcing properties of gambling behaviours and thus decrease the urge to gamble.

Kim & Grant (2001a) treated 17 individuals who had a DSM–IV diagnosis of pathological gambling for 6 weeks with naltrexone and found significant decreases in gambling thoughts, urges and behaviour. The average dose of naltrexone in this study was 157 mg/day. In a much larger study (83 participants) they noted that 75% of gamblers treated with naltrexone improved significantly on a range of outcome measures (Kim & Grant,

2001*b*). The mean dose of naltrexone was again high (188 mg/day) and only half the sample completed the study. Many participants reported significant adverse effects and many had elevated liver function tests, a particular concern with high-dose naltrexone treatment.

Mood stabilisers

Some researchers have conceptualised pathological gambling as a bipolar-spectrum disorder, because of shared characteristics such as impulsivity. As the impulsive behaviours in mania are treated effectively with mood stabilisers, it has been suggested that these may also be effective in the treatment of pathological gambling.

Case reports have shown lithium and carbamazepine to be effective in the treatment of the disorder. Pallanti *et al* (2002) evaluated the efficacy of lithium and valproate in a randomised single-blind study. In all, 15 people on lithium and 16 on valproate completed the 14-week trial. Both groups improved significantly over the trial period (61% of those taking lithium and 68% of those taking valproate, with no significant differences in improvement between groups). A more recent study of sustained-release lithium carbonate treatment of a sample of 40 pathological gamblers with bipolar affective disorder found significant improvements in gambling and affective instability in the treatment group compared with placebo (Hollander *et al*, 2005).

Other drugs

Other drugs that have been used with some success in treating pathological gambling include olanzapine, bupropion, topiramate and nefazodone (which is no longer licensed in the UK).

Summary of pharmacological interventions

No drug has been approved for use in the UK or USA to treat pathological gambling and no clear guidelines are currently available. Trials have shown that selective serotonin reuptake inhibitors (SSRIs), naltrexone and mood stabilisers are all effective, although none has demonstrated superiority over the others. The existence of comorbidity might often help determine the choice of drug. For example, choose an SSRI if there is coexisting obsessive–compulsive-spectrum disorder or depression; choose a mood stabiliser in the presence of comorbid bipolar disorder; and prefer naltrexone if pathological gambling is associated with other impulse-control disorders. Doses of SSRIs and naltrexone required are often at the higher end of the therapeutic range and side-effects are therefore more common. As discontinuation studies are lacking, there is no clear evidence on how long to continue treatment: at least 4–6 months initially and then maybe maintenance treatment (Grant *et al*, 2003). Although empirical evidence is lacking, a combination of pharmacological and psychological therapies might be the best option.

More robust studies looking at augmentation strategies, continuation and maintenance treatment and combined pharmacotherapy and psychotherapy are warranted.

Psychological interventions

Behavioural treatments

Behavioural theorists view gambling as a learned maladaptive behaviour that can be unlearned through behavioural treatments derived from both classical and operant learning theories.

Much of the early work (in the 1960s) on evaluating behavioural treatments for pathological gambling focused on aversion therapy, which is no longer used. Barker & Miller (1966) were the first to report the successful use of electrical aversion therapy in a pathological gambler. Seager (1970) found that 5 out of 14 gamblers were abstinent for 1–3 years after aversion treatment. Koller (1972) reported significant improvement in gambling behaviour in 8 out of 12 individuals given aversion treatment. However, some participants in the study also received other interventions, such as attending Gamblers Anonymous.

Other behavioural treatments that have been used successfully include imaginal desensitisation, imaginal relaxation, behavioural monitoring, covert sensitisation and spousal contingency contracting.

McConaghy et al (1983) compared aversion therapy and imaginal desensitisation in 20 pathological gamblers and demonstrated both treatments to be effective. They also noted that the imaginal desensitisation group had significantly lower levels of state and trait anxiety, and fewer gambling behaviours and urges at 1-year follow-up, compared with the aversion therapy group.

In a much larger study ($n = 120$), McConaghy et al (1991) compared four behavioural treatments – aversion therapy, imaginal desensitisation, imaginal relaxation and in vivo desensitisation (real-life exposure) – and found individuals receiving imaginal desensitisation to have the best outcome. This study had a relatively long-term follow-up (5.5 years), but the drop-out rate was very high (nearly 50%).

Although a range of behavioural treatments have been found to be effective in the treatment of pathological gambling, these days behavioural therapy is more often administered in conjunction with cognitive treatment, as a cognitive–behavioural treatment package.

Cognitive treatments

Cognitive errors such as gamblers' beliefs about randomness and chance, and the false notion that they can control and predict outcome, play a key role in the development and maintenance of gambling. Cognitive therapy attempts to correct these cognitive errors, thus reducing the motivation to gamble.

Ladouceur *et al* (2001) randomly allocated 66 pathological gamblers to either a cognitive therapy group or a waiting-list control group and demonstrated that 86% of treatment completers no longer fulfilled the criteria for pathological gambling. They also found that after treatment, gamblers had increased perception of control over the problem and better self-efficacy. These positive effects were maintained at 1-year follow-up. Cognitive therapy has also been found to be effective when delivered in a group format to pathological gamblers.

As already mentioned, in clinical practice cognitive therapy is often administered as part of a cognitive–behavioural package.

Cognitive–behavioural treatments

These treatments combine cognitive and behavioural aspects and attempt to alter gamblers' cognitions and behaviours. Sharpe & Tarrier (1993) developed a cognitive–behavioural approach that involves identifying high-risk situations (through functional analysis) or internal and external triggers that lead to urges to gamble and then working on effective coping strategies. Other treatments often incorporated in cognitive–behavioural packages include training in assertiveness, problem-solving, social skills, relapse prevention and relaxation. Specific cognitive–behavioural treatment models have been developed and evaluated by Petry (2002) and Ladouceur *et al* (2002).

Sylvain *et al* (1997) evaluated the efficacy of cognitive–behavioural treatment in a sample of 29 male pathological gamblers. The treatment incorporated cognitive restructuring, problem-solving training, social skills training and relapse prevention. Results indicated statistically and clinically significant improvement on many outcome measures and the gains were maintained at 1-year follow-up.

In a randomised study, Echeburua *et al* (1996) compared four treatments: individual stimulus control and real-life exposure; group cognitive restructuring; a combination of the two; and a waiting-list control. At 12-month follow-up, the rates of abstinence or minimal gambling were 69% for the individual treatment arm, 35% for the group treatment and 35% for the combined treatment. The same research group also evaluated the efficacy of providing a relapse prevention treatment after a 6-week individual intervention (Echeburua *et al*, 2000). At 12-month follow-up, less than 20% of those who received relapse prevention follow-up treatment had relapsed, compared with 50% of those who received no follow-up treatment.

Gamblers Anonymous

Gamblers Anonymous is a self-help group modelled on Alcoholics Anonymous. It was founded in 1957 in California and is currently one of the most popular and extensively accessed treatment models for pathological gambling. Gamblers Anonymous uses a medical model of pathological gambling and views total abstinence as the treatment goal. The 'twelve-step recovery program' (see chapter 1, p. 8) forms the cornerstone of this treatment and gamblers are assisted in working through steps 1 to 12 by regular attendance at and active participation in group meetings.

It is surprising that despite its popularity, very little research evidence exists to support the efficacy of Gamblers Anonymous. In a study of 232 attendees of Gamblers Anonymous groups, Stewart & Brown (1988) found abstinence rates of 7.5% at 1-year follow-up. They also found that nearly a quarter of new members did not attend a second meeting and nearly three-quarters attended fewer than 10 meetings.

Generally, those who regularly attend Gamblers Anonymous groups benefit from this intervention. From a clinical perspective it is more pragmatic to offer Gamblers Anonymous in conjunction with other treatments.

Summary of psychological interventions

Although a number of psychological interventions are effective in the treatment of pathological gambling, no one approach has clear superiority. Cognitive–behavioural treatments look particularly promising, but results need to be replicated in larger and more representative samples. Major limitations of psychological treatment studies are the lack of long-term follow-up and high drop-out rates. Studies comparing psychological and pharmacological interventions are warranted.

In clinical settings, multimodal treatments often tend to be used. In-patient treatment programmes have not yet been developed widely in the UK (probably because of the resources required to run them), but they are popular in the USA.

Conclusion

Pathological gambling has so far received scant attention in the psychiatric literature and this field is still in its infancy. With the deregulation of gambling in the UK, the prevalence of pathological gambling is likely to increase in the coming years. It is important to conceptualise pathological gambling as a heterogeneous entity, developed and maintained by a complex interplay of various biological, psychological and social variables. Preliminary research findings offer promising trends in pharmacological and cognitive–behavioural treatments. Improved awareness among health professionals of problem gambling can lead to early recognition and treatment, thus limiting the more severe adverse consequences. Gambling behaviour should therefore be routinely enquired about as part of all psychiatric assessments. Further research is needed to better understand the aetiological mechanisms that would inform effective treatment interventions for this disorder.

References

American Psychiatric Association (1994) *Diagnostic and Statistical Manual of Mental Disorders* (4th edn) (DSM–IV). APA.

Barker, J. C. & Miller, M. (1966) Aversion therapy for compulsive gambling. *Lancet, i*, 491–492.

Becona, E., Del Carmen, L. M. & Fuentes, M. J. (1996) Pathological gambling and depression. *Psychological Reports*, **78**, 635–640.

Black, D. W. & Moyer, T. (1998) Clinical features and psychiatric morbidity of subjects with pathological gambling behaviour. *Psychiatric Services*, **49**, 1434–1439.

Blanco, C., Petkova, E., Ibanez, A., *et al* (2002) A pilot placebo-controlled study of fluvoxamine for pathological gambling. *Annals of Clinical Psychiatry*, **14**, 9–15.

Crockford, D. N. & El-Guebaly, N. (1998) Psychiatric comorbidity in pathological gambling: a critical review. *Canadian Journal of Psychiatry*, **43**, 43–50.

Cunningham-Williams, R. M., Cottler, L. B., Compton, W. M., *et al* (1998) Taking chances: problem gamblers and mental health disorders – results from the St. Louis Epidemiological Catchment Area study. *American Journal of Public Health*, **88**, 1093–1096.

Echeburua, E., Baez, C. & Fernandez-Montalvo, J. (1996) Comparative effectiveness of three therapeutic modalities in psychological treatment of pathological gambling: long-term outcome. *Behavioural and Cognitive Psychotherapy*, **24**, 51–72.

Echeburua, E., Fernandez-Montalvo, J. & Baez, C. (2000) Relapse prevention in the treatment of slot-machine pathological gamblers: long-term outcome. *Behavior Therapy*, **31**, 351–364.

Gamblers Anonymous (2005) *Twenty Questions*. Gamblers Anonymous. http://www.gamblersanonymous.org/20questions.html

Grant, J. E., Kim, S. W., Potenza, M. N., *et al* (2003) Advances in the pharmacological treatment of pathological gambling. *Journal of Gambling Studies*, **19**, 85–109.

Griffiths, M. (2004) Betting your life on it. *BMJ*, **329**, 1055–1056.

Hollander, E., De Caria, C. M., Finkell, J. N., *et al* (2000) A randomised double-blind fluvoxamine/placebo crossover trial in pathologic gambling. *Biological Psychiatry*, **47**, 813–817.

Hollander, E., Pallanti, S., Allen, A., *et al* (2005) Does sustained-release lithium reduce impulsive gambling and affective instability versus placebo in pathological gamblers with bipolar spectrum disorders? *American Journal of Psychiatry*, **162**, 137–145.

Jacobs, D. F., Marston, A. R., Singer, R. D., *et al* (1989) Children of problem gamblers. *Journal of Gambling Behavior*, **5**, 261–267.

Johnson, E. E., Hamer, R., Nora, R. M., *et al* (1997) The Lie/Bet Questionnaire for screening pathological gamblers. *Psychological Reports*, **80**, 83–88.

Kausch, O. (2003) Patterns of substance abuse among treatment-seeking pathological gamblers. *Journal of Substance Abuse Treatment*, **25**, 263–270.

Kim, S. W. & Grant, J. E. (2001a) An open naltrexone treatment study of pathological gambling disorder. *International Clinical Psychopharmacology*, **16**, 285–289.

Kim, S. W. & Grant, J. E. (2001b) The psychopharmacology of pathological gambling. *Seminars in Clinical Neuropsychiatry*, **6**, 184–194.

Kim, S. W., Grant, J. E., Adson, D. E., *et al* (2002) A double blind, placebo-controlled study of the efficacy and safety of paroxetine in the treatment of pathological gambling. *Journal of Clinical Psychiatry*, **63**, 501–507.

Koller, K. M. (1972) Treatment of poker-machine addicts by aversion therapy. *Medical Journal of Australia*, **1**, 742–745.

Ladouceur, R., Sylvain, C., Boutin, C., *et al* (2001) Cognitive treatment of pathological gambling. *Journal of Nervous and Mental Disease*, **189**, 774–780.

Ladouceur, R., Sylvain, C., Boutin, C., *et al* (2002) *Understanding and Treating the Pathological Gambler*. John Wiley & Sons.

Lesieur, H. R. & Blume, S. B. (1987) The South Oaks Gambling Screen (SOGS): a new instrument for the identification of pathological gamblers. *American Journal of Psychiatry*, **144**, 1184–1188.

McConaghy, N., Armstrong, M. S., Blaszczynski, A., *et al* (1983) Controlled comparison of aversive therapy and imaginal desensitization in compulsive gambling. *British Journal of Psychiatry*, **142**, 366–372.

McConaghy, N., Blaszczynski, A. & Frankova, A. (1991) Comparisons of imaginal desensitisation with other behavioural treatments of pathological gambling. A two- to nine-year follow-up. *British Journal of Psychiatry*, **159**, 390–393.

Pallanti, S., Querciolli, L., Sood, E., *et al* (2002) Lithium and valproate treatment of pathological gambling: a randomised single-blind study. *Journal of Clinical Psychiatry*, **63**, 559–564.

Petry, N. M. (2002) *Pathological Gambling: Etiology, Comorbidity and Treatment*. American Psychiatric Association.

Raylu, N. & Oei, T. (2001) Pathological gambling: a comprehensive review. *JAMA*, **286**, 141–144.

Saiz-Ruiz, J., Blanco, C., Ibanez, A., *et al* (2005) Sertraline treatment of pathological gambling: a pilot study. *Journal of Clinical Psychiatry*, **66**, 28–33.

Seager, C. P. (1970) Treatment of compulsive gamblers by electrical aversion. *British Journal of Psychiatry*, **117**, 545–553.

Shaffer, H. J., Hall, M. N. & Vander Bilt, J. (1999) Estimating the prevalence of disordered gambling behavior in the US and Canada: a research synthesis. *American Journal of Public Health*, **89**, 1369–1376.

Sharpe, L. & Tarrier, N. (1993) Towards a cognitive–behavioural theory of problem gambling. *British Journal of Psychiatry*, **162**, 407–412.

Sproston, K., Erens, B. & Orford, J. (2000) *Gambling Behaviour in Britain: Results from the British Gambling Prevalence Survey*. National Centre for Social Research.

Stewart, R. M. & Brown, R. I. F. (1988) An outcome study of Gamblers Anonymous. *British Journal of Psychiatry*, **152**, 284–288.

Sylvain, C., Ladouceur, R. & Boisvert, J. M. (1997) Cognitive and behavioural treatment of pathological gambling: a controlled study. *Journal of Consulting and Clinical Psychology*, **65**, 727–732.

World Health Organization (1992) *The ICD–10 Classification of Mental and Behavioural Disorders. Clinical Descriptions and Diagnostic Guidelines*. WHO.

Zimmerman, M., Breen, R. B. & Posternak, M. A. (2002) An open-label study of citalopram in the treatment of pathological gambling. *Journal of Clinical Psychiatry*, **63**, 44–48.

CHAPTER 10

Use of investigations in the diagnosis and management of alcohol use disorders

Colin Drummond, Hamid Ghodse and Sanjoo Chengappa

Summary   A number of investigations are available for screening, diagnosing and monitoring people with alcohol use disorders. In research settings standardised alcohol self-report questionnaires perform well. However, in clinical settings haematological and biochemical markers are also used for their objectivity. Single tests on their own cannot be used for accurate diagnosis, and combinations of tests generally are more reliable. The strengths, drawbacks and care required in interpreting established markers, including liver enzymes, serum ethanol concentrations and mean corpuscular volume (MCV), are discussed here. The evidence for newer tests such as carbohydrate-deficient transferring (%CDT), high density lipoproteins, saliva and sweat ethanol measurements are also reviewed.

The purpose of this chapter is to familiarise the reader with the clinical utility of investigations in the diagnosis and management of alcohol use disorders. Many biochemical and haematological tests are widely available, and can improve significantly the quality of diagnosis and management. However, there is no single test that can detect alcohol use disorders with complete accuracy. Further, the validity of a test will vary depending on the clinical application. Such tests should never be relied on in isolation. Adequate clinical evaluation also needs to include a combination of interview and examination of the patient, and interview of other informants (Cantwell & Chick, 1994). In the research setting, self-report is generally a valid and reliable method of assessing alcohol consumption (Babor *et al*, 1987), particularly when it is elicited by a standardised method (e.g. Sobell *et al*, 1980) and the information is provided in confidence. In the clinical setting, however, the patient may report his or her version of past drinking to fit the situation, particularly if adverse consequences are likely to ensue (e.g. discharge from a treatment programme). Combinations of tests are likely to be more reliable than individual tests.

We are not concerned here with the full gamut of examinations available to investigate physical and psychiatric disorders associated with alcohol misuse. Rather, our review is intended to provide up-to-date information on biochemical and haematological markers of excessive drinking, and their application in clinical diagnosis and management.

Purpose of investigations

The choice and application of a test will depend on its purpose and the setting in which it will be used. Other factors include the cost and invasiveness of the procedure and the type of personnel conducting it.

Screening and diagnosis

The most typical and cost-effective method of screening in the primary care or general medical setting at present is the administration of standardised questionnaires. In the past, the CAGE questionnaire (Mayfield *et al*, 1974) and the Michigan Alcoholism Screening Test (MAST; Selzer, 1971) have been the most commonly used screening questionnaires. However, with the development of the theory and practice of screening methods, the World Health Organization's Alcohol Use Disorders Identification Test (AUDIT; Saunders *et al*, 1993) is now generally regarded as the standard approach in these settings. The AUDIT provides a measure of multiple dimensions of alcohol use disorders, including alcohol consumption, alcohol-related problems and symptoms of dependence. It has the advantage of being relatively short (10 items) and easy to administer by non-specialist personnel, and it has a relatively high sensitivity and specificity: 92% and 93% respectively. Our primary care screening study for alcohol use disorders in men found that the sensitivity of the AUDIT was 69% and its specificity 98% in hazardous drinking (Coulton *et al*, 2006) (Table 10.1) (for definitions

Table 10.1 Test results for 194 male attendees in primary care engaged in hazardous alcohol use (drinking more than 21 units per week)

	Area under ROC curve	Sensitivity % (95% CI)	Specificity % (95% CI)	Positive predictive value % (95% CI)	Negative predictive value % (95% CI)
AUDIT (≥8)	0.94	69 (57–81)	98 (97–100)	95 (91–99)	86 (78–94)
GGT (>55 IU/l)	0.64	37 (26–47)	72 (62–83)	41 (28–54)	69 (61–77)
AST (>50 IU/l)	0.53	20 (11–29)	80 (71–89)	34 (19–50)	66 (59–73)
%CDT (>2.5%)	0.68	47 (36–58)	71 (60–82)	46 (34–58)	72 (64–80)
MCV (95 fl)	0.62	32 (21–43)	71 (60–82)	36 (23–50)	67 (59–74)

AUDIT, Alcohol Use Disorders Identification Test; GGT, gamma-glutamyltransferase; %CDT, percentage of carbohydrate-deficient transferrin; AST, aspartate aminotransferase; MCV, erythrocyte mean cell volume. (Coulton *et al*, 2006. Reprinted with permission from the *BMJ*.)

Table 10.2 Characteristics of tests

	Sensitivity	Specificity	Duration
Aspartate aminotransferase	30–50%	80–86%	1–2 months
Alanine aminotransferase	30–50%	80–86%	1–2 months
Gamma-glutamyltransferase	50–70%	75–85%	1–2 months
Mean cell volume	25–52%	85–95%	1–3 months
Carbohydrate-deficient transferrin	40–70%	80–98%	1–3 weeks
AUDIT questionnaire	70–92%	93–98%	Past year

AUDIT, Alcohol Use Disorders Identification Test.

of sensitivity and specificity, see below). Other questionnaires based on the AUDIT are the AUDIT–C (Bush et al, 1998; Dawson et al, 2005) and the four-item Fast Alcohol Screening Test (FAST; Hodgson et al, 2002). The AUDIT–C consists of three consumption questionnaires from the AUDIT. The FAST questionnaire with one question can identify hazardous and non-hazardous use for >50% of most samples (Hodgson et al, 2002). The Paddington Alcohol Test (PAT; Smith et al, 1996; Patton et al, 2004) is another short tool that uses a four-item questionnaire and is recommended for use in accident and emergency settings. It has a sensitivity of 70% and a specificity of 85% in detecting early-onset hazardous drinkers (Patton & Touquet, 2002). A one-item quantity–frequency tool, the Single Alcohol Screening Question (SASQ; Canagasaby & Vinson, 2005) has also been recently developed. The advantage of shorter screening tools is that they are more likely to be used in practice by busy non-specialists. But shorter tools tend to have a slightly lower sensitivity and specificity.

Questionnaire screening methods are often supplemented with bio-chemical investigations, typically gamma-glutamyltransferase (GGT), erythrocyte mean cell volume (MCV) and alanine aminotransferase (ALT). Measurement of serum ethanol can also aid diagnosis, particularly if a high level is found in a morning specimen. The characteristics of these tests are described in Table 10.2.

Clinical management

Biochemical methods are particularly useful in the context of clinical management of alcohol use disorders. The most usual application is breath alcohol concentration measurement using a hand-held breath analyser, which can provide an immediate and accurate measurement. Often, alcohol detoxification programmes routinely include random breath alcohol testing.

115

It is not appropriate to continue to prescribe medication for detoxification in cases where an individual has relapsed to drinking, and breath testing provides a means of detecting this at an early stage. Further, feedback of improved biochemical test results can be used to good effect in enhancing motivation to maintain change (either abstinence or controlled drinking) and can be useful within a motivational interviewing framework (Miller & Rollnick, 1991).

Court proceedings

Psychiatrists are increasingly asked to provide assessment of individuals in both criminal and civil proceedings in relation to the presence or absence of an alcohol use disorder. Sometimes, this is to establish the contribution of alcohol in a criminal act (e.g. assault or murder). On other occasions, it may be to establish the contribution and treatability of an alcohol use disorder in a repeated pattern of offending (e.g. driving while intoxicated). Psychiatrists are also asked to provide an assessment of the contribution of an alcohol use disorder to problems in parenting (including child neglect and abuse). These are areas probably best dealt with by specialists in the field. Biochemical investigations often play a significant part in assessment and diagnosis. It is important to be able to inform the court of the likely limitations of recommended monitoring packages and of their cost.

Employee assistance programmes

A similar application for biochemical tests is in the context of employee assistance programmes. Increasingly, employers are becoming aware of the problems of alcohol misuse in the workplace, and in some occupations (e.g. airline pilots and doctors) alcohol misuse can be particularly hazardous. Psychiatrists are often asked to diagnose, treat and monitor alcohol-misusing employees, many of whom are reluctant patients.

Sensitivity and specificity of tests

Definitions

Sensitivity is the proportion of individuals with the target condition in a population who are correctly identified by a screening test. It is also referred to as the 'true positive rate'. In a screening study for alcohol misuse, for example, a test with a sensitivity of 60% would correctly identify 60% of persons who are truly misusing alcohol as diagnosed by a gold standard method (usually a standardised diagnostic interview). However, by the same token, the test would 'miss' the other 40% of true positives (i.e. it would classify 40% of alcohol misusers as not misusing – the false negatives). The higher the sensitivity of the test, the more effective it is as a screening tool.

Specificity is the proportion of individuals free of the target condition in a population who are correctly identified by a screening test. It is also referred to as the 'true negative rate'. In the same hypothetical screening study, a test that has a specificity of 90% will correctly identify 90% of persons who are truly not misusing alcohol as diagnosed by the gold standard method. However, it will falsely classify 10% of the people as alcohol misusers – the false positives.

In general, most blood tests used in screening for alcohol misuse (as in the hypothetical test above) have a relatively high specificity but a moderate sensitivity. In other words, they yield relatively few false positives at the expense of a relatively large number of false negatives (although there will be more false positives in the medical ward setting owing to, for example, liver disease or prescribed drugs). This is to some extent the result of a relatively large variation in the normal range in the non-alcohol-misusing population. Also the sensitivity and specificity of the tests will depend on the defined target population. For example, in our primary care study (Coulton *et al*, 2006) the sensitivity of the AUDIT for hazardous drinking was 69% but for the more severe disorder of alcohol dependence it was 84%. Conversely, specificity was higher for hazardous drinking (98%) than for alcohol dependence (83%).

Two other important measures of a test's performance are its positive predictive value (PPV) and negative predictive value (NPV). The positive predictive value is the proportion of individuals with a positive test result who have the target condition. The negative predictive value is the proportion of individuals who test negative who do not have the target condition. The closer the NPV and PPV are to the value of 1, the better the test performance, with 1 being the best possible result.

Normal ranges and measurement error

The setting of the upper limit of the normal range for a test is crucial in determining the sensitivity and specificity. As the cut-off point for the upper limit of the normal range increases, the specificity will increase as the sensitivity decreases. In other words, there will be fewer false positives but more false negatives. As the upper limit of normal is reduced, the converse applies – there will be fewer false negatives at the expense of more false positives. For any given test, a receiver operating characteristic (ROC) curve can be determined to provide the optimal cut-off point to maximise sensitivity and specificity. The total area under the curve (AUC) represents the probability that the test correctly identifies the true positives and the true negatives, i.e. it indicates the test's accuracy. Figure 10.1 shows ROC curves indicating the screening properties of a range of screening tests: the greater the AUC, the better the test's performance. The closer the AUC result is to 1, the better the performance of the test. So in Fig. 10.1 it can be seen that the AUDIT questionnaire has the AUC closest to the value of 1 and is therefore the best performing screening test.

Table 10.3   Laboratory reference ranges[1]

Substance	Range	Units
Sodium	135–145	mmol/l
Potassium	3.5–4.7	mmol/l
Urea	2.5–8.0	mmol/l
Creatinine	60–110	mmol/l
Bilirubin	0–17	mmol/l
Alanine aminotransferase	5–40	u/l
Alkaline phosphatase	30–100	u/l
Albumin	38–48	g/l
Gamma-glutamyltransferase		
Women	0–30	u/l
Men	0–60	u/l
Serum B_{12}	150–1000	ng/l
Red cell folate	150–750	µg/l
Serum folate	2.5–10	µg/l
Mean cell volume		
Women	78–95	fl
Men	80–95	fl
Mean cell haemoglobin	27–32.5	pg
Mean cell haemoglobin concentration	32–35.8	g/dl
White cell count	4–11	$10^9/l$
Neutrophils	1.8–8.0	$10^9/l$
Lymphocytes	1–4	$10^9/l$
Monocytes	0.4–1.1	$10^9/l$
Eosinophils	0.1–0.8	$10^9/l$
Basophils	0–0.4	$10^9/l$
Platelets	150–450	$10^9/l$
Haemoglobin		
Women	12–16	g/dl
Men	13–17	g/dl
Haematocrit		
Women	0.37–0.47	
Men	0.41–0.52	
%Carbohydrate-deficient transferrin (%CDT)[2]	0–6	%

1. All values have been provided by the Biochemistry and Haematology Departments, St George's Hospital, London. Normal ranges were established in donor specimens from the South West London Blood Transfusion Service. In clinical practice it is important to compare all results with the reference ranges provided by the laboratory in which the tests were conducted.

2. %CDT was determined using the Axis-Shield assay kit (Kimbolton, UK).

subject to wide individual variation and is dependent on body mass, gender and alcohol tolerance (Holford, 1987). Thus, it is easy to see how a person drinking 15 units of alcohol in an evening (about eight pints of beer) could remain above the legal limit for driving the following morning. However, even in very heavy drinkers, serum ethanol is unlikely to be positive after about 24 h following the last intake of alcohol.

Serum ethanol concentration is the most accurate method used in estimation. Several other body fluids have been studied and are relatively highly correlated with serum ethanol concentrations. Urine can be used as an alternative and is commonly used in cases of driving while intoxicated. Urine and blood ethanol measures are subject to similar metabolic factors. Breath ethanol is highly correlated with serum ethanol, and breath ethanol concentration measurement using a hand-held electronic analyser is rapid and less invasive. The manufacturer's instructions must be carefully followed, including obtaining an adequate specimen of alveolar air, regular calibration of the analyser, and not taking measurements immediately after consumption of alcohol or other chemicals, including cigarettes and some mouthwashes containing alcohol. The best method is to wash the mouth with water and then wait for 15 min before taking a measurement. Serum and breath ethanol concentrations are, however, markedly different in absolute terms. In the UK, the legal limit for driving is 35 μg/100 ml breath, equivalent to 80 mg/100 ml blood (the blood:breath ratio is assumed to be 2300:1 in the UK). However, most hand-held analysers convert breath measurements into serum ethanol equivalent concentrations.

Ethanol can also be measured in saliva and sweat. For saliva, dipsticks have been developed that have a correlation of 0.90–0.98 with serum and breath ethanol measurements (Bates & Martin, 1997). As saliva tests become more widely available, they may prove more cost-effective than buying a breath analyser (about £3 per test compared to an analyser costing about £650), particularly for practitioners who need to measure ethanol infrequently.

Only about 0.1% of ethanol is excreted in sweat (compared with 0.7% excreted in breath, 0.3% in urine and over 99% metabolised by the liver). It is possible to measure ethanol in sweat using sweat patches or biosensors. Transdermal alcohol sensors can be used for continuous, passive monitoring of blood alcohol levels. Typically, they use electrochemical technology that produces a current proportional to ethanol concentrations in the vapour at the surface of the skin (Swift, 2003). These devices could be used in abstinence monitoring, alcohol misuse assessments and alcohol treatment research. Other non-invasive methods are being developed that measure blood alcohol levels through infrared spectroscopy scanners. All these newer methods need further trials before being accepted into use in clinical settings.

Overall, most methods of ethanol measurement are useful in detecting recent alcohol intake, with the less invasive techniques such as breath alcohol testing providing a reliable, valid and more acceptable way of repeated analysis in the clinical setting. The sensitivity of ethanol measures as screening methods for alcohol misuse is low because of the short half-life of ethanol in the body. Further, their specificity is relatively low as a means of detecting alcohol use disorders, as about 90% of the UK population drinks alcohol. Nevertheless, a very high serum ethanol concentration (200 mg/100 ml or more) or a high level in the morning or when there is little clinical evidence of intoxication, is indicative of a significant degree of alcohol dependence.

In terms of monitoring progress in the clinical setting, breath ethanol provides the most rapid and easily repeated measure, particularly for monitoring abstinence during detoxification. In this context, breath ethanol should be monitored on a daily or random basis, and detoxification discontinued and the treatment plan reformulated if a positive specimen is returned. It should be noted, however, that it may be hazardous to insist that severely alcohol-dependent individuals can only commence detoxification when no ethanol is detectable in their breath, since they can develop severe withdrawal symptoms even with a high, but falling, serum ethanol concentration (relative withdrawal).

Liver enzymes

Three liver enzymes are commonly used in screening for alcohol use disorders: aspartate aminotransferase (AST), alanine aminotransferase (ALT) and gamma-glutamyltransferase (GGT). Some laboratories do not routinely provide all three tests and it is sometimes necessary to request them specifically.

The aminotransferases (AST, ALT) are found in many body tissues apart from the liver (including the heart, skeletal muscle, kidney, brain, erythrocytes and lungs), but it is the ability of alcohol to damage liver cells that provides their utility as a marker of excessive drinking. Early elevations of liver enzymes (including GGT) may be due to enzyme induction by alcohol. Alanine aminotransferase is more specific for liver damage than AST, and hence is a more useful test of excessive drinking. There are many possible causes of liver disease other than alcohol, and a range of factors gives rise to increases in aminotransferases (Box 10.1). However, an AST:ALT ratio >2 in a patient with liver disease diagnosed on clinical grounds is highly suggestive of alcohol as a cause (Marshall & Bangert, 1995).

The sensitivities of AST and ALT tests are relatively low for alcohol use disorders, typically between 30% and 50%. One study comparing the sensitivity and specificity of different biochemical screening tests in 502 medical patients found the sensitivities of AST and ALT tests to be 50% and 35%, respectively (Bell *et al*, 1994). Specificities are generally higher (80–86%).

Gamma-glutamyltransferase is a microsomal enzyme mainly found in the liver, although it is distributed widely in most organs except muscle. It adds little information to AST and alkaline phosphatase (ALP) screening in the diagnosis of liver disease; however, it can help to locate the origin of elevated ALP to the liver. In excessive drinkers GGT is more sensitive to enzyme induction by alcohol than AST or ALT, but levels can also be elevated owing to liver damage. False-positive results can be due to enzyme-inducing drugs (e.g. anticonvulsants). Box 10.1 shows other possible sources of false positives. Nevertheless, the sensitivity and specificity of GGT tests are typically higher than for AST and ALT. The sensitivity of GGT tests ranges between 40% and 70%, and the specificity between 70% and 85%. The upper limit of the normal range for GGT levels is typically higher for men than for women (at St George's Hospital, London, the normal range for men is 0–60 u/l compared with 0–30 u/l for women). However, in patients attending an alcohol treatment clinic, it is not unusual to see GGT levels of 300 u/l or more in the absence of evidence of hepatocellular damage. The GGT level is moderately correlated with the quantity and frequency of heavy drinking.

In practice, of the three liver enzyme screening tests, GGT is the most useful, widely available test for the detection of alcohol use disorders. If AST, ALT or GGT are elevated owing to alcohol misuse, they normally return to normal after 1–2 months of abstinence, although this is subject to individual variation and is dependent on the starting level. A higher initial level will take longer to return to normal, and the tests will take longer to return to normal where there is significant hepatocellular damage or cholestasis. However, it is safe to assume that the results of these tests only refer reliably to excessive drinking in the preceding month. Finally, it is also important to note that liver enzymes can be affected by factors complicating alcohol use disorders, including drug-induced liver damage, paracetamol overdose and disulfiram toxicity. The last is relatively rare, with the number of disulfiram adverse reactions being 1 per 200–2000 treatment years (Wright et al, 1988; Enghusen et al, 1992). In these cases there is evidence of gross liver impairment (hepatitis), with a distinct peak incidence after 2 months of treatment, but occasionally, isolated minor increases in aminotransferases have been reported. It is therefore important to monitor liver function, particularly in the initial stages of disulfiram treatment.

Mean cell volume

Mean cell volume is commonly used as a marker for excessive drinking. The precise mechanism for macrocytosis (increased corpuscular volume) in alcohol misuse is unclear, but is believed to be related to a toxic effect of alcohol on bone marrow, leading to the release of immature and abnormally large cells. Sometimes other evidence of bone marrow toxicity will be evident in alcohol misuse, with reduction in the number and function of granulocytes and macrophages, and in the number and function of platelets (thrombocytopenia, or occasionally thrombocytosis) (Estruch, 1996). Low platelet count can occur in alcohol use disorders in the absence of significant liver disease. However, chronic excessive drinking is also associated with various vitamin deficiencies, notably vitamins B_{12} and folate, which in turn are associated with macrocytic anaemia. Thus, it is important to examine the full range of haematological results and request serum B_{12} and folate levels to exclude macrocytic anaemia as a cause of macrocytosis. Disorders that may lead to false-positive MCV results are shown in Box 10.1.

The sensitivity of MCV screening is typically less than for GGT. Sensitivities of between 25% and 52% have been found, but specificity is typically 70–95%. The MCV takes longer than liver enzymes to return to normal with abstinence, owing to the relatively long half-life of red blood cells. As with liver enzymes, the speed of recovery depends on the initial starting level but it can take between 1 and 3 months.

Carbohydrate-deficient transferrin

Carbohydrate-deficient transferrin (CDT) is an isoform of transferrin and, in comparison with liver enzymes, appears to be relatively unaffected by liver disease. Early research with CDT in the detection of alcohol use disorders suggested a high sensitivity and specificity, of 82% and 97% respectively (Stibler, 1991). However, more recent studies have found lower sensitivity, ranging from 40% to 70%. Specificity is typically high across a range of studies, at 80–98%. It has also been suggested that CDT screening is more sensitive compared with GGT in detecting relapse in alcohol-dependent patients in treatment than as a screening method to detect alcohol use disorders in moderately heavy drinkers (Rosman *et al*, 1995; Mitchell *et al*, 1997; Schmidt *et al*, 1997).

The sensitivity of CDT screening is lower in women than in men, with some studies finding values as low as 44% (Anton & Moak, 1994). Specificity, however, is similar for both genders. It has been hypothesised that normal fluctuations in total transferrin during the menstrual cycle, and in pregnancy, may partly account for this. It has been found that the ratio of carbohydrate-deficient transferrin to total transferrin (%CDT) has a higher sensitivity and specificity than CDT alone, particularly in women and in patients vulnerable to fluctuations in transferrin (Keating *et al*, 1998). For this reason %CDT screening (Axis Biochemicals) is currently the method of choice (Sorvajarvi *et al*, 1996; Keating *et al*, 1998; Viitala *et al*, 1998). Our primary care study showed specificity for %CDT of 68% and sensitivity of 71% for hazardous drinking (Coulton *et al*, 2006). It has been reported that CDT increases and recovers more rapidly than GGT in response to a drinking binge, increasing within 1 week of onset of heavy drinking, and recovering typically in 1–3 weeks, compared with 1–2 months with GGT (Stibler, 1991). As with GGT, there is evidence that CDT is moderately correlated with alcohol consumption.

At present, CDT screening is available only in a small number of laboratories in the UK, and is relatively expensive compared with other routinely available measures. If, as seems likely, CDT screening becomes more widely used, its cost and availability should improve. However, for the time being, the use of CDT is likely to be restricted to medico-legal applications – as an investigative method where other markers are positive but there is doubt as to the cause of the elevation (e.g. liver disease) – and potentially as a measure to detect relapse, particularly in patients who do not show raised GGT levels after heavy drinking.

High-density lipoproteins

The relationship between alcohol consumption and high-density lipoproteins (HDL) is complex, but correlations between the two have been found (Skinner *et al*, 1985). The sensitivity and specificity of HDL testing are relatively low compared with other available markers, and it is therefore seldom used as a screening method.

Newer tests

Sharpe (2001) evaluated a number of new markers for alcohol. Serum mitochondrial aspartate aminotransferase appears to have low sensitivity in screening for hazardous drinking in the community and primary care. Serum beta-hexosaminidase (β-hex) can be measured inexpensively, offering a sensitive test for excessive alcohol consumption. However, many other conditions affect its level, so it is not useful in detecting lower but still harmful levels of drinking in unselected populations. The 5-hydroxytryptophol (5-HTOL) to 5-hydroxyindoleacetic acid (5-HIAA) ratio in serum or urine has a high sensitivity and specificity, but gas or high-performance liquid chromatography is required to measure these metabolites, thus limiting their utility.

Other markers include acetaldehyde adducts, ethylglucoronide (urine and hair), fatty acid esters (hair), phosphatidylethanol, sialic acid and erythrocyte aldehyde dehydrogenase. However, because of their variability in normal range across individuals and/or complex measurement methods these have not yet been adopted in clinical use.

Combinations of tests

So far we have examined the utility of individual biochemical tests in isolation. In practice, such tests are most often used in combination, and consequently the sensitivity of the combined tests is greater than that of any individual test alone (Leigh & Skinner, 1988). Sensitivity can be further improved by combining biochemical tests with interviews, questionnaires or physical examination methods. Box 10.2 shows our recommended testing package.

Usually, the way in which combined tests are interpreted is by counting one or more positive results as being indicative of a positive 'case'. However, it should also be noted that if multiple tests are positive, greater weight can be placed on the 'caseness'. Further, the higher the values are above the normal reference range, the greater the likelihood of caseness and the higher the likely level of drinking. As noted above, the specificity of a test typically increases with an increasing cut-off point.

It has been suggested that combined GGT and CDT screening, or CDT and MCV, be used to increase sensitivity, but neither has been widely accepted (Sharpe, 2001). It should be noted that combination usually leads to loss in specificity and increased costs (Niemela, 2007).

Box 10.2 Recommended testing package

The following approach to investigations is recommended

Initial assessment	Liver function tests (including ALT and/or AST, and GGT) Full blood count (including MCV) Serum B_{12} and folate (or red cell folate) Serum ethanol concentration (in medico-legal cases or cases with otherwise normal results consider %CDT)
During detoxification	Breath ethanol measurement Frequency: daily or randomly
Clinical follow-up	Liver function tests (including ALT and/or AST, and GGT) Full blood count (including MCV) Serum ethanol concentration (supplemented in research studies with %CDT) Frequency: monthly
Monitoring abstinence in medico-legal cases	Liver function tests (including ALT and/or AST, and GGT) Full blood count (including MCV) Serum ethanol concentration Frequency: monthly Breath, saliva or urine (depending on the availability of trained personnel) Frequency: random (approximately weekly) (supplemented, if necessary, with %CDT, monthly)

Individual baselines

Given that the sensitivity of all the tests described here is lower than their specificity, they are less useful in general screening than in monitoring treatment response and in the early detection of relapse in alcohol misusers who have abnormal results on entry to treatment. Even when a test is within the normal range following excessive drinking, it can show changes in response to abstinence and subsequent relapse. Thus, in treatment, it is useful to establish baseline measures at initial assessment from which to monitor subsequent progress. Indeed, some studies have shown that blood markers may increase in advance of a patient's self-reported relapse (Rosman *et al*, 1995). Often, patients are reluctant to report relapse for fear of losing face or 'disappointing' their therapist. Biochemical investigations can provide a way of helping the patient to look objectively at unpalatable truths.

Other disorders associated with alcohol dependence

Throughout this chapter, it has been assumed that physical illnesses that give rise to biochemical and haematological abnormalities are a confounding factor in screening for alcohol use disorders. This is true. However, the tests that we have discussed can also be valuable in the clinical identification and management of physical complications of alcohol dependence. Many physical disorders are more common in alcohol dependence, including hepatitis and cirrhosis, nutritional deficiency, pancreatitis, diabetes and gastrointestinal haemorrhage (Dinan & O'Flynn, 1994; Edwards *et al*, 1997). The addiction specialist has an important role in the early diagnosis of serious physical pathology. On occasions, alcohol misusers are not treated or investigated with the same vigour as other patients, perhaps owing to negative attitudes in the medical profession towards alcohol use disorders (Farrell & David, 1988).

Often the diagnosis of an alcohol use disorder will be made on the basis of a combination of findings, as noted above. The presence of physical stigmata typically associated with excessive drinking (e.g. spider naevi, rhinophyma, plethoric facies and pseudo-Cushing's syndrome), despite not being diagnostic in isolation, may add weight to the diagnosis in association with other evidence.

Another aspect of clinical assessment is the inclusion of urine screening for drugs, given that an increasing number of people presenting to treatment use a range of drugs in addition to alcohol. Therefore, it is important for the addiction specialist to investigate patients with alcohol use disorders adequately (Edwards *et al*, 1997).

Conclusion

Biochemical and haematological tests can add important precision to the diagnosis and management of alcohol use disorders. The approaches recommended here should form an important part of routine clinical practice. Specialist addiction services should routinely conduct blood investigations as part of an initial comprehensive clinical assessment to obtain measures of the nature and severity of the alcohol use disorder and associated clinical conditions. These investigations play a major role in enhancing patients' motivation to change their drinking behaviour. They Such measures also provide a baseline from which to monitor clinical improvement and/or subsequent relapse.

Biochemical and haematological tests also have a key role to play in medico-legal and employee assistance cases, when the client's self-reporting may be especially unreliable. However, as no individual test can provide total certainty, it is important to be aware of the limitations of the methods currently at our disposal.

Further, there is a need to encourage greater use of investigations in screening in the primary care, general hospital and general psychiatric service settings, where alcohol use disorders are common but seldom detected. In doing so, a greater proportion of alcohol misusers can be identified and can be offered early interventions. While the search for more sensitive and specific markers needs to continue, it is important to bear in mind that existing measures, if used correctly and more extensively, could significantly improve the quality of diagnosis and management of alcohol use disorders.

References

Anton, R. F. & Moak, D. H. (1994) Carbohydrate-deficient transferrin and gamma-glutamyltransferase as markers of heavy alcohol consumption: gender differences. *Alcoholism: Clinical and Experimental Research*, **18**, 747–754.

Babor, T. F., Stephens, R. S. & Marlatt, G. A. (1987) Verbal report methods in clinical research on alcoholism: response bias and its minimization. *Journal of Studies on Alcohol*, **48**, 410–424.

Bates, M. E. & Martin, C. S. (1997) Immediate, quantitative estimation of blood alcohol concentration from saliva. *Journal of Studies on Alcohol*, **58**, 531–538.

Bell, H., Tallaksen, C. M., Try, K., *et al* (1994) Carbohydrate-deficient transferrin and other markers of high alcohol consumption: a study of 502 patients admitted consecutively to a medical department. *Alcoholism: Clinical and Experimental Research*, **18**, 1103–1108.

Bush, K., Kivlahan, D. R., McDonell, M. B., *et al* (1998) The AUDIT alcohol consumption questions (AUDIT–C): an effective brief screening test for problem drinking. *Archives of Internal Medicine*, **158**, 1789–1795.

Canagasaby, A. & Vinson, D. C. (2005) Screening for hazardous or harmful drinking using one or two quantity–frequency questions. *Alcohol and Alcoholism*, **40**, 208–213.

Cantwell, R. & Chick, J. (1994) Alcohol misuse: clinical features and treatment. In *Seminars in Alcohol and Drug Misuse* (eds J. Chick & R. Cantwell), pp. 126–155. Gaskell.

Coulton, S., Drummond, C., James, D., *et al* (2006) Opportunistic screening for alcohol use disorders in primary care: comparative study. *BMJ*, **332**, 511–517.

Dawson, D. A., Grant, B. F. & Stinson, F. S. (2005) The AUDIT–C: screening for alcohol use disorders and risk drinking in the presence of other psychiatric disorders. *Comprehensive Psychiatry*, **46**, 405–416.

Dinan, T. & O'Flynn, K. (1994) Medical aspects of drug and alcohol abuse. In *Seminars in Alcohol and Drug Misuse* (eds J. Chick & R. Cantwell), pp. 202–222. Gaskell.

Edwards, G., Marshall, E. J. & Cook, C. C. H. (1997) *The Treatment of Drinking Problems: A Guide to the Helping Professions* (3rd edn). Cambridge University Press.

Enghusen, P. H., Loft, S., Andersen, J. R., *et al* (1992) Disulfiram therapy-adverse drug reactions and interactions. *Acta Psychiatrica Scandinavica Supplementum*, **369**, 59–65.

Estruch, R. (1996) Alcohol and nutrition. In *Alcohol Misuse: A European Perspective* (ed. T. J. Peters), pp. 41–61. Harwood.

Farrell, M. P. and David, A. S. (1988) Do psychiatric registrars take a proper drinking history? *BMJ (Clinical Research Edition)*, **296**, 395–396.

Hodgson, R., Alwyn, T., John, B., *et al* (2002) The FAST Alcohol Screening Test. *Alcohol and Alcoholism*, **37**, 61–66.

Holford, N. G. H. (1987) Clinical pharmacokinetics of ethanol. *Clinical Pharmacokinetics*, **13**, 273–292.

Jones, A. W. (1995) Pharmacokinetics of ethanol. In *Encyclopaedia of Drugs and Alcohol* (ed. J. H. Jaffe), vol. 2, pp. 803–808. Macmillan Library Reference.

Keating, J., Cheung, C., Peters, T. J., *et al* (1998) Carbohydrate deficient transferrin in the assessment of alcohol misuse: absolute or relative measurements? A comparison of two methods with regard to total transferrin concentration. *Clinica Chimica Acta*, **272**, 159–169.

Koch-Weser, J., Sellers, E. M. & Kalant, H. (1976) Alcohol intoxication and withdrawal. *New England Journal of Medicine*, **294**, 757–762.

Leigh, G. & Skinner, H. A. (1988) Physiological assessment, In *Assessment of Addictive Behaviours: A Reference Book for the Caring Professions* (eds D. M. Donovan & G. A. Marlatt), pp. 112–136. Hutchinson.

Marshall, W. J. & Bangert, S. K. (eds) (1995) *Clinical Biochemistry: Metabolic and Clinical Aspects*. Churchill Livingstone.

Mayfield, D., McLeod, G., and Hall, P. (1974) The CAGE questionnaire: validation of a new alcoholism screening instrument. *American Journal of Psychiatry*, **131**, 1121–1123.

Miller, W. R. & Rollnick, S. (1991) *Motivational Interviewing: Preparing People to Change Addictive Behaviour*. Guilford Press.

Mitchell, C., Simpson, D., and Chick, J. (1997) Carbohydrate deficient transferrin in detecting relapse in alcohol dependence. *Drug and Alcohol Dependence*, **48**, 97–103.

Niemela, O. (2007) Biomarkers in alcoholism. *Clinica Chimica Acta*, **377**, 39–49.

Patton, R. & Touquet, R. (2002) The Paddington Alcohol Test. *British Journal of General Practice*, **52**, 59.

Patton, R., Hilton, C., Crawford, M. J., *et al* (2004) The Paddington Alcohol Test: a short report. *Alcohol and Alcoholism*, **39**, 266–268.

Rosman, A. S., Basu, P., Galvin, K., *et al* (1995) Utility of carbohydrate-deficient transferrin as a marker of relapse in alcoholic patients. *Alcoholism: Clinical and Experimental Research*, **19**, 611–616.

Saunders, J. B., Aasland, O. G., Babor, T. F., *et al* (1993) Development of the Alcohol Use Disorders Identification Test (AUDIT): WHO Collaborative Project on Early Detection of Persons with Harmful Alcohol Consumption–II. *Addiction*, **88**, 791–804.

Schmidt, L. G., Schmidt, K., Dufeu, P., *et al* (1997) Superiority of carbohydrate-deficient transferrin to gamma-glutamyltransferase in detecting relapse in alcoholism. *American Journal of Psychiatry*, **154**, 75–80.

Selzer, M. L. (1971) The Michigan alcoholism screening test: the quest for a new diagnostic instrument. *American Journal of Psychiatry*, **127**, 1653–1658.

Sharpe, P. C. (2001) Biochemical detection and monitoring of alcohol abuse and abstinence. *Annals of Clinical Biochemistry*, **38**, 652–664.

Skinner, H. A., Holt, S., Schuller, R., *et al* (1985) Identification of alcohol abuse: trauma and laboratory indicators. In *Early Identification of Alcohol Abuse* (eds N. C. Chang & H. M. Chao), pp. 285–302. National Institute of Alcohol Abuse and Alcoholism/Government Printing Office.

Smith, S. G., Touquet, R., Wright, S., *et al* (1996) Detection of alcohol misusing patients in accident and emergency departments: the Paddington Alcohol Test (PAT) *Journal of Accident and Emergency Medicine*, **13**, 308–312.

Sobell, M. B., Maisto, S. A., Sobell, L. C., *et al* (1980) Developing a prototype for evaluating alcohol treatment effectiveness. In *Evaluating Alcohol and Drug Abuse treatment Effectiveness: Recent Advances* (eds L. C. Sobell, M. B. Sobell & E. Ward), pp. 129–150. Pergamon.

Sorvajarvi, K., Blake, J. E., Israel, Y., *et al* (1996) Sensitivity and specificity of carbohydrate-deficient transferrin as a marker of alcohol abuse are significantly influenced by alterations in serum transferrin: comparison of two methods. *Alcoholism: Clinical and Experimental Research*, **20**, 449–454.

Stibler, H. (1991) Carbohydrate-deficient transferrin in serum: a new marker of potentially harmful alcohol consumption reviewed. *Clinical Chemistry*, **37**, 2029–2037.

Swift, R. (2003) Direct measurement of alcohol and its related metabolites. *Addiction*, **98** (suppl. 2), 73–80.

Viitala, K., Lahdesmaki, K. & Niemela, O. (1998) Comparison of the Axis %CDT TIA and the CDTect method as laboratory tests of alcohol abuse. *Clinical Chemistry*, **44**, 1209–1215.

Wright, C., Vafier, J. A. & Lake, C. R. (1988) Disulfiram-induced fulminating hepatitis: guidelines for liver-panel monitoring. *Journal of Clinical Psychiatry*, **49**, 430–434.

CHAPTER 11

Laboratory investigations for assessment and management of drug problems

Kim Wolff, Sarah Welch and John Strang

Summary Much of the drug testing available today is able to determine the presence or absence of a variety of psychoactive substances in a range of body fluids and tissues. For the results of such tests to be confidently interpreted, additional information is required, including general assessment and history-taking. In a wide range of large psychiatric surveys, substance dependence emerges as one of the most common mental health-related disorders, and it is also the one that is least likely to be treated. The range of available tests can be best considered as acting to support and complement a broader assessment and diagnostic procedure.

The aim of this chapter is to outline the variety of laboratory investigations available that could be considered as biological indicators of substance use and misuse. We will review the strengths and weaknesses of different approaches and different body matrices (urine, blood/plasma monitoring, oral fluid and hair testing), along with other possible materials not usually considered, with a focus on the clinical usefulness of these procedures.

A drug may be detected in any body fluid or tissue, but there are practical limitations to the extent to which samples can be and are used, and the mechanism of collection and supervision of samples are critical to the procedure.

Chain of custody

The procedure of ensuring that an identified sample was provided by a specified individual (chain of custody), and has subsequently been correctly labelled to ensure accuracy, must be properly documented. In the case of urine samples, chain of custody procedures usually require the collection to be witnessed by a designated member of staff (clinician, nurse, drug worker, therapist, etc.) and written confirmation of its validity from the individual voiding the sample, as detailed in Box 11.1 (Wolff *et al*, 1999a).

Box 11.1 Chain of custody procedures for urine samples

- Before, during and after urination, collection site personnel must keep the urine specimen in sight
- The urine container must be tightly capped, properly sealed and labelled with the patient/client's name and the time and date of collection
- To maintain accountability the approved chain of custody form must be used and it must accompany the sample from initial collection to final disposition
- Reliable transportation (courier system) to the laboratory must be used

---

Legal and ethical issues

Legal issues that have surfaced in the development of workplace drug-testing programmes have been reviewed by Long (1989). The legal cornerstone of drug testing is a policy agreement, which usually takes the form of a contract between employers and employees and may include the points listed in Box 11.2 (Osterloh & Becker, 1990).

Those who oppose drug testing usually argue around issues concerned with civil rights. The courts have generally ruled that mandatory drug testing is a form of search and in some cases falls under constitutional protection. However, the potential value of testing to public health, safety and security in certain professions has led to wider legal support for testing programmes (Macdonald, 1990).

Rationale

The rationale for performing analytical tests varies depending on the question(s) to be answered. Drug treatment services vary in the way that they practise drug screening. Services may use test results to gauge the efficacy of therapy, or residential units requiring abstinence may use random checks of residents. Clinicians may use drug tests to make the initial diagnosis of

---

Box 11.2 Key elements of a drug-testing policy agreement

- The need for drug testing and why (e.g. critical safety environment)
- Conditions of testing (e.g. random selection, health check, location of test and who will conduct it)
- Procedures for collecting specimens
- Consequences of a positive test result
- Availability of treatment if substance misuse is revealed

---

substance misuse, for screening as a requirement of a treatment programme when measuring adherence to treatment, or for screening as a useful adjunct to a full drug history to gauge drug exposure over time.

Major challenges for testing procedures include the vast array of drugs that may be consumed, the hugely different clinical and legal significance of test results (which may not always be obvious in the laboratory) and the need for specific approaches for the different substances. One of the limitations of drug testing is that it can give no indication of the presence or absence of physical dependence.

Conducting the tests

Selecting the biological matrix and the challenge of interpretation

The choice of body fluid is influenced by the pharmacokinetics of the drugs being tested for, and by the period of time that the clinician wishes to consider. Blood and, to a lesser degree, oral fluid are likely to give the most accurate measurement of drugs currently active in the system, whereas urine provides a somewhat broader time frame, but with less quantitative accuracy. Hair provides a substantially longer time frame.

Routine drug testing

The standard procedure for routine analysis for drugs of misuse is an initial screening test using an automated commercial immunoassay kit such as an enzyme-mediated immunoassay technique (EMIT), followed by thin-layer, gas or liquid chromatography for confirmation of a specific drug (Braithwaite *et al*, 1995; Simpson *et al*, 1997). In light of the implications of a positive finding, it is usually recommended that a positive initial screening be followed by a confirmatory test (which should be qualitatively different from the first) specifically to identify the compound detected. Initial screening tests identify only the class of drug (opiate, benzodiazepine, etc.). The need to confirm the identity of the actual drug present will vary depending on whether this is in a legal, employment or clinical setting. The most sophisticated drug testing approach is gas or liquid chromatography coupled with mass spectrometry (GC–MS, LC–MS). The use of mass spectrometry is currently regarded as the gold standard for confirming the presence of a drug in a biological fluid.

Although drug testing can be easily undertaken, there remains the problem of interpreting the results for clinical use. The picture is often complex; a drug may be present as metabolites and the parent drug may be present in only relatively low concentrations (buprenorphine, lysergic acid diethylamide (LSD) and Δ^9-tetrahydrocannabinol) or not detected at all. Heroin (diamorphine), for instance, is seldom detected in blood as it is rapidly converted to an intermediary metabolite 6-monoacetylmorphine (MAM) and thus is not excreted into the urine.

Interpretation is also complicated by the relationship between compounds from the same drug class, which may share common metabolic end-products. For example, the benzodiazepine oxazepam, a prescription-only medication, is also a metabolic by-product of chlordiazepoxide, diazepam, clorazepam and temazepam. A similar problem exists with opiate drugs. The principal metabolite of heroin is morphine, but morphine is also a metabolite of codeine. Consequently, the detection of MAM is generally considered to be a more specific indication of heroin consumption. In contrast, dihydrocodeine (which should not be confused with codeine) has its own distinct metabolic pattern. The clinical explanation of drug-testing results is a challenging and often critical issue, particularly when establishing legitimate v. illegal use and all of its attendant complications.

False positives and false negatives

In qualitative screening tests, each sample is reported either positive or negative for a particular drug or drug group. There are four possible interpretations of the test result, as shown in Table 11.1. The two true test results accurately reflect the clinical situation. However, a true positive on a screening test may not itself indicate the specific drug and cannot indicate the dose, time or route of administration. A true negative indicates that no drug was taken within the time required for its use to be detected. Clinicians should be aware of the time taken for drugs to be eliminated from the body (Table 11.2), since a negative test could result from not sampling soon enough after drug consumption. False negatives can also occur when the threshold of sensitivity of the analytical procedure is set above the limit of detection of the drug.

Clinically, a false negative may be defined as a negative finding in a sample from a patient known to have recently taken the drug of interest. Chemically, a false negative report on a sample known to contain a particular substance may occur because the altered composition of the sample or endogenous components in it mask the presence of the drug of interest. Aspirin ingestion and its presence in urine interferes with the analytical process in all EMIT assays, potentially yielding false-negative results for drug screens (Linder & Valdes, 1994).

In the laboratory, a positive test report from the analysis of a biological sample that does not contain the drug in question is called a false positive.

Table 11.1 Interpretation of test result

	Person has taken drug	Person has not taken drug
Test result positive	True positive	False positive
Test result negative	False negative	True negative

Table 11.2 Approximate duration of detectability of commonly used substances and some of their metabolites in urine (based on common laboratory cut-off values)

Substance	Duration of detectability
Stimulants	
Amphetamine	2–3 days
Methylenedioxymethamphetamine (MDMA, ecstasy)	30–48 h
Methamphetamine	48 h
Cocaine[1]	6–8 h
Cocaine metabolite/benzoylecgonine	2 days
Barbiturates	
Short-acting (cyclobarbitone)	24 h
Intermediate-acting (pentobarbitone)	48–72 h
Long-acting (phenobarbitone)	>7 days
Benzodiazepines	
Short-acting (triazolam)	24 h
Intermediate-acting (temazepam, chlordiazepoxide)	40–80 h
Long-acting (diazepam, nitrazepam)[2]	>7 days
Opioids	
Methadone (maintenance dosing)	7–9 days
Codeine/morphine[3]	24 h
Morphine glucuronides	48 h
Codeine glucuronides	3 days
Propoxyphene/norpropoxyphene	6–48 h
Dihydrocodeine	24 h
Buprenorphine[4]	48–56 h
Buprenorphine conjugates	7 days
Cannabinoids (marijuana)	
Single use	3 days
Moderate use	4 days
Heavy use (daily)	10 days
Chronic heavy use[5]	?36 days
Other	
Methaqualone	>7 days
Phencyclidine (PCP)	8 days
Lysergic acid diethylamide (LSD)[6]	24 h

1. Cocaine is rapidly converted to benzoylecgonine in alkaline urine at room temperature.
2. The presence of nordiazepam, an active metabolite of diazepam, in urine may prolong detection when using immunoassay tests.
3. Morphine is rapidly oxidised at 4°C. Urine collection vessels should be filled to the top to minimise this effect.
4. New formulation (2–16 mg tablets) for maintenance and detoxification treatment has made detection easier, although testing is not always offered routinely.
5. The lipophilic nature of the cannabinoids may prolong detection in urine with chronic dosing (Dackis *et al*, 1982).
6. LSD is extremely photolabile and samples thought to contain this drug should be stored protected from light.

Box 11.3   Potential sources of urinary morphine

- Consumption of codeine
- Opiate drugs in foodstuffs, e.g. poppy seed strudel/danish pastry (Selavka, 1991), poppy seed cake (George, 1998)
- Analgesic prescription preparations, e.g. Gee's Linctus®, kaolin and morphine mixture
- Consumption of pharmaceutical diamorphine

It is an incorrect identification of the presence of the determined compound. One cause of false-positive results is the presence in the sample of artefacts or compounds of similar structure to the drug of interest. An analytical method that can be subject to such interference is said to have low specificity.

Clinical misinterpretations of the results of immunoassay (often used as an initial screening test) are a common source of false-positive reporting. Immunoassays, as a measurement technique, are generally the most susceptible to interference from compounds similar to the drug in question, since they commonly recognise all compounds belonging to a particular drug class, including metabolites. An opiate-positive test report using immunoassays, for instance, can be indicative of the presence of any number of opiate-type drugs and not necessarily illicit substances. Similarly, failure to acknowledge medication taken legitimately that is chemically similar to the drug of interest (e.g. pseudoephedrine in cough medicine with immunoassays for amphetamine) may lead to a false-positive interpretation.

A positive result due to passive drug exposure (e.g. to cannabis or nicotine) can also be falsely interpreted in the clinic. This is a particular issue for the detection of drugs in hair. Another cause of false interpretation of the result may be the presence (as already mentioned) of a compound that is actually a metabolite of other compounds. For example, the presence of morphine in urine is often assumed to be indicative of heroin use, but it is important to recognise that urinary morphine may result from several sources (Box 11.3). The 'poppy seed defence' has been shown to be a plausible explanation of a positive test result (as little as half a slice of poppy seed cake will give a positive immunoassay response). Thus, each case should be interpreted on its own merits and with caution (George, 1998).

Clearly, the more information that the clinician or drug worker can gather during sample collection, the better. Although self-reports of drug use have been criticised as an inaccurate source of information, carefully presented questions can produce a wealth of valuable information. Self-report interviews are all too often disregarded by workers in the field although they could be used as an important component of the screening test.

Currently available laboratory investigations

Urine

For those responsible for carrying out screening for drugs of abuse urine is the preferred biological fluid (Wolff *et al*, 1999b). Urinalysis is a well-known technology in which most of the analytical problems have been discovered and resolved. The significant advantage of urine for drug testing is that it is generally available in sufficient quantity and the drugs or their metabolites tend to be present in relatively high concentrations (Moffat *et al*, 1986).

A variety of methodological techniques have been employed for screening urine samples, and many comparative studies have been carried out to determine the most efficient system (Wilson *et al*, 1994). Automation has enabled mass screening of urine samples by a variety of techniques. Enzyme-linked immunosorbent assay (ELISA) is potentially the most cost-effective in terms of sample turnover and it can also be used for whole blood, serum, oral fluid and hair (Simpson *et al*, 1997).

A recent innovation has been the introduction of self-contained drug testing kits for on-site testing. These are marketed for testing for a variety of drugs in urine and are designed to provide rapid results without the need for laboratory facilities (Armbruster & Krolak, 1992). Those that test for cannabis (see Jenkins *et al*, 1993, 1995) are among the most commonly used. These tests offer several advantages (simplicity, ease of performance and rapid access to results), but potential drawbacks include the subjective and qualitative nature of the kits and, in some instances, the lack of a positive control (Armbruster & Krolak, 1992). There is a paucity of data on the validity of the 'stick tests' produced by some manufacturers. The main problem with most self-contained urine tests is interpretation of the results (George & Braithwaite, 1995). Detecting colour change is a highly subjective process and difficult for the inexperienced eye. Another problem is the cost, which can be prohibitive.

It is often thought that detection times for drugs in urine will vary with drug dosage, but this is not usually the case (certainly not to any great extent) since chronic drug consumption extends the detection time of the parent drug only slightly. A three-days-per-week urinalysis schedule has been reported as the most efficient to pick up illicit cocaine or heroin use (Cone *et al*, 1992). However, the cost of conducting such frequent tests would be prohibitive for most services and the schedule is recommended only in exceptional circumstances.

The benefits of using urine to screen for drugs of misuse are well known, but it has also been widely recognised that the collection of urine for drug screening has limitations. Care should be observed by those who collect the samples. For instance, morphine is rapidly oxidised at 4°C, so urine collection vessels should be filled to the top, where possible, to minimise this effect.

Drug addicts at times attempt to influence the results of a screening test to produce either a positive (prerequisite for pharmacotherapy) or negative (implied abstinent) test result. Various methods have been reported to achieve a false-negative result. Household detergents added to urine prior to testing cause false-negative results for amphetamine, cocaine, morphine and cannabis. Ibuprofen in urine has been associated with false-negative GC–MS confirmation results for cannabis (Brunk, 1988), while sodium chloride may lead to false-negative results with basic drugs such as opiates (Kim & Cerceo, 1976). Commercially available products for 'flushing' illicit substances from the body are used to achieve a negative result in a urine sample that is otherwise positive for one or more drugs (Wu et al, 1994).

Other steps taken include drinking copious amounts of fluid to dilute the urine; substituting weak black tea for urine; submitting a urine sample collected previously (when abstinent) or a sample from a drug-free friend; or diluting the sample with water from a tap or the toilet (Widdop & Caldwell, 1991). To help prevent dilution of the sample at the collection site, a blue dye can be added to the water in the toilet bowl.

A false-positive result can be achieved by adding the drug in question to the urine sample after voiding. This can be detected by checking that metabolites of the drug are also present, e.g. methadone should not be present without its main metabolite 2-ethylidene-1,5-dimethyl-3,3-diphenylpyrrolidine (EDDP)).

The best way to ensure sample validity is to witness the collection of the sample. This may raise several issues regarding infringements of a patient's privacy, more practical matters of staffing (e.g. female staff to observe female clients) and availability of facilities. There are, however, simple physical tests that may be taken to check the validity of a urine sample (Table 11.3).

The disadvantages of using urine to test for the presence of drugs of misuse have to be weighed up against the advantages of having a fluid that requires little pre-analysis preparation and can be collected non-invasively in large volumes. Urinalysis remains the most reliable tool for identification of the presence of most illicit substances.

Table 11.3 Physical tests employed for collecting a valid urine specimen

Suspected manipulation	Physical test
Diluted urine sample	Measure the specific gravity: normal range is 1.016–1.025. A specific gravity <1.003 clearly indicates dilution
	Measure creatinine level: normal range is 1.5–2.0 g/24 h for men and 0.8–1.5 g/24 h for women. A creatinine level <0.2 g/dl clearly indicates dilution
Substituted sample (tea/ water/someone else's urine)	Check temperature is 33–37°C: measure within 4 min of voiding
Adulterated sample (bleach, detergents, etc.)	Check pH: normal range is 4.5–7.8

Blood

Blood is the most useful biological matrix for the quantitative measurement of drugs and for interpretation by comparison with known blood concentrations corresponding to therapeutic, toxic and fatal levels (Moffatt *et al*, 1986). Also, because drugs leave the blood fairly rapidly, blood is most useful for identifying very recent drug use. At therapeutic levels, the concentration of drugs in the blood is usually low, typically in the 5 ng/ml to 5 µg/ml range. Psychoactive substances when used for illicit purposes are usually consumed in doses exceeding therapeutic recommendations, but there are exceptions, notably LSD and flunitrazepam. However, there is the advantage that in misuse, drug concentrations in blood may be 2–3 times higher than normal levels observed with therapeutic dosing.

Since most drugs of misuse (cocaine, ecstasy – methylenedioxymethamphetamine – heroin, etc.) leave the blood fairly rapidly (within a few hours of intake), blood concentrations will probably have fallen below detection levels applied in routine drug screening. The period of elimination of a drug from blood (the half-life) is determined by the physiological and chemical characteristics of the particular drug and the route by which it is administered. It usually takes 5–7 half-lives for a drug to be totally eliminated from the body (Table 11.4).

Until analytical assays are available to assess the biological effects of substance misuse, or until drug receptor concentrate can be estimated to indicate potential drug response, there is an increasing need for therapeutic drug monitoring to predict clinical outcomes of therapeutic regimes (Flanagan, 1995). Blood collection, however, is probably the least favoured procedure for routine drug testing, and the mechanics of storage of blood samples collected for routine drug screening presents additional problems for the clinician (Box 11.4).

Monitoring blood levels in maintenance therapy

Although clinical pharmacology is a well-established discipline, its influence on substance misuse treatment has been minimal. Dosage control has been the traditional tool for defining efficacy, safety and dose response in

---

Box 11.4 Issues to be overcome for blood collection

- Requires trained personnel
- Is an invasive procedure
- Involves the attendant risk of needle-stick injury and possible transmission of either HIV or hepatitis B/C virus
- Is difficult to obtain in large volumes
- Is difficult in intravenous drug users who may have thrombosed or sclerosed surface veins

---

Table 11.4 Approximate plasma elimination half-lives for drugs of misuse

Drug	Half-life (mean value)
Heroin	2 min
Morphine	3 h
Morphine glucuronides[1]	7.5 h
Dihydrocodeine	4 h
Codeine	3 h
Codeine glucuronides[1]	12 h
Buprenorphine[2]	8 h
Buprenorphine glucuronides[2]	24 h
Methadone[3]	36 h
Amphetamine	12 h
Cocaine	1 h
Benzoylecgonine (cocaine metabolite)[4]	7.5 h
Methylenedioxymethamphetamine (MDMA, ecstasy)	6 h
Nitrazepam	28 h
Flunitrazepam	25 h
Temazepam	10 h
Diazepam	48 h
Nordiazepam[5]	40–100 h
Cannabis[6]	20 h
Cannabinoid metabolites[7]	25–28 h

1. Cone *et al* (1991).
2. Hanks (1987).
3. Wolff *et al* (1997).
4. Ambre (1985).
5. Nordiazepam is an active metabolite of diazepam (Moffat *et al*, 1986).
6. Hunt & Jones (1980).
7. Lemberger *et al* (1971) and Law *et al* (1984).

prescribing programmes for drug dependence. However, there is mounting evidence, particularly for methadone treatment, that monitoring plasma drug concentrations may represent a better approach to achieving optimal dosing (Wolff & Hay, 1994).

Therapeutic drug monitoring is the science that combines measurement of blood drug concentrations with clinical pharmacokinetics. One of its major benefits is that it allows monitoring of adherence to pharmacotherapy regimens. The study of patient adherence is not new, and non-adherence is recognised to be common, occurring in all kinds of medical conditions. Drug dependence is no exception. Urinalysis drug screening is an important way of assessing illicit drug use by patients during methadone treatment, but, unlike therapeutic drug monitoring, it sheds no light on whether a patient is taking all their medication (at the correct time and in the correct amount – individuals may be selling some of their prescription), or is using extra medication (obtained illicitly). There is growing evidence that plasma methadone measurements can provide answers to these questions (Wolff *et al*, 1992) (Fig. 11.1).

Studies of methadone treatment response have shown that patients who adhere to the recommended course of treatment have longer-lasting post-treatment benefits (Allison & Hubbard, 1985). Thus, it is discouraging for many practitioners that opiate addicts in treatment are frequently poorly adherent or non-adherent clients. Dosage alterations based on interpretation of plasma measurements may help more individuals to do well on methadone (Wolff *et al*, 1991a, 1997).

Hair

Testing of scalp hair is a further biological tool for drug screening. The obvious advantage of hair testing is that this technique offers the potential for information over a much longer time scale than can be obtained with blood, urine and oral fluid analysis. The analysis of misused substances in hair is complicated because they are found in very low concentrations, usually within a range of 10 pg/mg to 10 ng/mg hair. Nevertheless, most illicit substances can be detected, yet it is noticeable that there is little in the way of a comprehensive drug screening methodology for this matrix.

Advocates of scalp hair analysis have emphasised the ease with which samples can be collected, but there has been a tendency to gloss over the many technical and even practical difficulties involved (Cone, 1996). The mechanism by which a substance is deposited in hair remains poorly defined (Joseph *et al*, 1996), but it is likely that the amount and type of melanin is important in determining how much drug enters hair from systemic circulation. This has led to research that has demonstrated that there may be a racial bias in hair analysis.

The physicochemical properties of each particular substance play an important role in the incorporation of a drug into hair. Lipophilicity and basicity (alkalinity) are clearly important in the blood-to-hair route. Alkaline drugs (such as opiates, amphetamine and cocaine) are incorporated easily into hair (Nakahara *et al*, 1995), acidic drugs (aspirin or methaqualone) much less so. Cannabis appears to be particularly difficult to detect in human scalp hair, although analytical procedures have been reported (Kintz *et al*, 1995; Uhl & Sachs, 2004).

Perhaps a unique problem with scalp hair analysis is passive contamination of the external surface of the hair, which presents an obvious interpretational problem. It has been known for some time (Dupont & Baumgartner, 1995) that exogenous false positives due to contamination of hair by drugs present in the environment present a real problem when screening for cannabis use.

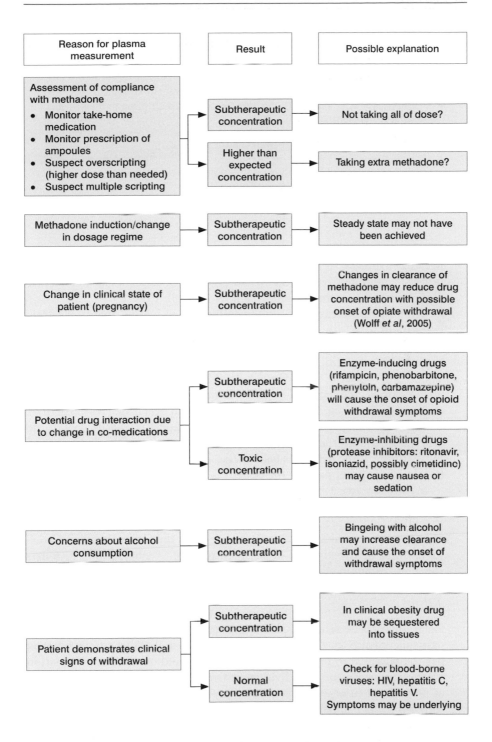

Fig. 11.1 Indications for plasma methadone measurements.

Box 11.5 Additional potential uses of hair analysis

- In post-mortem examination (Kintz *et al*, 1992)
- Forensic cases (Moeller, 1996)
- Medico-legal work in establishing a history of past exposures to therapeutic or abused substances (Huestis, 1996)
- Hair samples from children may help in child protection cases by providing evidence of previous drug exposure (Lewis *et al*, 1997)
- Neonatal hair analysis may (if present in sufficient quantity) be a useful biological marker for fetal exposure to drugs (Klein *et al*, 1994)

Decontamination of hair to exclude external interferants from analysis has become an integral step in most methodological procedures, but the process is very labour intensive and some hair types, such as thick black hair, seem more resistant to it than others (Blank & Kidwell, 1995).

While hair collection for drug screening is non-invasive, there are certain precautions to be taken into account. Marsh (1997) reports that maintaining alignment of, securing and identifying the cut ends of hair are critical if segmentation (quantification of time with drug concentration) is required. The style in which the hair is worn is also a source of variability. Hair growing from a closely cropped head may not contain the same concentration, after the same dose of drug, as hair that has not been cut over a long period of time. Variations in the expected concentration can exceed 20% (Sachs, 1995), and it is not clear from the literature how one corrects for these discrepancies. Furthermore, if the patient is bald or has a shaved head, hair samples must be taken from other parts of the body.

In regular practice in the addiction field, the clinician may be better served by urinalysis (Strang *et al*, 1993). Hair analysis should be seen as an adjunct to other screening procedures, for obtaining information regarding patterns of drug use, for establishing a drug history over time, or as a research tool, for example in investigation of passive exposure to tobacco. Box 11.5 lists some less common uses for hair analysis.

Oral fluid

Determination of drug concentrations in oral fluid is a newer territory, particularly since the collection of samples is non-invasive and this matrix has the potential to provide both quantitative and qualitative information on the drug status of an individual (Allen *et al*, 2005). The measurement of illicit drugs in oral fluid has been studied for more than a decade, but early work was hampered by inconsistent collection procedures (Haeckel & Hanecke, 1996).

Sample collection time is also an important variable. For drug addicts who self-administer by oral, intranasal and smoking routes, 'shallow depots' of the drug can result, which contaminate the oral cavity (Cone, 1993). This produces elevated oral fluid concentrations for several hours after ingestion and, although potentially useful in cases of overdose or accidental poisoning, should be borne in mind when interpreting results for routine drug screening. The presence of tetrahydrocannabinol (THC) in oral fluid, for example, appears to be due primarily to contamination of the oral cavity following smoking of marijuana cigarettes (Crouch, 2005). Being highly protein-bound, cannabinoids do not readily pass from blood into oral fluid and cannabis itself inhibits salivary excretion (Karlsson & Strom, 1988).

Oral fluid testing for drugs of misuse can, however, provide information on the drug status of the individual. Generally, once drugs have been eliminated from the buccal cavity, there is a high correlation between salivary and plasma drug concentrations for many compounds (Huestis & Cone, 1998), such as cotinine (Curvall et al, 1990) and methadone (Wolff et al, 1991b).

Oral fluid for drug analysis has the advantage of being relatively easy to obtain and collection can be carried out by non-clinical personnel (Gorodischer et al, 1994). Commercially available tools have allowed the collection of oral fluid in a more standardised manner than has been possible previously. The use of oral fluid in substance misuse treatment services is thought to be particularly advantageous with intravenous drug users, in whom it is often extremely difficult to find venous access. It would also enable more objective measurement and corroboration of self-reported drug use in a variety of social survey situations. The major drawback with oral fluid is that detection times for drugs are considerably shorter, ranging from 5 to 48 h, compared with 1.5–4 days for urine (Verstraete, 2004).

Despite the fact that drugs are detectable in oral fluid for a shorter period than in urine, it is possible that oral fluid detection procedures will expand significantly in the next few years, owing to the particular advantage over blood of the non-invasive nature of collection.

Breath

The analysis of human breath has been extensively used for the measurement of ethanol as a gauge of alcohol consumption (Cowan et al, 1996). Generally, the variety of instruments used to monitor breath are portable, economical and easy to use (Grote & Pawliszyn, 1997). Some drugs, such as anaesthetic gases (e.g. nitrous oxide) and inhalants (e.g. correction fluid and solvents), are naturally volatile compounds that mix freely with air. Others (e.g. tobacco, marijuana and crack cocaine) require combustion. Although tetrahydrocannabinol was identified in the breath of marijuana smokers by using radioimmunoassay and gas chromatography more than 20 years ago (Manolis et al, 1983), procedures for drug testing using breath remain underdeveloped. The increasing sophistication of technology is likely to improve both the availability and accuracy of such tests for wider clinical application.

Sweat

In recent years, remarkable advances in the sensitivity of analytical procedures have enabled the analysis of drugs in unconventional samples such as sweat. Sweat is collected by means of a 'sweat patch', which can be applied to various skin sites (biceps, torso or back). All of the commonly used illicit substances, including buprenorphine and ecstasy, have been detected in sweat using precision chromatographic techniques (Kintz et al, 1996a; Skopp et al, 1996). Sweat patches have been used in drug treatment services to monitor patients prescribed methadone and have been reported to compare favourably with urine drug tests (Kintz et al, 1998; Taylor et al, 1998). Intrasubject variability and the influence of the application site have been reported to be significant (Kintz et al, 1996b), and it is possible to adulterate the sweat patch by injection into or under it to cause a false-positive (Fay et al, 1996) or false-negative (Fogerson et al, 1997) test response.

However, little information is available on the characteristics of drug excretion in sweat under controlled dosing conditions, and sweat analysis is open to misinterpretation because of the difficulty of excluding topical contamination. Given the reported between-dose and between-subject variability, sweat patch test results cannot as yet be used to determine either the dose or the time of use (Burns & Baselt, 1995). Nevertheless, the sweat test does appear to offer an alternative non-invasive means of obtaining a cumulative estimate of drug exposure over a period of 7–21 days (Kintz, 1996). From a clinical viewpoint the sweat patch could serve as a useful monitoring device in surveillance of individuals on treatment and probation programmes. If applied to the skin with a tamper detection device, it could provide a more continuous monitor of drug exposure.

Body fluids and childbirth

The high increase in the number of pregnant substance users presenting at drug treatment agencies for treatment for their addiction, and at antenatal clinics, has led to a demand for improved technology to assess the extent of drug ingestion by the fetus and/or neonate.

Breast milk

All drugs pass, to some extent, from plasma into human breast milk. The milk-to-plasma concentration ratio is the most commonly used index of drug distribution into milk, and is used to calculate the likely infant drug dose from a given maternal plasma concentration (Atkinson & Begg, 1990). The usefulness of human breast milk for assessing the extent of infant exposure to illicit substances has not been fully evaluated (Huestis & Cone, 1998). In Britain, drug-dependent nursing mothers are usually advised against breastfeeding. In many cases, this may be unnecessary as the total dose to which the baby is likely to be exposed is thought to be negligible (Atkinson &

Begg, 1990). A particularly important case for consideration may be nursing mothers prescribed methadone. Breastfeeding has been advocated for such women (Batey et al, 1990), and may assist in reducing the severity of neonatal abstinence syndrome (Mack et al, 1991), although polydrug use is likely to complicate decisions made regarding suitability for breastfeeding.

Reports indicate accumulation of tetrahydrocannabinol (Astley & Little, 1990), amphetamine (Steiner et al, 1984) and cocaine (Dickson et al, 1994) in breast milk. Steiner et al (1984) argued over 20 years ago that analysis of breast milk for drugs of misuse should be performed in cases of possible infant intoxication, but such tests have yet to become routinely available. Further research in this area is required since the extent to which the ingestion of illicit and psychotropic drugs by nursing infants may affect growth and development is unknown.

Meconium

Many substances have been detected in meconium, including cannabis (Moore et al, 1996), methadone (Skolk et al, 1997), nicotine (Eliopoulos et al, 1996) and cocaine (Martin et al, 1996). However, analysis of drugs in meconium is currently conducted only by researchers.

Conclusion

Analysis of urine is currently the biological tool of choice for qualitative detection of illicit drug use. Quantitative accuracy usually demands the collection of a blood sample, although oral fluid may be an alternative in the future. The advantage of hair sampling is its reflection of weeks rather than hours of recent use. Accurate interpretation of test results within a clinical setting, alongside other relevant information, remains the key to the usefulness of any screening test.

References

Allen, K. R., Azad, R., Field, H. P., et al (2005) Replacement of immunoassay by LC tandem mass spectrometry for the routine measurement of drugs of abuse in oral fluid. Annals of Clinical Biochemistry, 42, 277–284.

Allison, M. & Hubbard, R. I. (1985) Drug abuse treatment process: a review of the literature. International Journal of Addiction, 20, 1321–1345.

Ambre, J. (1985) The urinary excretion of cocaine and metabolites in humans: a kinetic analysis of published data. Journal of Analytical Toxicology, 9, 241–245.

Armbruster, D. A. & Krolak, J. M. (1992) Screening for drugs of abuse with the Roche On TRAK assays. Journal of Analytical Toxicology, 18, 172–175.

Astley, S. J. & Little, R. E. (1990) Maternal marijuana use during lactation and infant development at one year. Neurotoxicology and Teratology, 12, 161–163.

Atkinson, H. C. & Begg, E. J. (1990) Prediction of drug distribution into human milk from physicochemical characteristics. Clinical Pharmacokinetics, 18, 151–167.

Batey, R. G., Patterson, T. & Sanders, F. (1990) Practical issues in the methadone management of pregnant heroin users. Drug and Alcohol Review, 9, 303–310.

Blank, D. L. & Kidwell, D. A. (1995) Decontamination procedures for drugs of abuse in hair: are they sufficient? *Forensic Science International*, **5**, 13–38.

Braithwaite, R. A., Jarvie, D. R., Minty, P. S. B., *et al* (1995) Screening for drugs of abuse. I: Opiates, amphetamines and cocaine. *Annals of Clinical Biochemistry*, **32**, 123–153.

Brunk, S. D. (1988) False negative GC/MS assay for carboxy THC due to ibuprofen interference. *Journal of Analytical Toxicology*, **12**, 290–295.

Burns, M. & Baselt, R. C. (1995) Monitoring drug use with a sweat patch: an experiment with cocaine. *Journal of Analytical Toxicology*, **19**, 41–48.

Cone, E. J. (1993) Saliva testing for drugs of abuse. *Annals of the New York Academy of Sciences*, **20**, 91–127.

Cone, E. J. (1996) Mechanisms of drug incorporation into hair. *Therapeutic Drug Monitoring*, **18**, 438–443.

Cone, E. J., Welch, P., Paul, B. D., *et al* (1991) Forensic drug testing for opiates. III. Urinary excretion rates of morphine and codeine following codeine administration. *Journal of Analytical Toxicology*, **15**, 161–166.

Cone, E. J., Dickerson, S., Paul, B. D., *et al* (1992) Forensic drug testing for opiates. IV. Analytical sensitivity, specificity, and accuracy of commercial urine opiate immunoassays. *Journal Analytical Toxicology*, **16**, 72–78.

Cowan, J. M. Jr, Weathermon, A., McCutcheon, J. R., *et al* (1996) Determination of volume of distribution for ethanol in male and female subjects. *Journal of Analytical Toxicology*, **20**, 287–290.

Crouch, D. J. (2005) Oral fluid collection: the neglected variable in oral fluid testing. *Forensic Science International*, **150**, 165–173.

Curvall, M., Elwin, C. E., Kazemi-Vala, E., *et al* (1990) The pharmacokinetics of cotinine in plasma and saliva from non-smoking healthy volunteers. *European Journal of Clinical Pharmacology*, **38**, 281–284

Dackis, C. A., Pottash, A. L. C., Annitto, W., *et al* (1982) Persistence of urinary marijuana levels after supervised abstinence. *American Journal of Psychiatry*, **139**, 1196–1198.

Dickson, P. H., Lind, A., Studts, P., *et al* (1994) The routine analysis of breast milk for drugs abuse in a clinical toxicology laboratory. *Journal of Forensic Sciences*, **39**, 207–214.

Dupont, R. L. & Baumgartner, W. A. (1995) Drug testing by urine and hair analysis: complementary features and scientific issues. *Forensic Science International*, **70**, 63–76.

Eliopoulos, C., Klein, J., Chitayat, D., *et al* (1996) Nicotine and cotinine in maternal and neonatal hair as markers of gestational smoking. *Clinical Investigations in Medicine*, **19**, 231–242.

Fay, J., Fogerson, R. Schoendorfer, D., *et al* (1996) Detection of methamphetamine in sweat by EIA and GC–MS. *Journal of Analytical Toxicology*, **20**, 398–403.

Flanagan, R. J. (1995) The poisoned patient: the role of the laboratory. *British Journal of Biomedical Science*, **52**, 202–213.

Fogerson, R., Schoendorfer, D., Fay, J., *et al* (1997) Qualitative detection of opiates in sweat by EIA and GC–MS. *Journal of Analytical Toxicology*, **21**, 451–458.

George, S. (1998) The poppy-seed defence, *Syva Drug Monitor*, **3**, 1–3.

George, S. & Braithwaite, R. A. (1995) A preliminary evaluation of five rapid detection kits for on-site drugs of abuse screening. *Addiction*, **90**, 227–232.

Gorodischer, R., Burtin, P., Hwang, P., *et al* (1994) Saliva versus blood sampling for therapeutic drug monitoring in children: patient and parental preferences and an economic analysis. *Therapeutic Drug Monitoring*, **16**, 437–443.

Grote, C. & Pawliszyn, J. (1997) Solid-phase microextraction for the analysis of human breath. *Annals of Chemistry*, **69**, 589–596.

Haeckel, R. & Hanecke, P. (1996) Application of saliva for drug monitoring. An in-vivo model for transmembrane transport. *European Journal of Chemistry and Clinical Biochemistry*, **34**, 171–191.

Hanks, G. W. (1987) The clinical usefulness of agonist–antagonist opioid analgesics in chronic pain. *Drug and Alcohol Dependence*, **20**, 339–347.

Huestis, M. A. (1996) Judicial acceptance of hair tests for substances of abuse in the United States courts: scientific, forensic, and ethical aspects. *Therapeutic Drug Monitoring*, **18**, 456–459.

Huestis, M. A. & Cone, E. J. (1998) Alternative testing matrices. In *Drug Abuse Handbook* (ed. S. Karch), pp. 799–857. CRC Press.

Hunt, C. A. & Jones, R. T. (1980) Tolerance and deposition of tetrahydrocannabinol in man. *Journal Pharmacology & Experimental Therapeutics*, **215**, 35–44.

Jenkins, A. J., Mills, L. C., Darwin, W. D., *et al* (1993) Validity testing of the EZ-SCREEN cannabinoid test. *Journal of Analytical Toxicology*, **17**, 292–298.

Jenkins, A. J., Darwin, W. D., Huestis, M. A., *et al* (1995) Validity testing of the accuPINCH THC test. *Journal of Analytical Toxicology*, **19**, 5–12.

Joseph, R. E. Jr, Su, T. P. & Cone, E .J. (1996) In vitro binding studies of drugs to hair: influence of melanin and lipids on cocaine binding to Caucasoid and Africoid hair. *Journal of Analytical Toxicology*, **20**, 338–344.

Karlsson, I. & Strom, M. (1988) Laboratory evaluation of the TDX assay for detection of cannabinoids in urine from prison inmates. *Journal of Analytical Toxicology*, **12**, 319–321.

Kim, H. J. & Cerceo, E. (1976) Interference by NaCl with the EMIT method of analysis for drugs of abuse. *Clinical Chemistry*, **22**, 1935–1936.

Kintz, P. (1996) Drug testing in addicts: a comparison between urine, sweat, and hair. *Therapeutic Drug Monitoring*, **18**, 450–455.

Kintz, P., Tracqui, A. & Mangin, P. (1992) Detection of drugs in human hair for clinical and forensic applications. *International Journal of Legal Medicine*, **105**, 1–4.

Kintz, P., Cirimele, V. & Mangin, P. (1995) Testing human hair for cannabis. II. Identification of THC–COOH by GC–MS–NCI as a unique proof. *Journal of Forensic Science*, **40**, 619–622.

Kintz, P., Tracqui, A., Mangim, P., *et al* (1996a) Sweat testing in opioid users with a sweat patch. *Journal of Analytical Toxicology*, **20**, 393–397.

Kintz, P., Tracqui, A., Jamey, C., *et al* (1996b) Detection of codeine and phenobarbital in sweat collected with a sweat patch. *Journal of Analytical Toxicology*, **20**, 197–201.

Kintz, P., Tracqui, A., Marzullo, C., *et al* (1998) Enantioselective analysis of methadone in sweat as monitored by liquid chromatography spray-mass spectrometry. *Therapeutic Drug Monitoring*, **20**, 35–40.

Klein, J., Forman, R., Eliopoulos, C., *et al* (1994) A method for simultaneous measurement of cocaine and nicotine in neonatal hair. *Therapeutic Drug Monitoring*, **16**, 67–70.

Law, B., Mason, P. A., Moffat, A. C., *et al* (1984) Forensic aspects of the metabolism and excretion of cannabinoids following oral ingestion of cannabis resin. *Journal of Pharmacy and Pharmacology*, **36**, 289–294.

Lemberger, L., Tamarkin, N. R. & Alexrod, J. (1971) Δ^9-Tetrahydrocannabinol. Metabolism and disposition in long term marijuana smokers. *Science*, **178**, 72–74.

Lewis, D., Moore, C., Morrissey, P., *et al* (1997) Determination of drug exposure using hair: application to child protective cases. *Forensic Science International*, **17**, 123–128.

Linder, M. W. & Valdes R., Jr (1994) Mechanism and elimination of aspirin induced interference in Emit II d.a.u. assays. *Clinical Chemistry*, **40**, 1512–1515.

Long, K. L. (1989) The discovery process in drug use testing litigation. *Journal of Forensic Science*, **34**, 1454–1470.

Macdonald, D.I. (1990) The Medical Review Officer. *Journal of Psychoactive Drugs*, **22**, 429–434.

Mack, G., Thomas, D., Giles, W., *et al* (1991) Methadone levels and neonatal withdrawal. *Journal of Paediatrics and Child Health*, **27**, 96–100.

Manolis, A., McBurney, L. J. & Bobbie, B. A. (1983) The detection of delta-9-tetrahydrocannabinol in the breath of human subjects. *Clinical Biochemistry*, **16**, 229–232.

Marsh, A. (1997) Hair analysis for drugs of abuse. *Syva Drug Monitor*, **2**, 1–4.

Martin, J. C., Barr, H. M., Martin, D. C., *et al* (1996) Neonatal neurobehavioral outcome following prenatal exposure to cocaine. *Neurotoxicology and Teratology*, **18**, 617–25.

Moeller, M. R. (1996) Hair analysis as evidence in forensic cases. *Therapeutic Drug Monitoring*, **18**, 444–449.

Moffat, A. C., Jackson, J. V., Moss, M. S., *et al* (1986) *Clarks Isolation and Identification of Drugs*. Pharmaceutical Press.

Moore, C., Lewis, D., Becker, J., *et al* (1996) The determination of 11-nor-delta-9-tetrahydrocannabinol-9-carboxylic acid (THCCOOH) in meconium. *Journal of Analytical Toxicology*, **20**, 50–51.

Nakahara, Y., Takahashi, K. & Kikura, R. (1995) Hair analysis for drugs of abuse. X. Effect of physicochemical properties of drugs on the incorporation rates into hair. *Biological Pharmacology Bulletin*, **18**, 1223–1227.

Osterloh, J. D. & Becker, C.E. (1990) Chemical dependency and drug testing in the workplace. *Journal of Psychoactive Drugs*, **22**, 407–417.

Sachs, H. (1995) Theoretical limits of the evaluation of drug concentrations in hair due to irregular hair growth. *Forensic Science International*, **70**, 53–61.

Selavka, C. M. (1991) Poppy seed ingestion as a contributing factor to opiate-positive urinalysis results: the Pacific perspective. *Journal of Forensic Sciences*, **36**, 685–696.

Simpson, D., Braithwaite, R. A., Jarvie, D. R., *et al* (1997) Screening for drugs of abuse. II: Cannabinoids, lysergic acid diethylamide, buprenorphine, methadone, barbiturates, benzodiazepines and other drugs. *Annals of Clinical Biochemistry*, **34**, 460–510.

Skolk, L. M., Coenradie, S. M., Smit, B. J., *et al* (1997) Analysis of methadone and its primary metabolite in meconium. *Journal of Analytical Toxicology*, **21**, 154–159.

Skopp, G., Potsch, L., Eser, H. P., *et al* (1996) Preliminary practical findings on drug monitoring by a transcutaneous collection device. *Journal of Forensic Science*, **41**, 933–937.

Steiner, E., Villen, T., Hallberg, M., *et al* (1984) Amphetamine secretion in breast milk. *European Journal of Clinical Pharmacology*, **27**, 123–125.

Strang, J., Black, J., Marsh, A., *et al* (1993) Hair analysis for drugs: technological breakthrough or ethical quagmire. *Addiction*, **88**, 163–166.

Taylor, J. R,. Watson, I. D., Tames, F. J., *et al* (1998) Detection of drug use in a methadone maintenance clinic: sweat patches versus urine testing. *Addiction*, **93**, 847–853.

Uhl, M. & Sachs, H. (2004) Cannabinoids in hair: strategy to prove marijuana/hashish consumption. *Forensic Science International*, **145**, 143–149.

Verstraete, A. G. (2004) Determination of drugs of abuse in blood, urine and oral fluid. *Therapeutic Drug Monitoring*, **26**, 200–205.

Widdop, B. & Caldwell, R. (1991) The operation of a hospital laboratory service for the detection of drugs of abuse. In *The Analysis of Drugs of Abuse* (ed. T. A. Gough), pp. 429–452. John Wiley & Sons.

Wilson, J. F., Smith, B. L., Toseland, P. A., *et al* (1994) External quality assessment of techniques for the detection of drugs of abuse in urine. *Annals of Clinical Biochemistry*, **31**, 335–342.

Wolff, K. & Hay, A. W. M. (1994) Plasma methadone monitoring with methadone maintenance treatment. *Drug and Alcohol Dependence*, **36**, 69–71.

Wolff, K., Sanderson, M., Hay, A. W. M., *et al* (1991*a*) Methadone concentrations in plasma and their relationship to drug dosage. *Clinical Chemistry*, **37**, 205–209.

Wolff, K., Hay, A. & Raistrick, D. (1991*b*) Methadone in saliva. *Clinical Chemistry*, **37**, 1297–1298.

Wolff, K., Hay, A., Raistrick, D., *et al* (1992) Measuring compliance in methadone maintenance patients: use of a pharmacologic indicator to 'estimate' methadone plasma levels. *Clinical Pharmacological Therapeutics*, **50**, 199–207.

Wolff, K., Rostami-Hodjegan, A., Shires, S., *et al* (1997) The pharmacokinetics of methadone in healthy subjects and opiate users. *British Journal of Clinical Pharmacology*, **44**, 325–334.

Wolff, K., Welch, S. & Strang, J. (1999*a*) Specific laboratory investigations for assessments and management of drug problems. *Advances in Psychiatric Treatment*, **5**, 180–191.

Wolff, K., Farrell, M., Marsden J., *et al* (1999*b*) A review of biological indicators of illicit drug use, practical considerations and clinical usefulness. *Addiction*, **94**, 1279–1298.

Wolff, K., Boys, A., Hay, A. W. M., *et al* (2005) Changes in methadone clearance during pregnancy. *European Journal of Clinical Pharmacology*, **61**, 763–768.

Wu, A., Schmalz, J. & Bennett, W. (1994) Identification of UrinAid-adulterated urine specimens by fluorometric analysis. *Clinical Chemistry*, **40**, 845–846.

CHAPTER 12

Pharmacotherapy in dual diagnosis

Ilana B. Crome and Tracey Myton

Summary   The prevalence of coexisting substance misuse and psychiatric disorder (dual diagnosis, comorbidity) has increased over the past decade, and the indications are that it will continue to rise. There have simultaneously been unprecedented developments in the pharmacological treatment of alcohol, opiate and nicotine misuse. Here we evaluate the evidence on the use of some of these treatments in dual diagnosis (with psychotic, mood and anxiety disorders). The evidence base is limited by the exclusion of mental illness when pharmacological agents for substance misuse are evaluated and vice versa. We set the available information within the context of the psychosocial management of comorbid substance misuse and mental illness, and the framework for service delivery recommended by UK national policy.

In 1980, Robin Murray raised the question 'Why are the drug companies so disinterested in alcoholism?' (Murray, 1980). Since then, we have witnessed the evolution of a 'specialist addiction field' (Edwards, 2002), including rapid developments in pharmacological treatments for problem use of alcohol, opiates and nicotine. In this review we discuss some of these pharmacological agents and then summarise the evidence on the treatment of combined or coexisting disorders, also described as 'dual diagnosis' (e.g. Banerjee *et al*, 2002; Crawford *et al*, 2003).

Dual diagnosis: a definition (see also chapter 13)

'Dual diagnosis' is one of a number of terms and phrases (Box 12.1) used to refer to people who have coexisting problems of mental disorder and substance misuse (including alcohol, nicotine and illicit drugs). It is also applied to people with two coexisting conditions, for example learning disability and mental disorder (Banerjee *et al*, 2002), although it does not take that meaning in this chapter.

The group of people with dual diagnosis is heterogeneous, with complex, changing needs. They may have had previous traumatic experiences such

---

Box 12.1 Alternatives to the term 'dual diagnosis'

- Co-occurring problems of substance misuse and mental disorder
- Comorbidity of substance misuse and mental disorder
- Mental illness and chemical abuse (MICA)
- Chemical addiction and mental illness (CAMI)
- Co-occurring addictive and mental disorders (COAMD)

---

as childhood sexual abuse, bullying at school or a broken and dysfunctional family life. Furthermore, mental disorder and substance misuse sit on separate dimensions, each with its own continuum of severity. 'Dual diagnosis' covers someone with bipolar disorder who is also alcohol dependent, and someone who has schizophrenia and smokes cannabis a few times a week. As a result of this complexity, numerous operational definitions may be applied in different clinical and social settings, thus complicating and confusing communication.

A patient labelled with a dual diagnosis can face prejudice and stigma from healthcare and other professionals, who might question the capacity of dually diagnosed individuals to respond to care.

These difficulties raise the question of which definitions and terminology to use. While acknowledging the problems inherent in the term and concept of dual diagnosis, we have chosen to use it as shorthand to describe patients with coexisting problems of mental disorder and substance misuse (of drugs, alcohol or nicotine).

Prevalence

The classic Epidemiologic Catchment Area Study in the USA (Regier *et al*, 1990) demonstrated that 47% of people with schizophrenia misused substances: alcohol (37%), cannabis (23%) and stimulants or hallucinogens (13%). Of those with an affective disorder, 32% had a comorbid substance use disorder. Of those with social anxiety disorder, 22% had a lifetime prevalence of alcohol dependence or misuse, while among the opiate-dependent population, lifetime rates of anxiety disorders were 6.1% in men and 10.7% in women.

In the UK, clinically based population and longitudinal studies consistently demonstrate the prevalence of substance misuse in psychiatric patients (Crawford *et al*, 2003). In a national comorbidity study, the prevalence of dependence on any drug was 4%, and cannabis dependence was reported most often (3%) (Coulthard *et al*, 2002). The prevalence of drug-taking during the previous year by 16- to 64-year-olds had increased from 5% to

12% since 1993. An estimated 27% of the total population surveyed had ever used drugs, and 4% of this group had experienced an accidental overdose.

Men (11%) were more likely than women (7%) to report heavy smoking; those aged 20–24 had the highest prevalence, at 44%. Similarly, men (12%) were more likely than women (3%) to be dependent on alcohol. In general, people who engaged in substance misuse were more likely to be visiting their general practitioner, receiving treatment or accessing mental health services.

It should be noted that lifetime prevalence of substance misuse and mental illness does not necessarily indicate their coexistence at any time. In one of the few studies on comorbidity in primary care in the UK, Frisher *et al* (2004) addressed this point by counting patients whose diagnoses of substance misuse and psychiatric illness co-occurred within a calendar year. Over the study period (1993–1998) the annual prevalence of dual diagnosis in England and Wales increased by 62% (from 24 226 to 39 296). The rates of comorbid psychosis, schizophrenia and paranoia increased by 147%, 128% and 144% respectively. By 2003, in a typical general practice 11 potentially chronic comorbid cases were likely to be encountered during the year. This growing epidemic has major implications for general practitioners' workload, as primary care resources in mental health are already thinly spread and are not integrated to deal with comorbidity (Frisher *et al*, 2004).

Drug problems are associated with smoking and alcohol consumption, constituting dual, or even triple, dependencies (Best *et al*, 2000). These conditions result in multiple social, physical and psychological complications, which cluster together and with which patients present to accident and emergency, paediatric, geriatric, general medical and surgical, and general psychiatric departments, to primary care and, of course, to specialist addiction units (e.g. Gfroerer *et al*, 2003).

Government policy

Comorbid substance misuse leads to more frequent recurrence of the mental disorder, greater time spent in hospital, increased violence, homelessness and alienation from families and carers. Once abstinent, however, people with dual diagnosis may have a better prognosis than do non-substance misusers with similar rates of hospitalisation (Granholm *et al*, 2003).

'Drug problems', especially in young people, remain high on the UK political agenda. The national service frameworks for mental health, children, young people and families, older people, coronary heart disease and cancer are all directly or indirectly related to addiction problems (e.g. Abdulrahim *et al*, 2001). In addition, there is now a national anti-smoking strategy (Department of Health, 1998) and an alcohol harm reduction strategy (Cabinet Office, Prime Minister's Strategy Unit, 2004).

Policy guidance on the implementation of dual diagnosis services in England and Wales, and in Scotland, is available (Department of Health,

2002; Scottish Executive, 2003). The *Dual Diagnosis Good Practice Guide* (Department of Health, 2002) places responsibility for treatment of people with dual diagnosis, especially those with severe and enduring mental health problems, on mental health services. The Scottish Executive's document proposes a five-stepped graded approach to service provision, which would range from a community response, through generic and specialised services, to a highly specialised dual diagnosis service. The focus of this integrated policy is primary care, and it puts more responsibility on primary healthcare teams to diagnose and treat less complex substance problems.

Treatment works and is cost-effective

Over the past decade, confidence in the assertion that 'treatment works' has grown immeasurably. To date, over 300 randomised controlled trials (RCTs) have investigated alcohol misuse, 100 tobacco misuse and 60 opiate misuse. It should be noted that some of these studies do not include patients with mental illness: indeed, this diagnosis was often an exclusion criterion, an obvious limitation in evaluating their results.

Brief psychological therapies carried out by generalists are likely to reap benefits as first-line interventions. However, the more costly intensive psychological interventions (often combined with pharmacological treatment) are effective for those with more complex needs.

Specialist smoking cessation, which costs about £800 for an intensive 6-week course, is the most cost-effective intervention in medicine: smoking-related illnesses cost £16000 per patient per year (National Institute for Clinical Excellence, 2002). Successful treatment of drug misuse saves the health service £3 for every £1 spent. Comorbid mental illness further increases the cost.

The psychosocial context of treatment

Pharmacological treatment is carried out in the context of attracting, engaging and retaining patients, enhancing their motivation to seek further support, providing the range of specific psychological treatments and medications, and relapse prevention (see also chapter 16).

Treatment should be part of an individualised comprehensive plan following detailed assessment. It should also be noted that, although it is the responsibility of all doctors to provide care for both general health needs and substance-related problems to a reasonable standard, practitioners should be aware of their limitations and seek specialist support if necessary. This is especially the case when treating young people.

Depending on the age of the patient, parental responsibilities, consent to treatment and child protection issues may have to be considered. For young people under the age of 16, explicit consent from a parent or guardian is required.

Psychosocial interventions are relevant throughout because, once detoxification, reduction or maintenance is established, sustained improvement depends on behavioural change. Although most practitioners are, understandably, very concerned about prescribing aspects because of safety issues, in fact the majority of treatment interventions are psychological.

Most general psychiatrists and their teams are in a position to give patients 5–10 minutes of brief advice or information regarding a substance misuse problem. This might include information about the personal risks of substances or about 'safe levels' of drinking, or the provision of self-help materials on ways to stop smoking or on safer injecting practices. The practitioner might also offer the opportunity for the patient to express anxieties, or to discuss the results of screening or blood tests.

Although it is often difficult to elicit from the patient an initial indication of 'motivation to change', if this can be established it can contribute substantially towards forming a judgement on how to proceed with regard to pharmacological treatments. Patients need to be encouraged to decide whether abstinence or reduction is their goal.

If abstinence is the goal, and no pharmacological treatment is required, a date on which the patient will stop using substances should be set. Patients should be advised to get rid of any alcohol, cigarettes or drugs and to work on alternative strategies for coping. A number of coping strategies for which there is a substantial and growing evidence base of efficacy are listed in Box 12.2. Whether harm reduction, harm minimisation or abstinence is the priority, information about related social issues, such as immunisation, vaccination and contraception, must also form part of the treatment package.

The degree of substance misuse and dependence, as well as associated social, medical and psychiatric problems, may be such that specialist addiction input is required. The practitioner should help the patient to arrange this, and should continue sustained and integrated support and encouragement in collaboration with different agencies.

Box 12.2   Coping strategies for substance misuse

- Self-monitoring (keeping a diary about how much they are using)
- Setting limits for use
- Controlling consumption rates (e.g. the number of drinks an hour)
- Learning refusal skills, assertiveness and relaxation
- Making use of new or alternative rewards
- Identifying and challenging negative automatic thoughts that predispose to substance misuse

It should be emphasised to patients and families that 'treatment works', especially if they have had previous negative experiences. This may be pertinent at particular times, for example during pregnancy, or in relation to particular behaviours and lifestyle issues such as prostitution and sex-working. It may be necessary and appropriate to arrange, and even accompany patients to, the first (and maybe more) assessments and consultations with the specialist service(s).

Specialist treatment interventions encompass psychological and pharmacological options. In certain circumstances, patients may have to be admitted to a specialist in-patient unit. This is usually in the case of severe dependence on one or more substances, severe physical illness, serious psychiatric illness, misuse of multiple substances, frequently relapsing substance misuse or unstable social circumstances.

Thus, if more intensive psychological support for the individual or family is required, this will be organised by a specialist and/or general service, on an out-patient basis, in the community, or in conjunction with other services (e.g. general practice or general psychiatric services) or during an assessment or admission.

Treating the substance misuse

Over the past decade, the capacity to intervene pharmacologically in substance misuse has increased greatly (Box 12.3). Pharmacotherapy is now available for opiate, alcohol and nicotine misuse (Table 12.1). Although there is an increasing number of protocols and guidelines for comorbidity in adults (Department of Health, 2002; Scottish Executive, 2003; Slattery *et al*, 2003), there are few protocols and little guidance specifically related to dual diagnosis in young people, pregnant women and older people. For these special groups, clinical decisions on the potential benefits of pharmacological

---

Box 12.3   Pharmacological interventions for substance misuse

Pharmacological interventions may be used:
- in emergencies
- to alleviate withdrawal symptoms so as to achieve abstinence, i.e. detoxification
- to substitute for the drug misused and thus reduce drug-related harm, i.e. stabilisation, reduction, maintenance
- to prevent relapse by reducing alcohol craving
- to treat comorbid psychiatric conditions
- to treat physical consequences
- to treat coexisting physical problems

Table 12.1 Pharmacological treatments for substance misuse

Treatment	Misused substance		
	Alcohol	Opiates	Nicotine
Detoxification	Chlordiazepoxide Diazepam	Methadone Buprenorphine Lofexidine Clonidine	Nicotine replacement therapy Bupropion
Substitution		Methadone Buprenorphine	Nicotine replacement therapy Bupropion
Relapse prevention	Acamprosate Disulfiram Naltrexone	Naltrexone	

treatments need to be grounded in good practice, since there is a paucity of well-controlled trials. If medications are prescribed for younger people, this should certainly be initiated and monitored by specialists.

Alcohol

The drug of choice for alcohol detoxification is chlordiazepoxide (see chapter 7). This is a long-acting benzodiazepine and is administered in a withdrawal or detoxification (reduction) regime. A useful rule of thumb is that the initiating dose be the score on the Severity of Alcohol Dependence Questionnaire (SADQ; Stockwell et al, 1979). If, for example, the SADQ score is 30, then 30 mg chlordiazepoxide three or four times a day should contain withdrawal symptoms. It is important to give sufficient medication. If the patient is oversedated, one dose can be withdrawn. Some practitioners prefer to prescribe diazepam. Anti-epileptics and anti-emetics are rarely required, although the former should be given if there is an additional risk factor, for example a history of fits or head injury. Alcohol withdrawal can be monitored using the Clinical Institute Withdrawal Assessment for Alcohol (CIWA–Ar) scale (Sullivan et al, 1989), and the medication reduced over 5–10 days.

Fluids and food should be taken as soon as possible. If not properly controlled, withdrawal can be fatal. Wernicke–Korsakoff syndrome can be confused with delirium tremens, and therefore adequate vitamin supplementation should also be given intravenously. This should be continued for as long as there is clinical improvement. If the syndrome is suspected or diagnosed, doses of up to 500 mg thiamine three times a day for 3 days should be used if necessary, followed by 250 mg daily for 3–5 days (Cook & Thomson, 1997). Wernicke–Korsakoff syndrome is a potentially reversible condition in a young person. If a patient is at risk of vitamin deficiency, i.e. has weight loss, poor diet or malnutrition, 250 mg thiamine should be given intravenously once a day for 3–5 days (Lingford-Hughes et al, 2004).

The effects of thiamine deficiency during alcohol detoxification should be treated proactively, and intramuscular vitamin supplementation should be given where possible, as there may be poor absorption of oral vitamins. Patients at low risk should have oral thiamine 200 mg four times a day and vitamin B compound 30 mg/day.

Carbamazepine has been shown to be effective in preventing withdrawal-related seizures, and interactions with antipsychotic medication (e.g. a reduced seizure threshold) should be considered.

Acamprosate (calcium acetylhomotaurinate) is a relatively new drug which has been reported to reduce craving (Geerlings *et al*, 1997). Side-effects include skin rash and gastrointestinal problems.

Disulfiram, which interferes with the breakdown of alcohol, resulting in the accumulation of acetaldehyde, produces unpleasant – even fatal – effects (e.g. headache, flushing, nausea, vomiting and circulatory collapse) if alcohol is taken. Its long-term effectiveness in adults is not convincing, but this could be due to inadequate dosage and supervision (Besson *et al*, 1998).

Naltrexone can only be administered on a named patient basis, as it is not licensed for use for alcohol problems in the UK.

Apart from detoxification with benzodiazepines and vitamin supplementation, there is no evidence to support the routine use of other medications at the moment, although there are potentially interesting developments with combined medications, for example naltrexone and acamprosate (Kiefer *et al*, 2003).

Nicotine (see chapter 8)

Two products are available for the treatment of nicotine addiction: nicotine replacement therapy (as chewing gum, spray, skin patch, sublingual tablets and lozenges) and bupropion.

Nicotine replacement therapy (NRT) is available in the UK over the counter or on prescription. For those under 18 years old it is available 'on the recommendation of a medical practitioner' (National Institute for Clinical Excellence, 2002). It is recommended that smokers who are pregnant or breastfeeding should discuss the use of nicotine replacement therapy with a relevant healthcare professional before it is prescribed (National Institute for Clinical Excellence, 2002). It may produce localised side-effects, and minor sleep disturbances are common.

Bupropion is available only on prescription. It is not recommended for young people under 18 years old, and it should be avoided in pregnant or breastfeeding women and in patients with a history of fits, with alcohol and other drug misuse problems or with cerebral trauma. Three per cent of those prescribed develop mild reactions (e.g. rash, urticaria or pruritus) and 0.1% develop hypersensitivity reactions.

Smokers of 10 or more cigarettes a day should normally be encouraged to use nicotine replacement therapy; combinations of nicotine replacement preparations are more effective than a single type. The agreement of the patient's physician should be obtained before nicotine replacement therapy is given to patients who have associated serious medical conditions.

Illicit drugs

Opiates

A range of medications are available for detoxification, stabilisation and reduction (see chapter 1). These includes methadone, buprenorphine, clonidine, lofexidine, naltrexone, as well as combinations (e.g. lofexidine and naltrexone). Naloxone is, of course, prescribed as an antidote to opioid overdose, but since it is short-acting, regular monitoring and supervision of the patient's state of consciousness and withdrawal are necessary. Although heroin can be prescribed by licensed practitioners in the UK, this is still an area of controversy which needs to be resolved by RCTs.

A definite diagnosis of dependence is invariably required before substitute medication is initiated. This should take into account clinical examination, history, with corroborating evidence, and results of investigations. In young people, it is extremely important that specialist assessment be organised at the earliest possible stage.

If substitute drugs are prescribed, the consensus is that they should be available on a 'daily pick-up' basis, at least at the start, supervised by the pharmacist or, failing that, by a reliable carer or parent (in the case of those under 18 years old). At present, pharmacists appear more willing to supervise methadone than buprenorphine therapy.

Stimulants and cannabis (see chapter 3)

Since substitute medication is not available for cocaine and cannabis, and not commonly used for amphetamines, the administration of general treatment measures is advised. In stimulant withdrawal, patients may become drowsy and depressed, and even suicidal. Regular monitoring of mental state and physical examination are therefore very important. Urine screening should be frequently and randomly carried out. Cannabis withdrawal may result in insomnia, and hypnotic sedatives should be prescribed cautiously.

Special groups

Young people

Apart from buprenorphine and, in some instances, nicotine replacement therapy (if recommended by a physician), no drug in the management of alcohol, nicotine or opiate dependence is licensed for use in those under 18 years old. Thus, as mentioned earlier, specialist assessment is essential.

Pregnant women

In pregnancy, alcohol consumption usually decreases as a matter of course. The first RCT of comprehensive assessment and brief interventions demonstrated reductions in both groups (assessment alone and assessment with intervention), but prior abstinence in addition to a brief intervention had the better outcome (Chang et al, 1999). Randomised controlled trials for nicotine replacement therapy in pregnancy are required. Guidance from the National Institute for Health and Clinical Excellence has stated that nicotine replacement therapy can be prescribed for pregnant or breastfeeding mothers with caution (National Institute for Clinical Excellence, 2002). Methadone treatment as part of a prenatal package for opiate-dependent women has been shown to improve birth outcomes and maternal psychosocial function. A neonatal withdrawal syndrome may develop if methadone is used, whereas buprenorphine has been found to be safe and effective in mother, foetus and neonate (Fischer et al, 2000).

Prisoners

Great care must be taken when prescribing substitute medication for someone who has just been released from prison. It is likely that their drug use has been markedly reduced while in custody and therefore their tolerance may have decreased. In other words, a previously prescribed dose of medication may be too high and even fatal.

Treating the psychiatric disorder

The vast range of pharmacological treatments for psychiatric disorders has been collated by the World Health Organization (Andrews & Jenkins, 1999). Here, we consider just a few for specific disorders comorbid with substance misuse. However, given the prevalence of such comorbidity and the wide range of psychiatric conditions involved, few studies have investigated pharmacological treatments for dual diagnosis (Table 12.2).

Schizophrenia and schizoaffective disorder

Treatment with clozapine

There is good evidence to suggest that clozapine reduces substance misuse in people with schizophrenia. The response to clozapine of patients with treatment-resistant illness and a current or previous history of substance misuse is comparable with that of patients with treatment-resistant illness who do not misuse substances: both groups show reduced psychopathology and improved psychosocial functioning (Buckley et al, 1994; Zimmet et al, 2000). This response may result from an improved mental state or a direct anti-craving effect produced by the drug. The mesolimbic dopamine system is associated with motivational states and is implicated in the reinforcing actions of most drugs of misuse. Nicotine, alcohol and cocaine increase extracellular dopamine levels. Clozapine's greater affinity for D_1 and lesser affinity for D_2 receptors may modulate the activity of the receptors involved in craving.

Table 12.2 Selected studies on the pharmacological treatment of psychosis and substance misuse

Study	Substance	Medication
Buckley *et al*, 1994	Various	Clozapine
Conley *et al*, 1998	Various	Olanzapine
Levin *et al*, 1998	Cocaine	Flupentixol
Drake *et al*, 2000	Alcohol Cannabis	Clozapine
Zimmet *et al*, 2000	Various	Clozapine
Littrell *et al*, 2001	Various	Olanzapine
George & Vessicchio, 2002	Nicotine	Clozapine

Clozapine and nicotine dependence

Clozapine is particularly beneficial when the drug of comorbid dependence is nicotine. Eighty per cent of people with schizophrenia are smokers, and this contributes to the considerable increase in standardised mortality rate seen in schizophrenia. Nicotine produces a transient improvement in sensory gating and other neuropsychological deficits associated with schizophrenia (George & Vessicchio, 2002). Clozapine produces similar improvements, but the effects are sustained

Clozapine and alcohol dependence

In people with a diagnosis of either schizophrenia or schizoaffective disorder and comorbid alcohol misuse, clozapine has been shown to decrease severity of alcohol use and number of drinking days and increase remission of alcohol-use disorders (Drake *et al*, 2000). This reduction was strongly correlated with a decrease in symptoms of anergia, but not with reduced positive symptoms of schizophrenia. Another study demonstrated that clozapine treatment was associated with a reduction in alcohol use in 83% of patients with comorbid alcohol misuse and schizophrenia (Zimmet *et al*, 2000). None of the group increased their alcohol consumption while on clozapine. There was a correlation between decreased alcohol use and a reduction in global clinical symptoms.

Clozapine and cannabis misuse

Drake *et al* (2000) also examined clozapine in comorbid cannabis use. The findings were less consistent than those with alcohol, but a reduction in use was demonstrated.

Treatment with other antipsychotics

Clozapine treatment has disadvantages in terms of adverse effects and the need for regular full blood count monitoring. There is less evidence for the use of olanzapine in dual diagnosis (Conley *et al*, 1998), although Littrell *et al* (2001) demonstrated that olanzapine improved both psychosis and substance misuse. A small pilot study examined the effects of flupentixol treatment in schizophrenia complicated by cocaine misuse (Levin *et al*, 1998). It reported a reduction in both positive and negative symptoms and a decrease in cocaine use in the majority of participants. Flupentixol may be the typical antipsychotic of choice if treatment with an atypical is not possible.

Mood disorders

In substance misuse, depressive and anxiety symptoms (as well as many psychological symptoms) are often transient and related to the effects of the substances misused, to withdrawal from them or to psychosocial stress associated with the individual's lifestyle. Detoxification often leads to an improvement in mood, as does maintenance therapy in opiate dependence. It is therefore preferable to delay diagnosis of clinical depression until the patient has had a period of abstinence, when it should also be easier to distinguish clinical depression from feelings of misery and unhappiness. Such a delay should be possible in most cases, although if patients report suicidal ideation a judgement may be needed regarding initiation of antidepressant medication before abstinence has been achieved.

Depression and alcohol dependence (see chapter 14)

Thirty per cent of those dependent on alcohol fulfil the criteria for a major depressive disorder, and 80% experience some depressive symptoms. Comorbidity has been shown to increase the risk of suicide. Schuckit *et al* (1994) demonstrated that few patients presenting with alcohol and depression have a major depressive disorder. It is generally believed that depressive symptoms should not be treated for 2–4 weeks following detoxification from alcohol. It is important to recognise that depressive symptoms increase the risk of relapse, either as a cue to drinking or by causing patients to disengage with relapse-prevention treatment. Studies investigating the benefits of prescribing antidepressants to this population have relatively short follow-up times, given that uncomplicated depression should be treated with medication for at least 6 months to reduce relapse.

Most of the available studies (some of which are listed in Table 12.3) are not standardised for dependent or harmful drinking, or for primary or secondary depression. There are no studies comparing the efficacy of tricyclics with selective serotonin reuptake inhibitors (SSRIs), or comparing differing doses of an individual medication. In a population at high risk of suicide, SSRIs have advantages over tricyclics in terms of safety profile.

Table 12.3 Selected studies on the pharmacological treatment of mood and anxiety disorders comorbid with substance misuse

Study	Disorder	Substance misused	Treatment/medication
Kranzler et al, 1995	Depression	Alcohol	SSRI
McGrath et al, 1996	Depression	Alcohol	Imipramine
Mason et al, 1996	Depression	Alcohol	Desipramine (withdrawn in the UK)
Cornelius et al, 2000	Depression and alcoholism	Marijuana	SSRI (fluoxetine)
Petrakis et al, 1994	Depression	Opiates	SSRI
Hamilton et al, 1998	Depression, methadone maintenance	Opiates	Nefazodone (withdrawn in the UK)
Nunes et al, 1998	Depression	Opiates	Imipramine
Schmitz et al, 2001	Major depressive disorder	Cocaine	Fluoxetine
Malec et al, 1996	Anxiety	Alcohol	Buspirone
Charney et al, 2000	Anxiety	Benzodiazepines	Reduction regime
Hertzman, 2000	Bipolar disorder	Alcohol	Valproate
Brown et al, 2002	Bipolar disorder	Cocaine	Quetiapine

Tricyclic antidepressants in alcohol misuse

Desipramine and imipramine have both been shown to be effective medications for depression comorbid with alcohol misuse. A double-blind, placebo-controlled trial of desipramine was carried out by Mason *et al* (1996) in alcohol-dependent patients who had been abstinent for at least a week. Both depressed and non-depressed individuals were recruited to see whether desipramine had an effect on relapse rate, irrespective of its antidepressant properties. Desipramine showed significant benefits over placebo in relapse rate (8.3% *v.* 40%) and also in time to relapse. However, desipramine is no longer licensed in the UK.

A randomised placebo controlled trial of imipramine followed patients with depression who were drinking excessively but who did not necessarily have a history of dependence (McGrath *et al*, 1996). Participants were required to have had depression prior to the alcohol misuse or during at least 6 months of sobriety. Treatment lasted 12 weeks, with maximum doses of 300 mg of imipramine. Depression improved in the imipramine-treated group, but there was no significant decrease in either drinking days or alcohol consumed per drinking day. There was no adverse interaction between imipramine and alcohol, but 13% of those treated with imipramine withdrew from the trial because of adverse side-effects.

SSRIs in alcohol misuse

Selective serotonin reuptake inhibitors (SSRIs) both decrease depressive symptoms and reduce alcohol consumption in people comorbid for depression and alcohol misuse.

A 1-year randomised, double-blind, placebo-controlled trial of fluoxetine in people with comorbid depression and alcohol dependence demonstrated the superiority of fluoxetine (Cornelius *et al*, 2000). The paper does not state the dose of fluoxetine prescribed, but no significant adverse effects were reported. The number of days of drinking to intoxication was reduced significantly. Total drinking days were also reduced by treatment with fluoxetine, but not statistically significantly so. None of the participants in either group was entirely abstinent. There was no improvement between 3- and 12-month outcomes. These findings suggest that continuing antidepressant medication for 12 months should be recommended in this group.

Kranzler *et al* (1995), however, report that fluoxetine in doses of up to 60 mg used for relapse prevention in the absence of depression was not effective in reducing drinking.

Bipolar affective disorder and substance misuse

The most common substance of misuse in bipolar disorder is alcohol. There is some evidence that treatment with sodium valproate is beneficial. Anticonvulsants may reduce membrane instability in the presence of substance misuse. A retrospective study of valproate used to treat bipolar disorder in people with concomitant substance misuse demonstrated that 50% reduced their substance misuse (Hertzman, 2000). A study by Brown *et al* (2002) reported improvement in cocaine users with bipolar disorder: see 'Cocaine and depression' below.

Depression and opiate dependence

The prescription of antidepressants should be undertaken very cautiously, and monitored regularly, particularly in light of recent findings on deaths due to antidepressants. Deaths involving antidepressants in combination with other drugs are significantly more likely to be those of drug misusers (Cheeta *et al*, 2004). Prescription should be undertaken within the context of a risk assessment that includes the potential for self-harm, suicidal ideation, intention or behaviour, risk of harm to others, and self-neglect. Predictors of risk behaviour include a previous history of harm to self or others, hopelessness, agitation, command hallucinations, social isolation, recent losses and recurrent psychiatric hospitalisation (Evans & Sullivan, 2000). A mental health or drug problem that impairs judgement may further heighten risk.

Tricyclic antidepressants

Imipramine has been shown to be effective in reducing depressive symptoms in a placebo-controlled study of opiate-dependent patients receiving methadone maintenance (Nunes *et al*, 1998). The participants had depression that either preceded the onset of regular substance misuse or had lasted at least 3 months after the start of misuse. Maximum doses of 300 mg imipramine were used (mean of 268 mg). It should be noted that methadone increases serum levels of tricyclics. Participants were followed for 12 weeks. Abstinence was achieved in 14% of the imipramine group and 2% of the placebo group. There was an association between improvement in depressive symptoms and reduced substance misuse, but causality could not be inferred. The substance misuse improved before the depression in more than half of responders, suggesting that mood is only one of several factors driving substance use.

SSRIs
Petrakis *et al* (1994) conducted a small pilot study to examine the effects of prescribing fluoxetine to opiate-dependent individuals in a methadone maintenance programme who had either comorbid depression or persistent cocaine use. The mean dose of fluoxetine was 47 mg, and the follow-up period was 12 weeks. Frequency of self-reported drug use decreased significantly, and depressive symptoms decreased but not significantly. Participants reported anecdotally that fluoxetine reduced their subjective craving for cocaine. There have also been case studies describing success with nefazodone in treating depression in opiate-dependent individuals on methadone maintenance (Hamilton *et al*, 1998). Nefazodone has recently been withdrawn in the UK.

Cocaine and depression
Several studies have investigated the treatment of comorbid cocaine addiction and depression (Schmitz *et al*, 2001; Brown *et al*, 2002). Fluoxetine and quetiapine were administered, respectively. Fluoxetine failed to produce a response, but the findings were 'promising' for quetiapine in that psychiatric symptoms and cocaine craving improved.

Anxiety disorders

The relationship between alcohol use and anxiety disorders is not necessarily causal but may be a reflection of neurophysiological factors that give rise to both disorders (Lingford-Hughes *et al*, 2002) (see chapter 15). Neurotransmitter and receptor function in the gamma-aminobutyric acid (GABA), serotonin and noradrenaline systems are altered in both. Thus, as with associated depressive symptoms, a period of abstinence following withdrawal or intoxication should elapse, if feasible, before a diagnosis of anxiety is made.

Some of the key studies addressing anxiety disorders comorbid with substance misuse are listed in Table 12.3.

Comorbid alcohol dependence and anxiety

Anxiety is a common symptom of alcohol withdrawal, and many patients presenting for detoxification give a history of agoraphobia or panic disorder.

Even with the most thorough history, it is often difficult to distinguish between the disorders. Anxiety disorders cannot be successfully treated while a patient is drinking heavily and so detoxification should be the first stage of treatment, followed by reassessment of the anxiety symptoms. Psychological treatment in the form of anxiety management groups is part of the treatment offered by in-patient detoxification units and community alcohol teams.

In terms of medication, there is some evidence for the effectiveness of buspirone in this group. Malec *et al* (1996) reviewed five studies, which showed that the main effects of buspirone were an improvement in anxiety symptoms and greater retention in treatment. There was no consistent reduction in alcohol consumption, however.

Comorbid benzodiazepine dependence and anxiety

Benzodiazepines are used as hypnotics, sedatives or anxiolytics. It is important to recognise that they can produce a withdrawal syndrome even if low doses have been prescribed (or misused). If taken in combination with other drugs and alcohol, overdose can result (Hawton *et al*, 1998). Alternatives such as buspirone, zolpidem and zopiclone do not appear to lead to dependence.

There is little evidence concerning the pharmacological treatment of comorbid benzodiazepine dependence and anxiety. Charney *et al* (2000) examined the treatment of benzodiazepine dependence to evaluate predictors of successful outcome. Although their study did not target a comorbid population, 62% of the study population had a lifetime diagnosis of an anxiety disorder and 68% of these had been prescribed benzodiazepines to treat this disorder. It seemed that after chronic use patients no longer experienced any anxiolytic effect. Treatment consisted of out-patient detoxification with reducing doses of diazepam over a maximum of 10 weeks, followed by group and individual work. After 6 months of follow-up they reported a decrease in anxiety symptoms, despite having considerably reduced their benzodiazepine use. Fifty per cent of the participants had maintained abstinence. In terms of predictors of outcome, anxiety did not impede successful treatment.

Monitoring interventions

It is worth pointing out that some psychiatric patients with comorbid substance misuse achieve stabilisation rapidly. Furthermore, severe mental illness does not necessarily predict worse outcome. However, early unplanned discharge from treatment is common in this patient population. Monitoring and adherence, helped by motivational techniques, are vital components of ensuring the value of pharmacological interventions (Hunt *et al*, 2002).

Socio-economic and emotional aspects are the main challenges to recovery, and case management in the context of integrated community and residential services with assertive outreach has been shown to be increasingly successful at improving medication adherence. A newer approach is 'sensitive anticipatory action' (Tyrer & Weaver, 2004). This focuses on medication review as one component of relapse prevention, and on social care planning, which encompasses help with accommodation as well as forward planning to avoid crises.

The appropriateness of a model of service delivery depends on local arrangements. For this reason, the health, social care, housing, criminal justice and voluntary sector agencies of each local area need to reach an operational definition of the patient group and to identify service roles and capacity (see chapter 13).

Outstanding critical issues

There are few controlled studies for such a common and complex area as dual diagnosis. In those that have been published, the robustness of diagnosis varies and some report a reduction in psychiatric symptoms although there was no ICD or DSM diagnosis of psychiatric disorder. Furthermore, in general, primary outcome measures are usually related to the psychiatric disorder and secondary outcomes to the substance of misuse. Some studies do look at the effect of a particular medication on, for example, both mood and drug misuse and attempt to relate these, rather than make drug use secondary. There is also the need to identify whether the primary objective of the pharmacotherapy is to treat the mental health issue or to alleviate the substance misuse problem (e.g. SSRIs to counter the serotonergic dysfunction of alcohol dependence). Furthermore, some studies have evaluated efficacy once patients were drug-free, whereas others were concerned about safety issues, e.g. side-effects of antipsychotics.

Sample selection, small sample sizes, lack of control groups, lack of masking, different outcome measures, reliability of self-report, length of follow-up, and concomitant psychosocial or pharmacological treatments further complicate the extent to which findings are practically useful. In summary, since the number of standardised studies is limited, it is difficult to draw conclusions or to make recommendations.

Conclusion

This is undoubtedly a complicated area, where adequate robust research evidence is just beginning to emerge. An array of pharmacological interventions is available for the treatment of individual substance use disorders. However, these agents have usually been evaluated in patients without comorbid psychiatric disorders. Similarly, although there are a growing number of antipsychotics, antidepressants and anti-anxiety agents, surprisingly few have been tested on comorbid conditions.

It would appear, on the basis of the limited evidence, that clozapine and possibly olanzapine are useful for psychotic disorders complicated by substance misuse. Although imipramine, fluoxetine, doxepin and venlafaxine have been reported to be effective in depressive disorders complicated by different substances of misuse or dependence, it must be stressed that many of the findings of studies are inconsistent. Similarly, results on the effects of buspirone for anxiety and alcohol disorders are mixed.

Decisions need to be made on the basis of a thorough assessment (including risk assessment) of the nature and extent of the mental illness and the substance misuse, the psychosocial environment in which the patient is functioning, as well as of the local multi-specialist and multi-agency arrangements in place for the delivery of care. People with a dual diagnosis form a heterogeneous group of often complex individuals with negative experiences of the treatment system, and they are consequently at high risk of significant morbidity and mortality. Practitioners need to be especially vigilant with regard to safety. Keeping a close clinical eye on medication is critical, because the research evidence on risk/benefit and cost-effectiveness is not yet forthcoming.

References

*Abdulrahim, D., Annan, J., Cyster, R., et al (2001) Developing an Integrated Model of Care for Drug Treatment: Promoting Quality, Efficiency and Effectiveness in Drug Misuse Treatment Services. National Treatment Agency.

Andrews, G. & Jenkins, R. (eds) (1999) Management of Mental Disorders (vols 1 & 2). World Health Organization Collaborating Centres in Mental Health.

*Banerjee, S., Clancy, C. & Crome, I. B. (eds) (2002) Co-existing Problems of Mental Disorder and Substance Misuse (Dual Diagnosis): An Information Manual (2nd edn). College Research Unit and Royal College of Psychiatrists.

Besson, J., Aeby, F., Kasas, A., et al (1998) Combined efficacy of acamprosate and disulfiram in the treatment of alcoholism: a controlled study. Alcoholism: Clinical and Experimental Research, 22, 573–579.

Best, D., Rawaf, S., Rowley, J., et al (2000) Drinking and smoking as concurrent predictors of illicit drug use and positive drug attitudes in adolescents. Drug and Alcohol Dependence, 60, 319–321.

Brown, E. S., Nejtek, V. A., Perantie, D. C., et al (2002) Quetiapine in bipolar disorder and cocaine dependence. Bipolar Disorders, 4, 406–411.

Buckley, P., Thompson, P. A., Way, L., et al (1994) Substance abuse and clozapine treatment. Journal of Clinical Psychiatry, 55 (suppl. B), 114–116.

Cabinet Office, Prime Minister's Strategy Unit (2004) Alcohol Harm Reduction Strategy for England. Cabinet Office.

Chang, G., Wilkins-Hang, L., Berman, S. A., et al (1999) Brief interventions for alcohol use in pregnancy. A randomised trial. Addiction, 94, 1499–1508.

Charney, D. A., Paraherakis, A. M. & Gill, K. J. (2000) The treatment of sedative–hypnotic dependence: evaluating clinical predictors of outcome. Journal of Clinical Psychiatry, 61, 190–195.

Cheeta, S., Schifano, F., Oyefeso, A., et al (2004) Antidepressant-related deaths and anti-depressant prescriptions in England and Wales, 1998–2000. British Journal of Psychiatry, 184, 41–47.

Conley, R. R., Kelly, D. L. & Gale, E. A. (1998) Olanzapine in treatment refractory schizophrenic patients with a history of substance misuse. Schizophrenia Research, 33, 95–101.

Cook, C. C. H. & Thomson, A. D. (1997) B-complex vitamins in the prophylaxis and treatment of Wernicke–Korsakoff syndrome. British Journal of Hospital Medicine, 57, 461–465.

Cornelius, J. R., Salloum, I. M., Haskett, R. F., et al (2000) Fluoxetine versus placebo in depressed alcoholics: a one-year follow-up study. *Addictive Behaviour*, 25, 307–310.

Coulthard, M., Farrell, M., Singleton, N., et al (2002) *Tobacco, Alcohol and Drug Use and Mental Health*. TSO (The Stationery Office).

*Crawford, V., Clancy, C. & Crome, I. B. (2003) Co-existing problems of mental health and substance misuse (dual diagnosis): a literature review. *Drugs: Education, Prevention and Policy*, 10 (suppl.), S1–S74.

Department of Health (1998) *Smoking Kills: A White Paper on Tobacco*. TSO (The Stationery Office).

Department of Health (2002) *Mental Health Policy Implementation Guide: Dual Diagnosis Good Practice Guide*. Department of Health.

Drake, R. E., Xie, H., McHugo, G. J., et al (2000) The effects of clozapine on alcohol and drug use disorders among patients with schizophrenia. *Schizophrenia Bulletin*, 26, 441–449.

Edwards, G. (ed.) (2002) *Addiction: Evolution of a Specialist Field*. Blackwell Publishing.

Evans, K. & Sullivan, J. M. (2000) *Dual Diagnosis: Counseling the Mentally Ill Substance Abuser*. Guilford Press.

Fischer, G., Johnson, R. E., Eder, H., et al (2000) Treatment of opioid-dependent pregnant women with buprenorphine. *Addiction*, 95, 239–244.

Frisher, M., Collins, J., Millson, D., et al (2004) Prevalence of comorbid psychiatric illness and substance misuse in primary care in England and Wales. *Journal of Epidemiology and Community Health*, 58, 1036–1041.

Geerlings, P., Ansoms, C. & van den Brink, W. (1997) Acamprosate and prevention of relapse in alcoholics. Results of a randomised, placebo-controlled, double-blind study in out-patient alcoholics in the Netherlands, Belgium and Luxembourg. *European Addiction Research*, 3, 129–137.

George, T. P. & Vessicchio J. C. (2002) Treating tobacco addiction in schizophrenia: where do we go from here? *Addiction*, 97, 795–796.

Gfroerer, J., Penne, M., Pemberton, M., et al (2003) Substance abuse treatment need among older adults in 2020: the impact of the aging baby-boom cohort. *Drug and Alcohol Dependence*, 69, 127–135.

Granholm, E., Anthenelli, R., Monteiro, R., et al (2003) Brief integrated outpatient dual-diagnosis treatment reduces psychiatric hospitalizations. *American Journal on Addictions*, 12, 306–313.

Hamilton, S. P., Klimchak, C. & Nunes, E. V. (1998) Treatment of depressed methadone maintenance patients with nefazodone. *American Journal on Addictions*, 7, 309–312.

Hawton, K., Arensman, E., Townsend, E., et al (1998) Deliberate self-harm: systematic review of efficacy of psychosocial and pharmacological treatments in preventing repetition. *BMJ*, 317, 441–447.

Hertzman, M. (2000) Divalproex sodium used to treat concomitant substance abuse and mood disorders. *Journal of Substance Abuse Treatment*, 18, 371–372.

Hunt, G. E., Bergen, J., & Bashir, M. (2002) Medication compliance and comorbid substance abuse in schizophrenia: impact on community survival 4 years after a relapse. *Schizophrenia Research*, 54, 253–264.

Kiefer, F., Jahn, H., Tarnaske, T., et al (2003) Comparing and combining naltrexone and acamprosate in relapse prevention of alcoholism. *Archives of General Psychiatry*, 60, 92–99.

Kranzler, H. R., Burleson, J. A., Korner, P., et al (1995) Placebo-controlled trial of fluoxetine as an adjunction to relapse prevention in alcoholics. *American Journal of Psychiatry*, 152, 391–397.

Levin, F. R., Evans, S. M., Coomaraswammy, S., et al (1998) Flupenthixol treatment for cocaine abusers with schizophrenia: a pilot study. *American Journal of Drug and Alcohol Abuse*, 24, 343–360.

Lingford-Hughes, A., Potokar, J. & Nutt, D. (2002) Treating anxiety complicated by substance misuse. *Advances in Psychiatric Treatment*, 8, 107–116.

Lingford-Hughes, A., Welch, S. & Nutt, D. J. (2004) Evidence-based guidelines for the pharmacological management of substance misuse, addiction and comorbidity.

Recommendations from the British Association for Psychopharmacology. *Journal of Psychopharmacology*, **18**, 293–335.

Littrell, K. H., Petty, R. G., Hilligross, N. M., *et al* (2001) Olanzapine treatment for patients with schizophrenia and substance abuse. *Journal of Substance Abuse Treatment*, **21**, 217–221.

Malec, T. S., Malec, E. A. & Dongier, M. (1996) Efficacy of buspirone in alcohol dependence: a review. *Alcoholism: Clinical and Experimental Research*, **20**, 853–858.

Mason, B. J., Kocsis, J. H., Ritvo, E. C., *et al* (1996) A double-blind, placebo-controlled trial of desipramine for primary alcohol dependence stratified on the presence or absence of major depression. *JAMA*, **275**, 761–767.

McGrath, P. J., Nunes, E. V., Stewart, J. W., *et al* (1996) Imipramine treatment of alcoholics with primary depression. *Archives of General Psychiatry*, **53**, 232–240.

Murray, R. M. (1980) Why are the drug companies so disinterested in alcoholism? *British Journal of Addiction*, **75**, 113–115.

National Institute for Clinical Excellence (2002) *Guidance on the Use of Nicotine Replacement Therapy (NRT) and Bupropion for Smoking Cessation. Technology Appraisal Guidance no. 39.* NICE.

Nunes, E. V., Quitkin, F. M., Donovan, S. J., *et al* (1998) Imipramine treatment of opiate-dependent patients with depressive disorders. A placebo-controlled trial. *Archives of General Psychiatry*, **55**, 153–160.

Petrakis, I., Carroll, K., Gordon, L., *et al* (1994) Fluoxetine treatment for dually diagnosed methadone maintained opioid addicts: a pilot study. *Journal of Addictive Diseases*, **13**, 25–32.

Regier, D. A., Farmer, M. E., Rae, D. S., *et al* (1990) Comorbidity of mental disorders with alcohol and other drug misuse: results from the Epidemiologic Catchment Area Study. *JAMA*, **264**, 2511–2518.

Schmitz, J. M., Averill, P., Stotts, A., *et al* (2001) Fluoxetine treatment of cocaine-dependent patients with major depressive disorder. *Drug and Alcohol Dependence*, **63**, 207–214.

Schuckit, M., Irwin, M. & Smith, T. L. (1994) One-year incidence rate of major depression and other psychiatric disorders in 239 alcoholic men. *Addiction*, **89**, 441–445.

Scottish Executive (2003) *Mind the Gaps: Meeting the Needs of People with Co-occurring Substance Misuse and Mental Health Problems.* Scottish Executive.

*Slattery, J., Chick, J., Cochrane, M., *et al* (2003) *Prevention of Relapse in Alcohol Dependence. Health Technology Assessment Report No. 3.* Health Technology Board for Scotland.

Stockwell, T., Hodgson, R., Edwards, G., *et al* (1979) The development of a questionnaire to measure severity of alcohol dependence. *British Journal of Addiction to Alcohol and Other Drugs*, **74**, 79–87.

Sullivan, J. T., Skykora, K. & Schneiderman, J. (1989) Assessment of alcohol withdrawal: the revised Clinical Institute Withdrawal Assessment for Alcohol Scale (CIWA–Ar). *British Journal of Addiction*, **84**, 1353–1357.

Tyrer, P. & Weaver, T. (2004) Desperately seeking solutions: the search for appropriate treatment for comorbid substance misuse and psychosis. *Psychiatric Bulletin*, **28**, 1–2.

Zimmet, S. V., Strous, R. D. & Burgess, E. S. (2000) Effects of clozapine on substance use in patients with schizophrenia and schizoaffective disorder. *Journal of Clinical Psychopharmacology*, **20**, 94–98.

*Key reviews.

CHAPTER 13

Dual diagnosis: management within a psychosocial context

Mohammed T. Abou-Saleh

Summary Recent developments in UK government policy have highlighted the unmet needs of people with dual diagnosis (comorbidity of substance misuse and psychiatric disorder, particularly severe mental illness). Advances in assessment techniques and diagnostic practice have informed the treatment of comorbidity and improved its outcome. There is growing evidence for the effectiveness of psychosocial interventions such as motivational interviewing and cognitive-behavioural therapy, mostly from US studies. However, within the secondary care provided by addiction and general psychiatric services there are serious implementation barriers related to service organisation, staffing levels, training and – most importantly – the difficulties of engaging people with severe mental illness and comorbid substance misuse in treatment. The evidence for the effectiveness of psychosocial treatments and models of service is reviewed and challenges for optimal practice in the UK are highlighted.

The co-occurrence of substance misuse with other psychiatric disorders is increasingly recognised as a major public health problem. The term 'dual diagnosis' has been introduced to describe this phenomenon, but 'comorbidity' might be a better term. Community-based surveys in the USA and the UK have reported high rates of comorbidity, particularly in people with serious mental illness (Harrison & Abou-Saleh, 2002). Farrell *et al* (2001), in a national household survey, reported prevalence rates of psychiatric disorder of 22% in nicotine dependence, 30% in alcohol dependence and 45% in drug dependence, compared with 12% prevalence in the non-dependent population.

The pattern of this comorbidity varies between comorbid mood, anxiety and personality disorders in patients accessing addiction services, and comorbid alcohol, cannabis and cocaine misuse in patients accessing general psychiatric services (Abou-Saleh, 2000). Comorbidity is associated with increased risk of violence, suicide and worse clinical and social outcomes. The National Confidential Inquiry into Suicide and Homicide has reported substance misuse as a factor in over half of homicides and suicides by people with serious mental illness (Department of Health,

169

2001). Moreover, people with comorbidity have high rates of criminality and blood-borne infections, including HIV infection and hepatitis B and C.

The severity of this morbidity also varies between these specialist settings: severe psychiatric disorder is associated with non-dependent use of substances (problematic substance misuse), whereas severe addiction is associated with personality disorder with or without minor psychiatric disorder. The pattern and severity of this comorbidity are therefore related to the clinical setting in which it presents, which may not be representative of comorbidity occurring in the community.

My aim in this chapter is to describe the policy context, define dual diagnosis, identify meaningful subgroups and describe key aspects of their assessment and treatment, with emphasis on psychosocial approaches in the context of integrated service models.

Policy context

The National Service Framework (NSF) for Mental Health (Department of Health, 1999), while emphasising the importance of tackling dual diagnosis, failed to include standards and service models to address the challenges posed by patients with dual diagnosis, including those with severe mental illness. It was in the context of this gap in policy that the *Dual Diagnosis Good Practice Guide* (Department of Health, 2002a) was launched. The NSF also omitted to provide standards and service models for people with substance use disorders, an omission that was addressed by the complementary guidance on models of care launched by the National Treatment Agency for Substance Misuse (2002).

The key message in the *Dual Diagnosis Good Practice Guide* is that substance misuse is usual rather than exceptional among people with severe mental health problems, and that the relationship between the two disorders is complex. Individuals with dual diagnosis have varied and complex needs and require high-quality, comprehensive and integrated care that should be delivered within the mainstream mental health services. The guide recognises that mainstreaming will not reduce the role of drug and alcohol services, which will continue to treat the majority of people with substance misuse problems and to advise on substance misuse issues. The guide summarises good practice in relation to treatment and sets out a programme for local implementation of the appropriate service model. It is concluded that integrated care by a single team delivers better outcomes than serial care (sequential referrals to different services) or parallel care (more than one service engaging with a patient at the same time). The guide recommends that more UK-based research be conducted to establish the evidence base, and that well-organised parallel care can be used as a stepping stone to integrated treatment delivered by existing mental health services following training and support from substance misuse services.

It should be noted that the *Dual Diagnosis Good Practice Guide* was launched at the same time and place as two other guidelines: *Adult Acute Inpatient Care Provision Guidance* (Department of Health, 2002b) and *National Minimum Standards for Psychiatric Intensive Care Units and Low Secure Environments* (Department of Health, 2002c). Neither of these other publications emphasises the importance of dual diagnosis. The intensive care guidance specifies substance misuse as an exclusion criterion on two counts, and falls into the trap of emphasising the primacy of one diagnosis over another in the acute situation, potentially perpetuating the passing of patients with complex disorders from 'pillar to post' – the title of a video produced by the mental health charity Mind in Croydon (2004) – because of the recognised diagnostic uncertainty and tautology. It is simplistic to adopt a dualist approach to behaviour where the relationship between the two conditions is properly comorbid, with shared aetiological factors.

Models of Care

The National Treatment Agency document *Models of Care* provides a treatment framework and process intended to support the move towards consensus about the essential components of specialist substance misuse services and the importance of links with other health, social care and criminal justice agencies (National Treatment Agency, 2002, 2006). The guidance structures substance misuse services into broad tiers, from non-specialist services, including general psychiatric services, to specialist community and residential services specifically for substance misusers and highly specialised services unrelated to substance misuse, such as forensic psychiatric services and specialist personality disorder services (see chapter 2). The guidance also stipulates the development of integrated care pathways as the preferred method of applying packages of care in a coordinated and integrated way. The integrated care pathways provide a means of agreeing local referral and treatment protocols to define where and when a particular service user needs to be referred.

Treatment of personality disorder

The national guidance *Personality Disorder: No Longer a Diagnosis of Exclusion* (Department of Health, 2003) has highlighted the inadequate provision for people with personality disorders. This is related to the reluctance of clinicians to treat these people because they do not have the skills, the training or the resources. A survey of NHS trusts in England found that only 17% provide dedicated services for patients with personality disorders and 28% provide no identified service. The guidance aims to increase specialist provision for patients with personality disorders within mainstream and specialist psychiatric services, including forensic and addiction psychiatry, and to introduce the necessary education and training of mental health practitioners in these services. In view of the common occurrence of alcohol and drug misuse in patients with personality disorders, referral pathways and protocols need to be agreed between general, forensic and addiction services for the provision of treatment, training and support.

Defining dual diagnosis (see chapter 12)

Currently recognised subgroups of patients with dual diagnosis are defined by presumed aetiological mechanisms: primary psychiatric disorder with secondary substance misuse, substance misuse with secondary psychiatric disorder, and psychiatric symptoms related to substance intoxication or withdrawal. These categories are consistent with the operationally defined corresponding categories in DSM–IV (American Psychiatric Association, 1994), in which a distinction is made between independent (primary psychiatric comorbidity) and substance-induced (organic) psychiatric comorbidity and the category of expected symptoms of substance use or withdrawal. The evidence base for these subgroups has identified two key aetiological factors for dual diagnosis: the presence of underlying antisocial personality disorder and the vulnerability of people with severe mental illness to non-dependent problematic substance misuse (the supersensitivity model; Mueser *et al*, 1998). The self-medication hypothesis has not been sustained despite its plausibility and popularity with users and clinicians alike. In the case of schizophrenia, it has been suggested that the emergence of comorbid substance misuse is integral to the disorder and is related to the disconnection in the neural networks that occurs in the schizophrenia disease process (Chambers *et al*, 2001). An important piece of the jigsaw that is often missing is the underlying personality disorder, offering a triple diagnosis. This absence is related to the difficulties of reliably diagnosing personality disorder in the context of comorbidity. An inclusive and pragmatic approach would offer the typology of:

- severe psychiatric disorder with problematic substance misuse, with or without an underlying personality disorder
- substance-induced psychiatric disorder
- substance dependence with personality disorder, without comorbid psychiatric disorder.

Assessment

As comorbidity is the rule rather than the exception, it is crucial that all patients are routinely screened to detect substance misuse in those presenting to general psychiatric services and to detect psychiatric problems in those presenting to addiction services. Detection is based on self-report, informant report and laboratory tests. Hair analysis carries a major advantage over urine testing in that it covers much longer periods than a single urine test (McPhillips *et al*, 1997) (see chapter 11). Those with comorbidity are

---

Box 13.1 Essential assessments for patients with dual diagnosis (comorbidity)

- A detailed assessment of the substance misuse and its interaction with the psychiatric disorder
- A functional assessment of the impact of substance misuse on relationships, housing, work, leisure and personal goals
- Assessment of risks of self-harm, harm to others, self-neglect and blood-borne viral infections
- Assessment of motivation to change and preferences for treatment
- Treatment planning to address motivation to reduce or stop substance misuse, and pressing needs, including social needs, risk, and medical and psychiatric conditions

---

then provided with a specialised assessment (Noordsy et al, 2003), which should include the items listed in Box 13.1.

Diagnostic assessment of comorbidity using DSM–IV criteria (see above) optimally takes place following detoxification, to disentangle substance-induced disorders from primary comorbid psychiatric disorders and expected effects of substance intoxication/withdrawal. Psychiatric symptoms or disorders that persist after 4 weeks of substance withdrawal indicate primary comorbidity. Similar considerations apply for the optimal assessment of personality disorders (Axis I), particularly in the setting of Axis II comorbidity.

Screening tests

A number of screening instruments have been introduced to assess comorbidity (Box 13.2) (Crawford & Crome, 2001), including the following.

- The Psychiatric Research Interview for Substance and Mental Disorders (PRISM) is a diagnostic interview based on DSM–IV. It is reported to be more reliable than previous instruments for assessing psychiatric disorders in those who have comorbid substance use disorders (Hasin et al, 1996).
- The Dartmouth Assessment of Lifestyle Instrument (DALI; available at http://dms.dartmouth.edu/prc/instruments/DALI.pdf) is an 18-item interviewer-administered tool that takes on average 6 min to complete (Rosenberg et al, 1998). It was formed as a composite of the most validated questions from ten established screening questionnaires for substance use disorder. It can be used as a screening instrument for substance use disorder in the psychiatric population. It was developed primarily to detect alcohol, cannabis and cocaine use disorders.

Box 13.2   Assessment and screening tests

- A thorough and ongoing assessment, which includes a comprehensive history, should underpin comorbidity treatment
- When diagnostic issues are complex, the improved reliability of the PRISM is worth the extra effort
- The DALI may be useful for assessing alcohol, cannabis and cocaine use disorders in people with severe mental illness
- The CUAD is potentially useful for detecting substance use disorders in severely mentally ill patients
- The SATS can be used to evaluate treatment progress or as an outcome measure
- Neurocognitive impairment will affect the assessment process
- Biochemical screening increases rates of identification of substance use
- Hair analysis covers much longer periods than a single urine specimen

(Based on Crawford & Crome, 2001)

- The Alcohol Use Disorders Identification Test (AUDIT; Babor *et al*, 1992) is a brief self-report questionnaire developed by the World Health Organization to identify people whose alcohol consumption is hazardous or harmful to their health. The questions asked (about consumption and problems associated with dependence, regular use or intoxication) enable practitioners to identify areas that require attention.
- The Drug Abuse Screening Test (DAST–10) (Skinner, 1982) is a self-report questionnaire for measuring the severity of drug (not alcohol) dependence.
- The Mini-Mental State Examination (MMSE; Folstein *et al*, 1975) is a brief, quantitative measure of cognitive status in adults. It can be used to screen for cognitive impairment, to estimate its severity, to follow cognitive changes over time and to document response to treatment.
- The Chemical Use, Abuse and Dependence (CUAD) scale is a brief (20 min to administer), reliable and validated tool for the identification of substance use disorders in severely mentally ill in-patients (Appleby *et al*, 1996).
- The Substance Abuse Treatment Scale (SATS; McHugo *et al*, 1995) can be used to evaluate treatment progress or as an outcome measure. The scale is intended for assessing a person's stage of substance misuse treatment.

Treatment models

People with comorbidity often fall into the cracks between general psychiatric and specialist addiction services. Whereas the culture of addiction services is dedication to 'clients' who want to be helped, general psychiatric services are obliged to treat all patients, including reluctant ones detained under the Mental Health Act. The plight of these patients is compounded by the lack of community care facilities, including residential care, while day centres and rehabilitation facilities often do not admit them. Several models for treatment of comorbidity have evolved.

The serial treatment model involves management of the psychiatric disorder and substance misuse in separate settings and services; for example, patients are treated first in the general psychiatric service, and when recovered are referred to the specialist addiction service.

The parallel treatment model involves the concurrent treatment of substance misuse and psychiatric disorder by different staff and in different settings. Both serial and parallel treatment models have serious limitations for optimal treatment of both disorders, with high rates of patient drop-out.

The preferred model is integrated treatment, in which the same staff treat both disorders in the same setting. The limitation of this model, however, is that it may not provide the intensity of treatment for the substance misuse that is afforded to the psychiatric disorder. A review by Drake *et al* (1998*a*) of 36 studies of the effectiveness of integrated treatment for patients with dual diagnosis identified ten studies (six uncontrolled and four controlled) of comprehensive, integrated out-patient treatment programmes that were effective in engaging patients in services, reducing substance use and sustaining remission. Outcomes related to hospital use, psychiatric symptoms and other domains were less consistent. Several features of the programme appeared to be associated with effectiveness: assertive outreach, case management and a longitudinal, stage-wise, motivational approach to treatment of the substance misuse.

The integrated approach involves individually tailored treatments and differs from traditional substance misuse treatment in several respects:

- the focus is on preventing anxiety, rather than breaking through denial
- it emphasises trust, understanding and learning, rather than confrontation and criticism
- it emphases reducing harm from substance use, rather than abstinence
- it uses slow-paced and long-term management, rather than rapid withdrawal and short-term treatment
- it provides staged and motivational counselling, rather than confrontation
- it employs supportive clinicians readily available in familiar settings, rather than only during working hours and at clinics
- 12-step groups (such as Alcoholics Anonymous and Narcotics Anonymous: see chapter 1, Box 1.2) are available for those who choose and can benefit from them, rather than being required for all patients.

Box 13.3 Principles of treatment of substance misuse in people with severe mental illness (Drake *et al*, 1993)

- Assertive outreach to facilitate engagement
- Close monitoring to provide structure and social reinforcement
- Integrated concurrent service
- Comprehensive, wide range of interventions
- Stable living situation
- Flexibility and specialisation (modified approaches)
- Stages of treatment: engagement, persuasion, active treatment and relapse prevention
- Longitudinal perspective for relapsing and chronic disorder
- Optimism – instilling hope in patients and carers

Drake *et al* (1993), using an evidence-based approach, identified nine principles for the treatment of substance misuse in people with severe mental illness (Box 13.3).

A Cochrane systematic review (Ley *et al*, 1999) of treatment programmes for those with both severe mental illness and substance misuse identified six relevant studies. It found no clear evidence supporting an advantage over standard care of any type of programme, including integrated assertive community treatment and a residential treatment programme.

Treatment considerations

The treatment of comorbidity is fraught with difficulties related to diagnostic assumptions and to the setting in which the comorbidity is encountered. One consideration is a tendency for the comorbid condition to be considered as being of secondary importance and hence to be ignored or insufficiently treated. This is based on the assumption that the comorbid disorder is secondary to the primary disorder – be it substance misuse or other psychiatric disorder – and that treatment of the primary disorder may resolve the secondary disorder, which is not considered to require specific treatment. Also, there is general reluctance to treat psychiatric patients who misuse substances. Reasons for this are multiple, and include concern about possible toxic interaction between the prescribed medication and the substances that are misused; the assumption that active substance misuse will cause worsening of comorbid psychiatric symptoms and impair response to treatment; and the fear that 'enabling' the patient by treating the psychiatric illness would diminish the patient's motivation to deal with the substance misuse problem (Weiss & Najavits, 1998).

Although assessment of comorbidity is best done after the substance of misuse has been withdrawn, complete withdrawal is rarely obtained in an out-patient setting and treatment of the psychiatric disorder often begins while the patient is still misusing the substance. There is evidence that treatment of the psychiatric disorder during active substance misuse is effective and occasionally also has a positive impact on the substance misuse itself. Saxon & Calsyn (1995) showed that outcome at the end of 1 year of treatment in a substance misuse programme was as favourable for patients with a dual diagnosis as for those with substance misuse alone. Controlled trials of antidepressants in patients with depression who misuse alcohol have demonstrated efficacy in treatment of the depressive disorder and modest effect on the substance misuse. These findings counter the assumption that treatment of the comorbid psychiatric disorder in those actively engaged in substance misuse represents a form of 'enabling' (Cornelius *et al*, 1997) (see chapter 14).

Specific treatment approaches

Treatment is guided by a comprehensive assessment, and in integrated settings it involves a number of interventions matching patients' needs. Treatment is normally provided in the community with assertive outreach, but is also given in in-patient settings, particularly when the patient needs to be stabilised, to be assessed following detoxification or to achieve abstinence. Importantly, staff should hold a realistic and longitudinal view of treatment of substance misuse, with different interventions matched to different stages of the treatment process:

- engagement – regular contact and development of a therapeutic alliance, and meeting basic needs
- persuasion – motivational techniques to enhance motivation to change (reduce substance use)
- active treatment – from harm reduction to abstinence-oriented approaches
- relapse prevention – identification of high-risk situations for relapse and management of future relapses.

Noordsy *et al* (2003) have mapped various interventions at different stages of treatment (Table 13.1).

Drake & Mueser (2000) identified the following common components of integrated treatment.

- Case management – multidisciplinary case management with assertive outreach to engage and retain patients in community services.
- Close monitoring – medication supervision, urine drug screening and coercive approaches.
- Substance misuse treatment – motivational approaches; harm reduction and cognitive–behavioural therapy in individual, group and family settings; self-help (12-step programmes) and social skills training.

Table 13.1 Potential interventions at different stages of treatment

	Stage of treatment			
	Engagement	Persuasion	Active treatment	Relapse prevention
Case management	✓	✓	✓	✓
Family work	✓	✓	✓	✓
Pharmacological treatment	✓	✓	✓	✓
Assertive outreach	✓	✓	✓	
Coerced or involuntary interventions	✓	✓	✓	
Residential programmes		✓	✓	
Motivational interviewing		✓	✓	
Persuasion groups		✓	✓	
Cognitive–behavioural counselling		✓	✓	✓
Social skills training		✓	✓	✓
Vocational rehabilitation		✓	✓	✓
Active treatment groups			✓	✓
Self-help groups			✓	✓

From Noordsy *et al* (2003). © John Wiley & Sons Ltd. Reproduced with permission.

- Rehabilitation – provision of long-term support in the community, whether day care or residential care, to enable restoration of social and occupational function (supported education and employment).
- Housing – both supported and independent.
- Pharmacotherapy – provision of antipsychotic medication (particularly clozapine) in those with schizophrenia, and improvement of adherence by providing education and medication supervision.

Evaluations of treatment interventions

General dual diagnosis

In the USA, Drake *et al* (1998*b*) conducted a randomised controlled trial of assertive community treatment in comparison with standard care for patients with dual diagnosis in the context of their integrated treatment services. Assertive community treatment (ACT) showed greater improvement in substance misuse and quality of life. Further analysis of the results showed that patients in high-fidelity programmes (with faithful implementation of and adherence to the ACT model) showed greater reductions in alcohol and drug use and achieved higher rates of remission from substance misuse than those in low-fidelity programmes (McHugo *et al*, 1999).

Dual diagnosis with bipolar disorder

Studies in the USA have shown that integrated psychoeducation group therapy for in-patients is effective in improving comorbidity (Galanter *et al*, 1994). A trial of integrated group therapy with a focus on rapid intervention for patients with bipolar disorder and substance misuse showed greater efficacy in improving drug use, manic symptoms and medication adherence than non-integrated group therapy (Weiss *et al*, 2000).

Dual diagnosis with psychosis

In Australia, Kavanagh *et al* (2003) evaluated a brief intervention for substance misuse in early psychosis and showed that motivational interviewing during acute in-patient treatment was associated with reduction in substance misuse at 6-month and 12-month follow-up compared with standard care.

In the UK, Barrowclough *et al* (2001) conducted a randomised controlled trial of family intervention in psychosis with substance misuse. The intervention, which comprised five weekly sessions of motivational interviewing, six sessions of cognitive therapy held every 2 weeks, and 10–16 sessions of family intervention was more effective than routine care in improving general functioning, symptoms and days of abstinence from substance misuse over 12 months. Another UK project, the Combined Psychosis and Substance Use (COMPASS) programme, has reported positive findings using cognitive–behavioural therapy techniques in the treatment of patients with dual diagnosis (Graham *et al*, 2003, 2006)

Dual diagnosis with personality disorders

The treatment of antisocial personality disorder by psychotherapy in patients with opiate addiction has yielded inconsistent results (Woody *et al*, 1985; Rounsaville *et al*, 1986). However, a study of methadone-treated patients with antisocial personality disorder reported that those who were rewarded quickly and frequently for not using drugs and were given progressively greater control over major aspects of their treatment had significantly lower rates of opiate and cocaine use than those who received standard treatment and who were only rewarded after they had achieved prolonged periods of abstinence (Brooner *et al*, 1998).

The national guidance on treatment of personality disorders (Department of Health, 2003) advocates a number of approaches, including scheme-based cognitive therapy, contingency management, dialectical behavioural therapy and the Henderson Hospital's therapeutic community approach. Although there is some evidence for the efficacy of these approaches, these treatments have not been evaluated in those with comorbid substance misuse except for a randomised controlled trial involving people with borderline personality disorder and substance misuse (van den Bosch *et al*, 2002). The study showed that dialectical behavioural therapy resulted in greater reductions in borderline symptoms and behaviours than treatment as usual, an effect that was not modified by the presence of comorbid substance misuse. Importantly, dialectical behavioural therapy had no effect on substance misuse, and it was advocated that specific treatment for substance misuse should be combined with dialectical behavioural therapy for dual therapeutic impact on borderline symptoms and substance misuse.

Optimal services

The optimal model of care for patients with comorbidity could be developed in the context of current service models and structures, provided minimum standards for quality are established (Abou-Saleh, 2000) (Box 13.4).

Johnson (1997) advocated the development of a dedicated, highly specialised service for patients with dual diagnosis along the lines of the integrated treatment model discussed above. She suggested integrated models of addiction workers working within community mental health teams (CMHTs); training and supervision of CMHT staff in substance misuse; and establishing dual diagnosis specialists in CMHTs. However, there is a risk that such a service could become too selective and exclusive, with two dangers: exclusion of the most difficult patients, and de-skilling of the staff working in addiction and general psychiatric services.

The national guidance on good practice in dual diagnosis (Department of Health, 2002a) is timely and welcome, and in so far as it focuses on the needs of patients with serious mental illness and comorbid substance misuse, it is a step in the right direction. It places lead responsibility with mainstream mental health services; provides 'joined-up thinking' at the policy level, standards of good practice in assessment and treatment, with good examples such as the Kingston Community Drug and Alcohol Team, the Haringey Dual Diagnosis Service and the COMPASS programme in Birmingham; and gives guidance on implementation and commissioning standards. However, the document fails to address important issues relating to social care, the resource implications of this major service development, and the interface between mainstream mental health services and addiction services, as well as implications for the future and the scope of addiction services.

Box 13.4   Quality standards for service planning

- Access to relevant services (crisis, support, housing, after-care, therapeutic and legal services)
- Responsive and flexible approaches (assessment, engagement, retention, managing chaos and crisis, individual responses)
- Continuous care and management (monitoring, liaison, involvement of carers, risk assessment and management)
- Adequately trained staff (access to staff with mental health training)

Concerning social care, particularly the housing needs of this vulnerable population, there is a lack of provision, with limited access to mainstream community care and residential care in mental health and addiction. It is a prime task for local implementation teams working with drug action teams to tackle this problem. The provision of housing is also important because the pooled budget for drug misuse is targeted towards meeting the rising demand for drug misuse services, and it is doubtful whether mainstream mental health funding could cater for the needs of this population.

A most important implication of the guidance on dual diagnosis is the role of addiction services vis-à-vis mainstream mental health services, which at present lack capacity to deal with this population. A survey of the training and support needs of staff working with patients with dual diagnosis showed that mental health service workers lacked the knowledge and skills for assessment and treatment of substance misuse and were insufficiently aware of the available resources and how to access substance misuse services (Maslin et al, 2001). The role of addiction services is paramount in providing training and support for development of capacity and, importantly, in sustaining this capacity with optimal supervision and the agreement of local shared care working arrangements and care pathways, including the care programme approach. Our experience at South West London and St George's Mental Health NHS Trust has been positive, with the introduction of shared-care working arrangements and protocols to ensure that patients with dual diagnosis who present to addiction services have optimum access to mental health services for assessment and treatment. However, one problem that has persisted is that of people with substance-induced psychiatric disorders who have a high risk of self-harm and harm to others and who are often not accepted by mainstream mental health services. From the perspective of addiction services, the introduction and implementation of the National Treatment Agency for Substance Misuse's Models of Care framework (2002) could address these difficulties. Commissioners and providers of services should consider how to integrate the guidance on dual diagnosis (Department of Health, 2002a) with the Models of Care framework to create a single policy document that also addresses referral to mental and addiction services from primary care.

References

Abou-Saleh, M. T. (2000) Substance misuse and comorbid psychiatric disorders. *CPD Bulletin in Psychiatry*, **2**, 61–67.

American Psychiatric Association (1994) *Diagnostic and Statistical Manual of Mental Disorders* (4th edn) (DSM–IV). APA.

Appleby, L., Dyson, V., Altman, E., et al (1996) Utility of the chemical use, abuse, and dependence scale in screening patients with severe mental illness. *Psychiatric Services*, **47**, 647–649.

Babor, T. F., de la Fuente, J. R., Saunders, J., et al (1992) *AUDIT: The Alcohol Use Disorders Identification Test*. World Health Organization.

Barrowclough, C., Haddock, G., Tarrier, N., et al (2001) Randomized controlled trial of motivational interviewing, cognitive behavior therapy, and family intervention for patients with comorbid schizophrenia and substance use disorders. *American Journal of Psychiatry*, **158**, 1706–1713.

Brooner, R. K., Kidorf, M., King, V. L., et al (1998) Preliminary evidence of good treatment response in antisocial drug abusers. *Drug and Alcohol Dependence*, **49**, 249–260.

Chambers, R. A., Krystal, J. H. & Self, D. W. (2001) A neurobiological basis for substance abuse comorbidity in schizophrenia. *Biological Psychiatry*, **50**, 71–83.

Cornelius, J. R., Salloum, I. M., Cornelius, M. D., et al (1997) Fluoxetine in depressed alcoholics: a double blind placebo-controlled trial. *Archives of General Psychiatry*, **54**, 700–705.

Crawford, V. & Crome, I. (2001) *Co-existing Problems of Mental Health and Substance Misuse (Dual Diagnosis): A Review of Relevant Literature.* Royal College of Psychiatrists.

Department of Health (1999) *National Service Framework for Mental Health: Modern Standards and Service Models.* Department of Health.

Department of Health (2001) *Safety First: Five-Year Report of the National Confidential Inquiry Into Suicide and Homicide by People With Mental Illness.* Department of Health.

Department of Health (2002a) *Mental Health Policy Implementation Guide: Dual Diagnosis Good Practice Guide.* Department of Health.

Department of Health (2002b) *Adult Acute Inpatient Care Provision Guidance.* Department of Health.

Department of Health (2002c) *National Minimum Standards for Psychiatric Intensive Care Units and Low Secure Environments.* Department of Health.

Department of Health (2003) *Personality Disorder: No Longer a Diagnosis of Exclusion.* Department of Health.

Drake, R. E. & Mueser, K. T. (2000) Psychosocial approaches to dual diagnosis. *Schizophrenia Bulletin*, **26**, 105–117.

Drake, R. E., Bartels, S. J., Teague, G. B., et al (1993) Treatment of substance abuse in severely mentally ill patients. *Journal of Nervous and Mental Disease*, **181**, 606–611.

Drake, R. E., Mercer-McFadden, C. & Mueser, K. T. (1998a) Review of integrated mental health and substance abuse treatment for patients with dual disorders. *Schizophrenia Bulletin*, **24**, 589–608.

Drake, R. E., McHugo, G. J., Clark, R. E., et al (1998b) Assertive community treatment for patients with co-occurring severe mental illness and substance use disorder: a clinical trial. *American Journal of Orthopsychiatry*, **68**, 201–215.

Farrell, M., Howes, S., Bebbington, P., et al (2001) Nicotine, alcohol and drug dependence and psychiatric comorbidity. Results of a national household survey. *British Journal of Psychiatry*, **179**, 432–437.

Folstein, M. F., Folstein S. E. & McHugh, P. R. (1975) 'Mini-Mental State': a practical method for grading the cognitive state of patients for the clinician. *Journal of Psychiatric Research*, **12**, 189–198.

Galanter, M., Egelko, S., Edwards, H., et al (1994) A treatment system for combined psychiatric and addictive illness. *Addiction*, **89**, 1227–1235.

Graham, H. L., Copello, A., Birchwood, M. J., et al (2003) Cognitive-behavioural integrated treatment approach for psychosis and problem substance use. In *Substance Misuse in Psychosis: Approaches to Treatment and Service Delivery.* John Wiley & Sons.

Graham, H., Copello, A., Birchwood, M., et al (2006) A preliminary evaluation of integrated treatment for co-existing substance use and severe mental health problems: impact on teams and service users. *Journal of Mental Health*, **15**, 577–591.

Harrison, C. & Abou-Saleh, M. T. (2002) Psychiatric disorders and substance misuse psychopathology. In *Dual Diagnosis*, pp. 43–57. Blackwell.

Hasin, D., Trautman, K., Miele, G., et al (1996) Psychiatric Research Interview for Substance and Mental Disorders (PRISM): reliability in substance abusers. *American Journal of Psychiatry*, **153**, 1195–1201.

Johnson, S. (1997) Dual diagnosis of severe mental illness and substance misuse: a case for specialist services? *British Journal of Psychiatry*, **171**, 205–208.

Kavanagh, D. J., Young, R., White, A., *et al* (2003) Start over and survive: a brief intervention for substance misuse in early psychosis. *Substance Misuse in Psychosis: Approaches to Treatment and Service Delivery*. John Wiley & Sons.

Ley, A., Jeffrey, D. P., McLaren, S., *et al* (1999) Treatment programmes for those with both severe mental illness and substance misuse. *Cochrane Library*, issue 4, 1–19. Update Software.

Maslin, J., Graham, H. L., Cawley, M., *et al* (2001) Combined severe mental health and substance use problems. What are the training and support needs of staff working with this client group? *Journal of Mental Health*, **10**, 131–140.

McHugo, G. J., Drake, R. E., Burton, H. L., *et al* (1995) A scale for assessing the stage of substance abuse treatment in persons with severe mental illness. *Journal of Nervous and Mental Disease*, **183**, 762–767.

McHugo, G. J., Drake, R. E., Teague, G. B., *et al* (1999) Fidelity to assertive community treatment and client outcomes in the New Hampshire dual disorders study. *Psychiatric Services*, **50**, 818–824.

McPhillips, M. A., Kelly, F. J., Barnes, T. E., *et al* (1997) Detecting co-morbid substance abuse among people with schizophrenia in the community: a study comparing the results of questionnaires with analysis of hair and urine. *Schizophrenia Research*, **25**, 141–148.

Mind in Croydon (2004) *Pillar to Post. A Film about Dual Diagnosis*. Video available from http://www.mindincroydon.org.uk/videos.asp

Mueser, K. T., Bellack, A. S. & Blanchard, J. J. (1998) Comorbidity of schizophrenia and substance abuse: Implications for treatment. *Journal of Consulting and Clinical Psychology*, **60**, 845–856.

National Treatment Agency for Substance Misuse (2002) *Models of Care for the Treatment of Drug Misusers*. National Treatment Agency.

National Treatment Agency for Substance Misuse (2002) *Models of Care for Treatment of Adult Drug Misusers: Update 2006*. National Treatment Agency.

Noordsy, D. L., McQuade, D. V. & Mueser, K. T. (2003) Assessment considerations. In *Substance Misuse in Psychosis: Approaches to Treatment and Service Delivery* (eds H. L. Graham, A. Copello, M. J. Birchwood, *et al*), pp. 159–180. John Wiley & Sons.

Rosenberg, S. D., Drake, R. E., Wolford, G. L., *et al* (1998) Dartmouth Assessment of Lifestyle Instrument (DALI): a substance use disorder screen for people with severe mental illness. *American Journal of Psychiatry*, **155**, 232–238.

Rounsaville, B. J., Kosten, T. R., Weissman, M. M., *et al* (1986) Prognostic significance of psychopathology in treated opiate addicts. A 2.5 year follow-up study. *Archives of General Psychiatry*, **43**, 739–745.

Saxon, A. J. & Calsyn, D. A. (1995) Effects of psychiatric care for dual diagnosis patients treated in a drug dependence clinic. *American Journal of Drug and Alcohol Abuse*, **21**, 303–313.

Skinner, H. (1982) The Drug Abuse Screening Test. *Addictive Behavior*, **7**, 363–371.

Van den Bosch, L. M., Verheul, R., Schippers, G. M., *et al* (2002) Dialectical behavior therapy of borderline patients with and without substance use problems. Implementation and long-term effects. *Addictive Behavior*, **27**, 911–923.

Weiss, R. & Najavits, L. (1998) Overview of treatment modalities for dual diagnosis patients: pharmacotherapy, psychotherapy, and 12-step programmes. In *Dual Diagnosis and Treatment: Substance Abuse and Comorbid Medical and Psychiatric Disorders* (eds H. Kranzler & B. Rounsaville), p. 87–105. Marcel Dekker Inc.

Weiss, R. D., Griffin, M. L., Greenfield, S. F., *et al* (2000) Group therapy for patients with bipolar disorder and substance dependence: results of a pilot study. *Journal of Clinical Psychiatry*, **61**, 361–367.

Woody, G. E., Luborsky, L., McLellan, A. T., *et al* (1985) Psychotherapy for opiate dependence. *NIDA Research Monograph*, **58**, 9–29.

CHAPTER 14

Treating depression complicated by substance misuse

Claire McIntosh and Bruce Ritson

Summary Dependence on alcohol or other drugs is a depressing experience. The way of life of a person dependent on alcohol is replete with incidents that are demoralising, waking daily with a hangover or with tremor and retching, coupled with amnesia for events of the night before, a sense of inability to face the day ahead and awareness of recriminations at work and at home. Little wonder that depressed mood is common in such circumstances. Similarly, in drug addiction, when life is dominated by the daily problem of obtaining supplies of a substance that brings transient relief or pleasure but also an impoverished existence and low mood. Add to this the fact that the biological action of many commonly misused substances can induce depression, then it is hardly surprising that depression is common in this population. A smaller number use alcohol or illicit drugs to cope with primary depression. Teasing out the interplay of affect and substance misuse is a challenge for the general psychiatrist and the addiction specialist.

As many as 80% of alcoholics experience depressive symptoms, including 30% who fulfil criteria for a major depressive disorder (Raimo & Schuckit, 1998). A lifetime history of depressive disorder has been found in 48% of opiate addicts (Rounsaville *et al*, 2001). Thus, it is clear that substance misuse and depressive symptoms often occur together, but what is less clear is their true relationship. Box 14.1 shows three frequently asked questions concerning it.

The combination of depressive symptoms and substance misuse presents important management issues, both at the level of the individual patient and regarding service provision. In individual patients it is often difficult to disentangle all threads of the presentation. An unusual mental state may be due to intoxication, and substance misuse may be hidden. A frequent management dilemma is the intoxicated patient in the middle of the night, who has self-harmed, or is threatening to do so.

Although depressive symptoms and substance misuse commonly occur together, services for their joint management do so less frequently; one editorial talks of the 'medical model of psychiatric services [...] contrasting sharply with the psychosocial orientation of substance misuse services'

Box 14.1   The relationship between substance misuse and depression

Three frequently asked questions:

- Are the depressive symptoms and disorders caused by the substance misuse?
- Do depressive illnesses cause people to self-medicate with alcohol and drugs?
- Are there common predisposing factors linking the two presentations that account for their frequent co-occurrence?

(Weaver *et al*, 1999). In the UK patients with depression are cared for by generic psychiatric services and substance misusing patients by drug and alcohol services. Few examples of dual diagnosis services are in evidence. We should remember, however, that no similar distinction exists in primary healthcare and that the general practitioner plays a key role in which route is taken by the patient. It is also known that the majority in both categories do not come to specialist services. None the less, having more than one psychiatric diagnosis leads to an increased likelihood of presentation to treatment services (Wu *et al*, 1999), but there are rarely appropriately skilled services available, able to offer a multifaceted approach to care.

Epidemiology

The scale of the co-occurrence of the diagnoses of depression and drug and alcohol misuse has been examined by a number of large population-based studies.

The largest of these is the Epidemiologic Catchment Area (ECA) study (Regier *et al*, 1990). This showed that of people with an alcohol disorder, 13% met criteria for an affective disorder. More strikingly, 32% of those with affective disorder met criteria for a substance misuse disorder. Other studies support these figures and suggest higher correlations (Farrell *et al*, 1998; Kessler *et al*, 2001).

As would be expected, studies looking at groups of people in contact with treatment services give an even higher estimate of the co-occurrence of depression and substance misuse (Rounsaville *et al*, 1982).

There is also a body of work looking at suicide in this group; in fact, the most common mental disorders preceding suicide have consistently been found to be depressive illness and alcohol misuse. Comorbidity is more common in alcoholics who die by suicide than in alcoholics who do not, and it has been found to predict suicide risk (Driessen *et al*, 1998). Interestingly, severity of alcoholism seems not to be of importance (Berglund & Ojehagen,

1998). The extent to which substance misuse increases the likelihood of a fatal outcome also needs to be taken into account: drug overdoses are frequently taken in association with large quantities of alcohol.

The likelihood of suicide in conservatively diagnosed alcoholics has variously been estimated at between 60 to 120 times that for those without psychiatric illness. A number of life stressors have also been implicated, including interpersonal loss and conflict, which have been found more often in the 6 weeks preceding death in those suicides associated with substance misuse. Other associations include an increased likelihood of parental alcoholism and a younger age at which problem drinking started (Berglund & Ojehagen, 1998).

A strong predictor of completed suicide is previous self-harm. A consistent finding has been that suicide attempters who misuse alcohol have higher rates of substance misuse and depression, multiple psychiatric disorders and more encounters with law-enforcement agencies (Berglund & Ojehagen, 1998). In drug misusers there is also a high excess mortality from suicide. Prevalence rates of attempted suicide have been reported ranging from 15% to 45% (Rossow & Lauritzen, 2001).

Substance misuse and depressive symptoms

Is depression caused by substance misuse?

Alcohol intoxication can be accompanied by temporary but severe depressive symptoms. Long-term alcohol use is also associated with depressed mood, and almost all alcoholics report periods of intense sadness. A categorisation of the presentations of alcohol-associated mood disorders is given in Box 14.2. This suggests that substance-induced disorders are commonly phenomenologically indistinguishable from independent major depressive disorder. However, they will remit 2–4 weeks after alcohol drinking has ceased, without the need for antidepressants. At presentation to an alcohol

---

Box 14.2 Presentations of alcohol-associated mood disorders

Patients with alcohol-related mood disorders may be categorised as:

- those with a primary substance-induced disorder and secondary depressive symptoms
- those with underlying physical disorders, such as liver disease or medication effects (e.g. treatment with antihypertensives), who are remediable by treatment of the underlying disorder
- those with an independent major depressive disorder

(Raimo & Schuckit, 1998)

---

treatment programme, 42% of alcoholic men had significant depressive symptoms, but only 6% were clinically depressed after 4 weeks of abstinence (Brown & Schuckit, 1998).

In support of the validity of this distinct sub-category, Brown & Schuckit give the following evidence: both alcoholism and depression are highly familial disorders, but children of alcoholics, although showing increased problems with substance misuse, do not show an increased incidence of independent mood disorders, as would be expected if all depressive symptoms were attributable to independent mood disorder. Work looking at longitudinal follow-ups of adults who had had teenage depression demonstrated no increased incidence of alcohol dependence compared with controls. A longer-term follow up of alcoholic men also showed that with sobriety, the incidence of depression was similar to that for other men (Raimo & Schuckit, 1998). It is from such work looking at the differences in presentations over time that the concept of substance-induced depressive disorder came to be formulated.

Although the majority of work done has related alcohol and mood, other substances also have important mood effects. Amphetamine and cocaine may have dramatic intoxication presentations, including mood disturbance, which have been well documented. Post-intoxication effects, particularly depression, should also be borne in mind with these drugs, as they can be more devastating than acute effects. Depressed mood following the use of ecstasy (methylenedioxymethamphetamine, MDMA) is frequently described and sometimes severe.

Long-term studies have looked at depressive symptoms in opiate addicts. Overall, depressive symptoms were found to be common, particularly at presentation to services, but were generally in the mild to moderate category. The reasons prompting the contact, such as child custody or criminal justice involvement, may also lead to lowering of mood. During contact with drug treatment services substantial improvement occurred, with little difference between drug-free and methadone-maintained groups. Only 1% of this patient group required antidepressant treatment, showing that stabilisation of drug use and detoxification can have beneficial effects on the mood state, without formal treatment for depression (Rounsaville et al, 2001).

Do depressive illnesses cause self-medication?

It is very difficult to design studies to answer this question. A search for plausible explanations is a universal human characteristic, and patients seeking treatment will inevitably be involved in a search for cause and explanation, thus biasing their recall. The 'self-medication hypothesis', the proposal that people with psychiatric symptoms are motivated to take alcohol or drugs to relieve their symptoms, is a key concept in this field. Patients will often report that they drink or take drugs to alleviate stress or to help depressed feelings.

Prospective studies have found that a diagnosis of major depression at entry to in-patient treatment for alcohol dependence predicted a shorter time to first drink or relapse in both women and men (Greenfield *et al*, 1998).

Stimulants such as cocaine or amphetamines produce a transitory lifting of mood but with rebound depression. Alcohol relieves anxiety and gives some blunting of concern about depressing circumstances, but these effects are short lived. There are, however, no indications for the positive effects of alcohol in psychiatric disorder, and any effect may be explained more by positive expectations from alcohol than by any true effect (Berglund & Ojehagen, 1998). Indeed, the detrimental effect of alcohol and drug misuse on symptomatology is much more common.

Are there common predisposing factors linking the two presentations?

An alternative way of viewing these disorders is that there are factors, either genetic or environmental, that independently cause both conditions. Several genes involved in serotonin metabolism have been implicated in both depression and alcohol dependence. Research using twin studies has also been initially supportive of this hypothesis, although further studies are needed (Chick, 1999).

Recognition of comorbidity

As already stated, substance misuse plays a key role in the genesis of symptoms and has also been shown to worsen prognosis in mood disorders (Berglund & Ojehagen, 1998). It is therefore important to seek out its occurrence, especially in frequent users of psychiatric services, who have been found to be particularly at risk (Scott *et al*, 1998).

Assessment

The assessment process should ensure that mental health service staff can reliably detect alcohol and drug misuse and that addiction services can detect depressed mood. Ideally, both services should use similar guidelines for identifying and recording this information.

A cross-sectional prevalence survey in four urban UK centres found that 44% of community mental health team (CMHT) patients reported past-year problem drug use and/or harmful alcohol use (Weaver *et al*, 2003). Because these drugs may be relevant to the patient's mood, a history of drug use is an essential part of the initial examination. This should be backed up by urine testing for drugs in cases where suspicion is aroused. Many commonly misused substances are eliminated from the body within 24–48 h; therefore, if testing for toxicology is required, samples should be taken early after admission or at the time of first contact.

The close links between alcohol misuse and mood disturbance make it essential that a drinking history is taken in every case. It is still not uncommon to find psychiatric case records where there is no description of the patient's drinking pattern or it is given in a very cursory way, for example 'drinks socially' or 'moderate drinker'. What is required is a brief but clear picture of the patient's drinking habits. This can be achieved in a variety of ways; one of the simplest is to ask on how many days a week the patient normally drinks alcohol, and how much is typically drunk on those days. Calculate the answer in units and you have a rough estimate of that patient's weekly consumption. This information is augmented by asking whether alcohol has caused any problems.

There are a variety of screening tests for alcohol use, including the CAGE questionnaire (Mayfield et al, 1974), which reliably identifies drinkers with problems but often misses 'at-risk drinkers'. The latter are detected by the broader Alcohol Use Disorders Identification Test (AUDIT) questionnaire (Babor et al, 1989). Both the CAGE and the AUDIT are slightly more time consuming than very brief tests such as the Paddington Alcohol Test (Smith et al, 1996), developed for accident and emergency settings. These tests can be augmented by blood markers such as gamma-glutamyl transferase (GGT), mean corpuscular volume (MCV) and carbohydrate-deficient transferrin (CDT). These biological measures can also be used as a guide to progress (see chapter 10). Feedback concerning abnormal blood results can be powerful objective evidence demonstrating to the patient that alcohol is causing damage, an appreciation that is reinforced by signs that these figures gradually improve once drinking ceases.

The assessment interview should provide a clear picture of the level of current substance misuse, the amount taken on a daily basis, the pattern of use and the route of administration. Evidence of self-harm, violence to others, disturbed thoughts or moods, and their relationship to substance use should be noted. Assessment of mood should enquire into biological symptoms of depression, the duration of the depression and its particular relation to substance misuse.

The screening instruments for alcohol and drug use and those concerned with affective disorder have not been tested in patients with dual diagnosis. The influence of one condition on the other may give rise to misleading results; for example, many of the features of biological depression are mimicked by the consequences of repetitive excessive drinking, such as feeling ill and depressed in the morning, being unable to face the day, weight loss, impaired concentration and memory, and insomnia.

Depression is probably overdiagnosed in individuals with alcohol problems, as it often proves to be secondary to the drinking problem itself. A wrong diagnosis of depression may give rise to unnecessary prescribing of drugs or even electroconvulsive therapy. However, on some occasions, an underlying depressive disorder is missed. The lifetime risk of suicide is very much higher in problem drinkers than in the general population, and this risk is increased by the presence of a depressive illness.

Even at the stage of assessment it can be useful to include components of motivational interviewing (Miller & Rollnick, 1991) and to forge links in the patient's mind between increased substance misuse and worsening of symptoms. At assessment it is also important to create an open, non-judgemental attitude to try to encourage frankness about substance misuse.

If the patient is intoxicated it may be very difficult to obtain any form of coherent history. In these circumstances the importance of a collateral history cannot be overstated. In an ideal world a safe environment would be available, in which the patient could remain until the effects of intoxication have resolved, allowing a clearer assessment of mental state. Unfortunately, this is not always possible owing to lack of resources. Even an assessment on the following day is not always straightforward, as withdrawal symptoms are not without their own powerful influences.

Management

Safety is of prime importance in the management of comorbid substance misuse. In addition to the increased risks of self-harm, the disinhibiting effects of many substances, particularly alcohol, should be carefully considered. Within psychiatry, there prevails a culture of ignoring the threats of intoxicated patients, even though they are sometimes carried out. A risk assessment should be made of each individual patient's circumstances.

Pharmacological management

At initial presentation it will be very difficult to differentiate independent mood disorders from those due to continued substance misuse. A key message in all the literature in this area is the importance of treating the substance misuse, and the highly probable beneficial effects that this will have on the mood state.

Alcohol detoxification is covered in chapter 7, which recommends a period free from psychoactive drugs prior to starting treatment for depression. A wait of 2–4 weeks after cessation of drinking is advised before commencing antidepressant treatment, to ensure that the mood effects of the alcohol have cleared the system (Raimo & Schuckit, 1998).

With opiate misuse, a primary aim of treatment may be stabilisation and substitute prescribing, not detoxification (see chapter 1). This in itself has been shown to have a beneficial effect on mood (Rounsaville et al, 2001).

In the past, antidepressants were considered as treatments for alcohol misuse in people without depressive symptoms. Current opinion does not support this. However, in an in-patient sample, detoxified patients with de-pression randomly allocated to fluoxetine or placebo showed that the active drug helped to reduce depressive symptoms (Cornelius et al, 1997). Other studies do not support this result, and work continues to clarify the benefits of antidepressants within alcoholic subtypes (Pettinati et al, 2000).

Mason *et al* (1996) found that desipramine reduced depressive symptoms and was associated with significantly longer abstinence from alcohol. However, they concluded that there was no support for desipramine in alcoholics without depression. In a review of this topic, Lynskey (1998) concludes that antidepressant treatment is not a stand-alone treatment for alcoholics with depression, but that pharmacological treatment of depression may help to optimise the outcome of treatment for alcohol dependence. The same paper also raises the important question of drug safety in this group.

Darke & Ross (2001) studied the safety of prescribing antidepressants to injecting drug users. They reported a strong association between antidepressants and non-fatal heroin overdose. The use of tricyclics was particularly hazardous. They recommended the use of selective serotonin reuptake inhibitors (SSRIs), but only where clearly indicated. They commented on the street value of antidepressants, noting that opiate misusers took them for a variety of reasons: to self-medicate depressive symptoms, to become intoxicated, to aid sleep and to manage heroin withdrawal. A further consideration is that methadone slows tricyclic metabolism, so tricyclic dosing must be carefully titrated.

There are few studies examining the positive effects of antidepressant use among drug misusers. Randomised controlled trials have been difficult to complete owing to high drop-out rates. There are mixed reports of efficacy, with some positive results reported (Scott *et al*, 1998). A study looking at fluoxetine concluded that it was not effective in treating depressive symptoms in opiate addicts on methadone maintenance, but commented that there were significant overall reductions in depression while patients were in contact with drug treatment services (Petrakis *et al*, 2001).

A variety of pharmacotherapies are available for treating alcohol problems. Disulfiram is a useful aid to abstinence of proven effectiveness when combined with supervision. In a small number of cases, psychotic episodes have been described as a side-effect of disulfiram, but in most respects it is safe to use. Unfortunately, it can have serious consequences if misused, and particular care should be taken in prescribing it to patients with depression who may be suicidal. Acamprosate and naltrexone have both produced improved outcomes in individuals who are alcohol dependent. We do not know about their efficacy in patients with dual diagnosis, but it seems reasonable to use one or the other when patients are particularly conscious of craving during the early months of abstinence. Either can be combined with antidepressants, if necessary.

Psychological therapies

Psychological therapies must be considered both in their own right and in combination with medication. There is a growing literature in this area, although most work has centred on motivational interviewing (Miller & Rollnick, 1991), which can be a useful technique throughout assessment and treatment (see chapters 16 and 17).

Trials of cognitive therapy have shown promising results that mirror antidepressant findings: an improvement in depressive symptoms can lead to a reduction in substance misuse (Lynskey, 1998). There has also been promising work incorporating facets of cognitive therapy and early work on interpersonal therapy (Scott *et al*, 1998).

Miller & Wilbourne (2002) have reviewed the literature on the treatment of alcohol misuse, deriving a methodological quality score; they listed a number of positive and negative results for each and gave a clinical effectiveness score for those methods that had been adequately investigated. Motivational enhancement showed consistent benefits, as did community reinforcement, acamprosate, naltrexone and social skills training. Again, it is not clear how well these approaches combine with other treatments for depression. None the less, it seems reasonable to think that that these psychological therapies for alcohol problems should be added to traditional therapies for depression.

Any treatment for substance misuse commonly relies heavily on the motivation or commitment of the patient. Bien *et al* (1993) listed the key features of brief psychological intervention as feedback about current mis-use, the patient's own responsibility for change and advice about making and maintaining this change. Therapy for substance misuse, and particularly alcohol dependence, places much greater responsibility for change on the patient and there is less reliance on a medical model. Patients with severe depression may find it hard to engage in this kind of therapy until their mood has lifted.

Although group therapy now has a less salient place in the treatment of alcohol problems than formerly, it is still widely used. Patients with depression may find group processes very threatening and they require careful introduction, usually after severe depression has lifted. Alcoholics Anonymous (AA) and Narcotics Anonymous (NA) are very effective self-help agencies but, again, individuals who are depressed may find it difficult to join them because they anticipate that the experience will be threatening. The first steps can often be made easier by introduction to an empathic member before attending the first meeting.

The risks of the interaction of antidepressant medication with alcohol and illicit drugs, and the associated special hazards of medication overdose and misuse, make psychological therapies an attractive proposition either as an alternative or additional treatment.

Prognosis

Comorbidity carries with it a worse prognosis, both for substance misuse and for depressive symptoms (Hall & Farrell, 1997). As already mentioned, a diagnosis of current major depression predicted a shorter time to first drink after in-patient treatment for alcohol dependence (Greenfield *et al*, 1998). Similarly, among patients addicted to opiates, a current major or minor depressive episode at entry to treatment was correlated with higher levels of illicit drug use during the subsequent 6 months (Rounsaville *et al*, 2001). The large increase in risk for attempted and completed self-harm implicit in a diagnosis of comorbidity has also been described above.

Service provision

Often, patients with dual diagnosis fall between services designed to treat either the depression or the substance misuse. The creation of 'super-specialist' services has been advocated, particularly in the USA, but UK services have suggested other strategies to try to improve practice. In a number of centres, combined psychosis and substance misuse teams have been created to treat patients with dual diagnosis and act as a consultancy and training resource for other agencies (see chapter 13).

There have been calls for improved staff training, in both mental health and addiction services, to try to improve recognition of comorbidity. Increased sharing of skills and support between the two services has also been recommended (Hall & Farrell, 1997). It is often helpful for staff in one agency to gain experience in the other, as this helps mutual understanding and knowledge of the issues involved. It has also been stated that services for drug misuse and mental health have tended to develop in ways determined more by public anxiety and political ideology than by research evidence (Weaver *et al*, 1999). Training an appropriate workforce, research into the efficacy of services and the development and testing of new models of service provision are required. Box 14.3 lists the attributes that should be present if both services are to achieve optimum efficacy.

Conclusion

Patients presenting with depression complicated by substance misuse pose particular challenges to treatment. Their depressive symptoms are very likely to be caused or exacerbated by their substance misuse. In alcohol misuse, a 1-month period of abstinence and then further evaluation are recommended before the commencement of pharmacotherapy. Opiate users should be stabilised before pharmacotherapy. Prescription of antidepressants to substance users must be very carefully considered, as they have a street value and might therefore be widely disseminated. If pharmacotherapy is indicated for this group, SSRIs should be the treatment of choice. Strong consideration should be given to psychological therapies such as motivational interviewing and cognitive–behavioural therapy, which are currently being further evaluated and hopefully should become more available to patients with comorbidity. Equally, treatment of depressive symptoms also yields benefit in managing substance misuse, with antidepressant treatment decreasing alcohol intake in alcoholics with depression.

Box 14.3 Requirements of services to ensure optimal treatment of depression in substance misuse

Psychiatric services

- Individuals who misuse substances must have the same right to treatment as other patients
- A substance-use history must be recorded in all cases
- Clear protocols should be in place to ensure treatment and follow-up when misuse is identified
- Regular liaison with addiction services and knowledge of services available are essential
- Care plans should identify a strategy for dealing with substance misuse
- The implications of interactions between prescribed medication and alcohol or illicit drugs must be considered

Addiction services

- The attitude that mental illness excludes patients from effective therapy must not be allowed
- Mood and suicidality must be assessed and monitored
- If mood disorder persists after 2 weeks of abstinence or stabilisation, a diagnosis of depressive illness should be considered
- Regular liaison with general psychiatric services is essential
- Follow-up plans should include regular mental state assessments

---

References

Babor, T. F., Hofman, M., Delboca, F. K., *et al* (1989) *The Alcohol Use Disorder Test: Guidelines for Use in Primary Health Care*. World Health Organization.

Berglund, M. & Ojehagen, A. (1998) The influence of alcohol drinking and alcohol use disorders on psychiatric disorders and suicidal behavior. *Alcoholism: Clinical and Experimental Research*, **22**, 333S–345S.

Bien, T. H., Miller, W. R. & Torigan, J. S. (1993) Brief interventions for alcohol problems: a review. *Addiction*, **88**, 315–335.

Brown, S. A. & Schuckit, M. A. (1998) Changes in depression among abstinent alcoholics. *Journal of Studies on Alcohol*, **49**, 412–417.

Chick, J. (1999) Alcohol dependence, anxiety and mood disorders. *Current Opinion in Psychiatry*, **12**, 297–301.

Cornelius, J. R., Salloum, I. M., Ehler, J. G., *et al* (1997) Fluoxetine in depressed alcoholics. *Archives of General Psychiatry*, **54**, 700–705.

Darke, S. & Ross, J. (2001) The use of antidepressants among injecting drug users in Sydney, Australia. *Addiction*, **95**, 407–417.

Driessen, M., Veltrup, C., Weber, J., *et al* (1998) Psychiatric co-morbidity, suicidal behaviour and suicidal ideation in alcoholics seeking treatment. *Addiction*, **93**, 889–894.

Farrell, M., Howes, S., Taylor, C., *et al* (1998) Substance misuse and psychiatric comorbidity: an overview of the OPCS National Psychiatric Morbidity Survey. *Addictive Behaviours*, **23**, 909–918.

Greenfield, S. F., Weiss, R. D., Muenz, L. R., *et al* (1998) The effect of depression on return to drinking. *Archives of General Psychiatry*, **55**, 259–265.

Hall, W. & Farrell, M. (1997) Comorbidity of mental disorders with substance misuse. *British Journal of Psychiatry*, **171**, 4–5.

Kessler, R. C., McGonach, K. A., Zhoa, S., *et al* (2001) Lifetime and 12 month prevalence of DSM–III–R psychiatric disorders in the United States. *Archives of General Psychiatry*, **51**, 8–19.

Lynskey, M. T. (1998) The comorbidity of alcohol dependence and affective disorders: treatment implications. *Drug and Alcohol Dependence*, **52**, 201–209.

Mason, B. J., Kocsis, J. H., Ritvo, E. C., *et al* (1996) A double blind placebo-controlled trial of desipramine for primary alcohol dependence stratified on the presence of absence of major depression. *JAMA*, **275**, 761–767.

Mayfield, D., McCleod, G. & Hall, P. (1974) The CAGE questionnaire: validation of a new alcoholism screening instrument. *American Journal of Psychiatry*, **131**, 1121–1123.

Miller, W. R. & Rollnick, S. (1991) *Motivational Interviewing: Preparing People to Change Addictive Behavior.* Guilford Press.

Miller, W. R. & Wilbourne, P. L. (2002) Mesa Grande: a methodological analysis of clinical trials of treatments for alcohol use disorders. *Addiction*, **97**, 265–277.

Petrakis, I., Carroll, K. M., Nich, C., *et al* (2001) Fluoxetine treatment of depressive disorders in methadone maintained opiate addicts. *Drug and Alcohol Dependence*, **50**, 221–226.

Pettinati, H. M., Volpicelli, J. R., Kranzler, H. R., *et al* (2000) Sertraline treatment for alcohol dependence: interactive effects of medication and alcoholic subtype. *Alcoholism: Clinical and Experimental Research*, **24**, 1041–1049.

Raimo, E. B & Schuckit, M. A. (1998) Alcohol dependence and mood disorders. *Addictive Behaviours*, **23**, 933–946.

Regier, D. A., Farmer, M. E., Rae D. S., *et al* (1990) Comorbidity of mental disorders with alcohol and other drug misuse: results from the Epidemiologic Catchment Area Study. *JAMA*, **264**, 2511–2518.

Rossow, I. & Lauritzen, G. (2001) Shattered childhood – a key issue in suicidal behaviour in drug addicts? *Addiction*, **96**, 227–240.

Rounsaville, B. J., Weissman, M. M., Kleber, H., *et al* (1982) Heterogenicity of psychiatric diagnosis in treated opiate addicts. *Archives of General Psychiatry*, **39**, 161–166.

Rounsaville, B. J., Weissman, M. M., Crits-Cristoph, K., *et al* (2001) Diagnosis and symptoms of depression in opiate addicts. *Archives of General Psychiatry*, **39**, 151–156.

Scott, J., Gilvarry, F., & Farrell, M. (1998) Managing anxiety and depression in alcohol and drug dependence. *Addictive Behaviours*, **23**, 919–931.

Smith, S. G. T, Touquet, R., Wright, S., *et al* (1996) Detection of alcohol misusing patients in accident and emergency departments. The Paddington Alcohol Test (PAT). *Journal of Accident and Emergency Medicine*, **13**, 380–312.

Weaver, T., Renton, A., Stimson, G., *et al* (1999) Severe mental illness and substance misuse. *BMJ*, **318**, 138–139.

Weaver, T., Madden, P., Charles, V., *et al* (2003) Comorbidity of substance misuse and mental illness in community mental health and substance misuse services. *British Journal of Psychiatry*, **183**, 304–313.

Wu, L. T., Kouzis, A. C. & Leaf, P. J. (1999) Influence of comorbid alcohol and psychiatric disorders on utilization of mental health services in the National Comorbidity Survey. *American Journal of Psychiatry*, **156**, 1230–1236.

CHAPTER 15

Treating anxiety complicated by substance misuse

Anne Lingford-Hughes, John Potokar and David Nutt

Summary   Anxiety and substance misuse often coexist, particularly with alcohol disorders. Anxiety can either lead to or arise from substance misuse, and determining the relationship between the two is key to their management. It is essential to establish whether a discrete anxiety disorder is present in patients with possible comorbidity. The neurobiology of anxiety and substance misuse, again particularly of alcohol, overlap with similar changes seen in especially the GABA, serotonin and noradrenaline systems. A combination of pharmacological and psychological approaches are available for both disorders separately, although few studies have examined approaches for such comorbidity.

The relationship between anxiety disorders and substance misuse is intimate. Here we concentrate on alcohol, although for completeness we also briefly mention other substances taken for anxiety relief or that cause anxiety.

The term 'misuse' is important and should be qualified. Many people drink alcohol or take illicit drugs without any apparent consequences. Once this use becomes problematic, at any level of consumption, misuse is a more appropriate term.

Recent research exploring the molecular underpinning of anxiety disorders, together with advances in our understanding of how alcohol affects brain neurochemistry, can help to explain this intimate relationship. We review the evidence and how this can provide a framework for both diagnosis and management in a patient with comorbid anxiety and substance misuse. Few studies address the best way of treating patients with dual diagnosis but several drugs are licensed for the treatment of individual anxiety disorders and are likely to be helpful in combination with alcohol treatment strategies.

Until recently, anxiety was used as an umbrella term that spanned the spectrum from normal human emotion to severe pathological states. The 1970s and 1980s heralded the beginning of a more rigorous approach to the discrete constellation of symptoms that make up the individual anxiety disorders. This has not only helped in tailoring therapeutic approaches but has also enabled researchers to explore the pathophysiological foundations of the various disorders. The ICD–10 (World Health Organization, 1992) categorises anxiety disorders as phobic (social, simple, agoraphobic), generalised, panic disorder and obsessive–compulsive disorder (OCD). Of these, the last is less robustly associated with substance misuse.

Although pharmacological and psychological treatments for anxiety disorders are effective, the most common response for an individual with anxiety is to use recreational drugs, principally alcohol, to alleviate the symptoms. The widespread availability and relatively low cost of alcohol means that although it is widely used as a social lubricant and for its short-term euphoriant effects, it is also frequently used as self-medication for anxiety disorders, low mood and sleep problems. Prospective studies show that alcohol dependence and anxiety disorders demonstrate a reciprocal causal relationship over time, with anxiety disorders leading to alcohol dependence and vice versa (Kushner et al, 1990).

Psychoactive substances and anxiety

The ICD–10 lists a number of behavioural and mental disorders (e.g. acute intoxication, dependence and withdrawal) that can result from misuse of psychoactive substances, including alcohol and other sedatives, opioids, cannabinoids, stimulants such as cocaine, amphetamine and caffeine, hallucinogens and tobacco. The interaction between anxiety and other substance misuse is described in Table 15.1.

Alcohol and other sedatives

Although alcohol is a fast-acting and effective anxiolytic, it can also lead to increased anxiety, particularly when consumption is excessive. Withdrawal is experienced as anxiety, thus fuelling more alcohol intake, which results in a vicious cycle of anxiety and alcohol consumption (Fig. 15.1). People with panic disorder who are alcohol dependent are usually unable to distinguish panic symptoms, with the exception of tremor, from alcohol withdrawal (George et al, 1988).

Anxiety commonly presents as a symptom of alcohol withdrawal, initially in the form of 'shakes and sweats' as the blood alcohol level declines. The management of alcohol withdrawal is reviewed in chapter 7.

Alcohol shares many similar pharmacological and behavioural actions with benzodiazepines and barbiturates. These drugs can be prescribed as sedatives, anxiolytics, hypnotics or anticonvulsants. Short-acting benzodiazepines have greater addictive potential than longer-acting formulations. Not surprisingly, anxiety is commonly associated with withdrawal from benzodiazepines. At what dose and after how long a benzodiazepine causes significant withdrawal is difficult to define in routine clinical practice, but current *British National Formulary* (BNF; British Medical Association & Royal Pharmaceutical Society

197

Table 15.1 Anxiety as a feature of substance misuse

Substance	Use	Intoxication	Withdrawal	Long-term effects
Alcohol	To overcome anxiety (especially social)		Pronounced anxiety (see text)	Panic disorder and GAD can emerge from misuse
Stimulants (cocaine, amphetamine)	To overcome social anxiety	Anxiety with tachycardia, pupillary dilation, psychomotor agitation, impaired judge-ment, impulsive behaviour	Yes	Panic disorder, phobias and GAD can emerge from misuse
Hallucinogens		Anxiety, with altered perceptions, hallucinations		Not clear, but flashbacks can be similar to symptoms of PTSD
PCP		Occasionally anxiety, with usually delirious psychotic state		
Inhalants				GAD and panic disorder can emerge from chronic use
Nicotine			Pronounced anxiety	
Caffeine		Anxiety	Anxiety	
Opioids	Rarely, for anxiety relief			
Cannabis			Can present like a panic attack but with paranoid thoughts; more likely in inexperienced smokers	

GAD, generalised anxiety disorder; PTSD, post-traumatic stress disorder; PCP, 1-(1-phencyclohexyl) piperidine, phencyclidine.

of Great Britain, 2007) guidelines suggest prescription only for 'disabling' conditions and for not longer than 4 weeks. However, it is important to note that benzodiazepines are far safer than alcohol and in patients with anxiety disorders long-term use is sometimes indicated where other medications have failed.

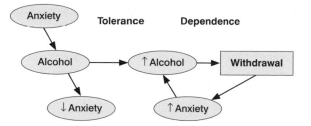

Fig. 15.1 Pathway from anxiety to self-medication with alcohol and consequent dependency; ↑, increase; ↓, decrease.

Alcohol misuse and anxiety: prevalence and incidence

Alcoholism and social anxiety disorder comprise the next most prevalent mental disorders after depression (Kessler *et al*, 1997). They are often present together, increasing the therapeutic challenge.

Several community prevalence studies have determined the comorbidity of anxiety and alcoholism. People with an anxiety disorder have approximately double the odds of also having a substance misuse disorder (Table 15.2). This typically equates to one-quarter to one-third of people with an anxiety disorder, with rates of comorbidity being higher in women. The anxiety disorder generally precedes alcohol or drug problems or dependence. This finding is consistent with but not confirmatory of the 'self-medication hypothesis'. The exception to this is panic disorder, which can emerge from alcohol misuse (Merikangas *et al*, 1998).

Table 15.2 Odds ratio of an additional diagnosis (alcohol or drug problems or dependence) with any anxiety disorder

Survey	Alcohol problems	Alcohol dependence	Drug problems	Drug dependence
ECA	1	1.8	2.3	2.4
NCS				
Male	0.95	2.2		
Female	1.78	3.08		
ICPE	1.78	2.5	2.95	4.78

ECA, Epidemiologic Catchment Area (Regier *et al*, 1990); NCS, National Comorbidity Survey (Kessler *et al*, 1997); ICPE, International Consortium in Psychiatric Epidemiology (Merikangas *et al*, 1998).

In patient populations, the lifetime prevalence of alcohol misuse or dependence in people with social anxiety disorder is 22%, with the prevalence of social anxiety disorder in people seeking treatment for alcohol problems around 15% (Regier *et al*, 1990). The rate of any anxiety disorder in in-patients with alcohol dependence ranges from 22.6 to 68.7%, with phobias typically highly represented (Kushner *et al*, 1990). Therefore about one-quarter to one-fifth of patients diagnosed with alcohol problems or social anxiety disorder will also suffer from the other disorder. In people with DSM–III–R alcohol abuse or dependence, the prevalence of social anxiety disorder in females is higher than in males (female:male ratio = 30%:19%; Kessler *et al*, 1994, 1997).

The rates of anxiety disorders in substance misusers are also quite high. In a survey of drug misusers in contact with treatment services, the lifetime prevalence of a phobic disorder was 26% in men and 45% in women (Krausz *et al*, 1998). For other anxiety disorders the rates were 10% for men and 22% for women. In out-patients on methadone maintenance, lifetime rates of any anxiety disorder were 6.1% for men and 10.7% for women. The most common disorders seen were simple phobia (women) and panic disorder (men) (Brooner *et al*, 1997).

Thus, in both substance misuse and anxiety disorder populations, rates of the other disorder are high. When comorbidity occurs it is likely that each disorder will be more difficult to treat and consequently the clinician needs to know not only why this relationship occurs but also how to recognise and manage this comorbidity.

Aetiological theories and issues

The co-occurrence of alcohol and anxiety has led to proposals of an aetiological link. Both biological and psychosocial factors have been described. The concept of alcohol as a provider of 'Dutch courage' to help people with social anxiety attend social occasions is widely held. This self-medication hypothesis receives support from prevalence surveys (Merikangas *et al*, 1998), showing that phobias and social anxiety tend to have preceded the onset of alcohol or drug misuse. On the other hand, panic disorder does not necessarily follow this pattern and in some patients it clearly emerges in alcohol dependence.

The association does not necessarily reflect a direct causal relationship. Instead, the vulnerability to both disorders may arise from another factor, perhaps genetic, familial or biological.

A number of research paradigms have been devised to study the anxiolytic effects of alcohol. Not all studies confirm that alcohol is anxiolytic, and factors such as how anxiety is defined (e.g. as tension, fear, frustration, stress), the amount of alcohol consumed, previous experience, situation and expectations play a role (Kushner *et al*, 1990). For example, in one group of individuals with social anxiety disorder, alcohol itself failed to reduce anxiety associated with public speaking but the belief that they had received alcohol did reduce anxiety (Himle et al, 1999).

From a psychiatric perspective the relationship between alcohol and anxiety disorders cannot be understood without knowledge of the effect of alcohol on brain neurotransmission and the role of neurotransmitters in these disorders. In the past it was thought that anxiety disorders were purely functional, with no real biological basis, and alcohol dependence was often perceived to be the result of constitutional weakness. It is now very clear that neurotransmitter and receptor function are altered in both anxiety disorders and alcohol dependence. Three neurotransmitter systems are likely to be especially important in this relationship: the gamma-aminobutyric acid (GABA), serotonin (5-HT) and noradrenaline systems.

The GABA-ergic system

Although alcohol acts on a variety of neurotransmitter systems (see Nutt, 1999), its effects on the GABA-benzodiazepine receptor (GBzR) are likely to be critical in its anxiolytic effect. This receptor also appears important in the tolerance, dependence and withdrawal that can occur through use of alcohol or benzodiazepines. GABA is the major inhibitory neurotransmitter system in the central nervous system and the GBzR has several functional forms, which differ in their sensitivity to alcohol or benzodiazepines. For instance, altering the α_1 subunit of the GBzR in mice renders diazepam no longer sedative and altering the α_2 subunit leaves it no longer anxiolytic (Rudolph et al, 2001).

As alcohol is a GBzR agonist, it has been proposed that hypofunction of this system is involved in vulnerability to alcoholism. Although short-term exposure to alcohol increases GABA-ergic function, long-term exposure is associated with reduced GBzR levels and function. It has been proposed that such a reduction is important as an underlying neurobiological mechanism of tolerance. Neuroimaging studies have shown reduced levels of the GBzR in abstinent alcohol-dependent patients, predominantly in the frontal lobes (e.g. Lingford-Hughes et al, 1998).

There is also evidence for altered GABA-ergic function in anxiety disorders. People with panic disorder appear to be sub-sensitive to the effects of benzodiazepines (Roy-Byrne et al, 1989), suggesting an alteration in the 'set-point' of the receptor. This, together with the panicogenic effects of the benzodiazepine antagonist flumazenil, points to altered GABA-ergic function, which may underpin the raised anxiety in these individuals. Chronic benzodiazepine use in people with anxiety disorders is associated with reduced GBzR sensitivity (Potokar et al, 1999) and we have some preliminary evidence that alcohol dependence is associated with grossly reduced GBzR sensitivity. Furthermore, Malizia et al (1998) have shown, using positron emission tomography, that there is a reduction in global GBzR binding in people with panic disorder compared with matched controls, emphasising the important role of this receptor system in this disorder.

The serotonergic system

Several lines of evidence point to an important role of 5-HT in anxiety and alcoholism (Nutt & Cowen, 1987; Heinz *et al*, 2001). Clinically, a number of serotonergic drugs are effective in treating anxiety disorders and many are licensed for this indication (see below and Table 15.3).

Table 15.3 Indications for pharmacotherapy and potential problems of prescribed drugs[1]

Drug	Anxiety disorder: indications	Potential problems
Selective serotonin reuptake inhibitors	Panic disorder Generalised anxiety disorder Obsessive–compulsive disorder Post-traumatic stress disorder Social anxiety disorder	Possibly less efficacious in type 2 alcoholism
Trazodone		Enhanced sedative effects with alcohol
Tricyclic antidepressants	Panic disorder Post-traumatic stress disorder	Enhanced sedative effects with alcohol Toxicity in overdose – often taken with alcohol Lowering of seizure threshold
Venlafaxine (SNRI)	Generalised anxiety disorder	
Reboxetine (NaRI)	No specific indication	
Mirtazapine (NaSSA)	No specific indication	Enhanced sedative effects with alcohol
Monoamine oxidase inhibitors	Social anxiety disorder	Potential interactions with alcohol
Benzodiazepines	Anxiety disorders (disabling, <4 weeks use)	Dependence with escalating use of alcohol/drugs; enhanced effects of alcohol
Buspirone	Generalised anxiety disorder	Enhanced sedative effects with alcohol
Pregabalin	Generalised anxiety disorder	Enhanced sedative effects with alcohol

SNRI, serotonin and noradrenaline reuptake inhibitor; NaRI, noradrenaline reuptake inhibitor; NaSSA, noradrenergic and specific serotonergic antidepressant.

1. Liver (and renal) impairment will affect the dosing regimen for most drugs, and severe impairment often results in the drug being contraindicated (see current *British National Formulary*). Since many patients with anxiety disorders are sensitive to side-effects, pharmacotherapy should be started at a low dose and slowly increased.

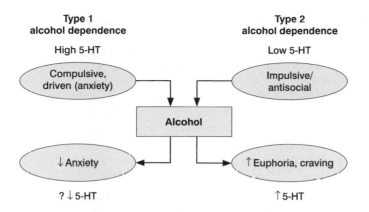

Fig. 15.2 Possible routes to alcohol dependence implicating the serotonergic (5-HT) system; ↑, increase; ↓, decrease.

In alcoholism, low 5-HT function is associated with type 2 alcoholism, in which early disease onset, impulsivity, antisocial personality traits and a positive family history are seen (Heinz *et al*, 2001). In this alcohol-dependent population, increased 5-HT (with m-chlorophenylpiperazine (mCPP), a mixed 5-HT agonist/antagonist) resulted in craving and an increased urge to drink alcohol (George *et al*, 1997) (Fig. 15.2).

The noradrenergic system

Enhanced noradrenergic activity is thought to underlie many symptoms of drug or alcohol withdrawal, including agitation, anxiety, sweating and tachycardia (George *et al*, 1990). These symptoms can be controlled with lofexidine, an α2 agonist, which reduces noradrenergic output from the brainstem. This drug is increasingly used to manage opiate withdrawal, but a recent study has suggested lack of efficacy in people undergoing in-patient alcohol detoxification (Keaney *et al*, 2001).

A dysfunctional noradrenergic system is also implicated in anxiety, providing another common biological substrate for both anxiety and substance misuse. Drugs such as amphetamines and cocaine, which increase noradrenaline, are anxiogenic, whereas the α2 agonist clonidine reduces anxiety and has some activity in reducing spontaneous and lactate-induced panic (Coplan *et al*, 1992).

In conclusion it is clear that anxiety and alcohol misuse can each give rise to the other, but the relationship is complex. Similarities in the underlying cause of substance misuse and anxiety disorders suggest that a common mechanism may be effective in ameliorating both disorders.

Management

Three factors are likely to be important in the symptomatic and functional improvement of a patient with anxiety and alcohol misuse: whether anxiety disorder is diagnosed, the degree of alcohol misuse (e.g. hazardous, harmful or dependent) and whether the relationship between the two has been explored.

There are many reasons why people with anxiety disorders initiate and maintain alcohol misuse and why current management is not optimum. These include the availability of alcohol, failure of patients and doctors to recognise pathological anxiety and uncertainty or lack of knowledge about treatment options. Education of both patients and doctors is obviously critical if some of these factors are to be addressed.

Diagnostic issues

Assessment of anxiety

It is essential to establish whether a discrete anxiety disorder is present in patients with possible comorbidity. Three questions should be asked when assessing a patient 'with anxiety': does the patient have an anxiety disorder; what type of anxiety disorder is it; and is there any comorbidity?

Anxiety is a normal human emotion that rises and falls in response to both external and internal cues. Pathological anxiety ('anxiety disorder') is characterised by its intensity, duration, autonomy (i.e. it has a life of its own) and functional impairment (often characterised by changes in behaviour).

If an anxiety disorder is suspected, are panic attacks present? Panic attacks are often not identified because the clinician asks only about the recent past, whereas the natural history of panic attacks frequently results in a reduction in their intensity with time. A useful question is to ask whether the patient has ever experienced a sudden surge in anxiety that felt overwhelming and was accompanied by the typical somatic and cognitive symptoms. If a positive answer is elicited, the clinician should ask about the first time that this ever happened – this will often be remembered in great detail and may also explain consequent avoidant (e.g. agoraphobic) behaviour. If a history of panic attacks is obtained, are these cued (social anxiety disorder, post-traumatic stress disorder (PTSD) or specific phobia) or spontaneous (panic disorder)?

Every patient who presents with anxiety symptoms should be asked about alcohol intake and, if a history of excessive alcohol use is obtained (hazardous, harmful or dependent), anxiety disorders should be screened for. A useful tool is the Alcohol Use Disorders Identification Test (AUDIT) questionnaire, which has been recommended for routine use by the World Health Organization (Saunders *et al*, 1993).

It is essential to try to establish the sequence of development of clinical problems. Was the anxiety disorder present before the alcohol misuse (e.g.

social anxiety disorder, agoraphobia) or secondary to it (e.g. panic disorder, general anxiety disorder)? Psychoeducation is useful. Often patients will never have discussed in detail their anxiety symptoms and may not relate their alcohol problem to anxiety.

Assessment of substance misuse

Clearly, a comprehensive assessment of any patient is critical. Although it is commonly thought that patients do not accurately reveal their true alcohol and drug consumption, this is not necessarily the case nor should it hinder a history being obtained. Evidence can also be obtained from a physical examination: needle or track marks may be indicative of intravenous drug misuse and palmar erythema of alcohol misuse. A urine drug screen will reveal recent drug use (see chapter 10); abnormal liver function tests and mean corpuscular volume are generally apparent in alcohol misuse (see chapter 10). In patients with anxiety disorder, the amount being consumed is not as relevant as the reliance on the substance.

Treatment

Anxiety disorders

The following is a brief summary of the principal treatments for uncomplicated anxiety disorders. Clinical guidelines for the management of anxiety have been produced by the National Institute for Health and Clinical Excellence (National Institute for Clinical Excellence, 2004) and the British Association for Psychopharmacology (Baldwin, 2005). Table 15.3 summarises pharmacological treatments and potential problems with them, and further information can be found in the review by Argyropoulos et al (2000).

Panic disorder

Pharmacological treatments
Results from several studies show that 70–80% of patients treated with anti-panic agents show moderate to marked improvement (e.g. Ballenger, 1993). Selective serotonin reuptake inhibitors (SSRIs) are efficacious, and of these citalopram, escitalopram and paroxetine are licensed for this use. Of the tricyclic antidepressants, clomipramine and imipramine are the most studied and are effective. There is slightly more evidence for clomipramine, which is the more serotonergic of these drugs. Improvement does not depend on the presence of depression. None of the tricyclics is licensed for this indication in the UK. Most studies of monoamine oxidase inhibitors (MAOIs) have been uncontrolled, and although many clinicians view them as effective, they are usually reserved for treatment-resistant patients. Reversible monoamine oxidase inhibitors (RIMAs) such as moclobemide have minimal side-effects and probably some efficacy. They are not licensed for use in panic disorder.

Benzodiazepines are efficacious but high doses of standard benzodiazepines or high-potency agents such as clonazepam are needed (presumably because of reduced GBzR sensitivity in these patients). Tolerance to therapeutic effects does not tend to occur. Their fast onset of action makes them ideal for co-prescribing when other agents (e.g. SSRIs) are initiated, thus preventing the initial exacerbation of symptoms that occurs with the latter. Relapse rates are high when they are withdrawn.

Psychological treatments

Behavioural (both exposure and relaxation), cognitive and cognitive–behavioural treatments are effective. Psychodynamic therapy has not been evaluated.

Post-traumatic stress disorder

Pharmacological treatments

Up to 80% of people with PTSD have comorbid conditions, including the high prevalence of substance misuse. Antidepressants have the most evidence supporting use, especially those with serotonergic activity. The SSRIs are useful and both paroxetine (UK) and sertraline (US) are licensed. Trazodone, which blocks 5-HT$_2$ receptors as well as 5-HT reuptake, may be useful, especially if there is pronounced sleep disturbance. The MAOIs may be useful for treatment-refractory illness. Although there are no controlled studies of benzodiazepines, clonazepam (which has a long duration of action and some serotonergic effects) is sometimes usefully prescribed.

Psychological treatments

Cognitive–behavioural strategies (usually employing exposure rather than systematic desensitisation) are effective in reducing symptoms. Several studies have shown eye movement desensitisation and reprocessing to be reasonably effective (Rothbaum, 1997; Carlson *et al*, 1998), although other studies report more modest effects (Pitman *et al*, 1996; Devilly & Spence, 1999).

Social anxiety disorder

Pharmacological treatments

The SSRIs are efficacious, tolerable and safe and are generally considered first-line treatment. Paroxetine is licensed for treatment of social anxiety disorder. The MAOIs are also effective but their relatively poor tolerability and safety means that they are reserved for refractory cases. Early studies (Versiani *et al*, 1992) suggested considerable efficacy for RIMAs, but results of subsequent research (Schneier *et al*, 1998) have been equivocal, although moclobemide is licensed.

Two controlled studies of benzodiazepines in social anxiety disorder have been carried out (Davidson *et al*, 1993). A response rate of 78%

was found for clonazepam (*v.* 20% for placebo). Although well-tolerated, concerns about dependence mean that they are usually reserved for resistant cases.

Beta-blockers are frequently prescribed, especially by general practitioners, but are generally not useful in social anxiety disorder. They are, however, effective in specific performance anxiety.

Psychological treatments

Both cognitive therapy and exposure therapy are effective and the combination probably has advantages over each therapy alone.

Generalised anxiety disorder

Pharmacological treatments

Both trazodone and imipramine have demonstrated efficacy in controlled trials. Of the newer agents, venlafaxine is effective and has recently been licensed for this use. Buspirone is effective and may be especially so when there are prominent psychic symptoms. Benzodiazepines are effective and have rapid onset of action. Although people with uncomplicated generalised anxiety disorder do not tend to run into problems with benzodiazepine use, concerns about dependence limit their prescription. Pregabalin, a calcium channel blocker, has recently been licensed for this disorder.

Psychological treatments

Cognitive–behavioural therapies (CBTs) incorporating relaxation training, cognitive therapy and image rehearsal have some efficacy.

Specific phobia

Generally, drug treatments are not useful unless the fear is so great that exposure therapy (the treatment of choice) is not possible.

Obsessive–compulsive disorder

Pharmacological treatments

Clomipramine is effective, as are the SSRIs. The relatively benign side-effect profile of the latter means that they are first-line treatments; paroxetine, fluoxetine, sertraline and fluvoxamine are licensed for this indication.

Psychological treatments

Behavioural therapy is superior to both relaxation therapy and placebo. Cognitive therapy (especially in CBT) appears to be effective.

Treating anxiety disorders in the presence of substance misuse

Treating comorbid substance misuse and anxiety can be tackled either by concentrating on one of the disorders first – but which one? – or by addressing them together. Psychological approaches are commonly applied to treat both substance misuse and many forms of anxiety, although lack of availability may be a limiting factor. Pharmacotherapy is frequently used to treat anxiety, but some form of psychological therapy is also usually required. In treating substance misuse, pharmacotherapy can be used as a substitute, for withdrawal or for maintaining abstinence.

Although both psychological and pharmacological treatments have been shown to be efficacious in treating either anxiety or a substance misuse disorder, there is limited knowledge about treating the comorbid condition (Scott *et al*, 1998). Most of the literature concerned with treating comorbid anxiety disorder concentrates on alcohol misuse, with little described on drug misuse. Clearly, if alcohol is being used to 'medicate' anxiety symptoms, then relapse after or during alcohol treatment is more likely if the anxiety disorder is not also treated. A pragmatic approach might be to target treatment on the patient's anxiety, even if he or she is still drinking, but in our experience this is more likely to have an impact if drinking is at non-dependent levels. Further details can be found in the British Association for Psychopharmacology guidelines (Lingford-Hughes *et al*, 2004).

Abstinence

Abstinence alone may improve anxiety symptoms. Although 40% of in-patients undergoing alcohol withdrawal had significantly elevated anxiety ratings in the first week, in the following week scores returned to normal (Brown *et al*, 1991). This emphasises the need to detoxify the patient first and then to reassess after 2–3 weeks of sobriety (see UK Alcohol Forum guidelines at http://www.ukalcoholforum.org). Even if abstinence is not achieved, minimising the contribution of alcohol or other drugs to the mental state is desirable.

Psychological treatment

Psychological strategies dominate treatment of alcohol and substance misuse, often involving group work. Inevitably, those with anxiety disorders, especially social anxiety disorder, find groups hard to attend. Thus, at best these individuals may not be able to benefit fully from the treatment offered for alcoholism and at worst the underlying cause of their alcoholism may be untreated. Many alcohol services run anxiety-management groups or tackle a patient's anxiety in individual therapy.

Given that achieving abstinence can be very difficult for patients because it involves removing their 'anxiolytic', is there any evidence to support concurrent treatment? Randall *et al* (2001) have addressed this question: people with alcoholism were randomly assigned to 12 weeks of CBT for their alcohol dependence alone or for alcohol and social anxiety disorder together. Drinking behaviour and social anxiety improved in both groups, but the group that received treatment for both anxiety and alcohol had poorer outcomes in drinking behaviour. Notably, no correlation was seen between improvement in anxiety and drinking behaviour. The reasons for this result were not clear, but alcohol may have been drunk in order to cope with the treatment programme for anxiety. This study did not explicitly address whether treatment for alcohol misuse or for anxiety should come first. Another study compared out-patient CBT with 12-step facilitation therapy in females with alcoholism and social anxiety disorder. Abstinence was achieved for longer with CBT than with 12-step therapy. However, the reverse was seen in males with the same disorder (Randall *et al*, 2000). These studies underscore the need for appropriate patient selection for treatment and that there is no universal panacea.

Pharmacological treatment

Imipramine was shown to improve panic disorder and drinking behaviour over 30 years ago (Quitkin *et al*, 1972), but few studies have been performed since. Buspirone, a 5-HT$_{1A}$ partial agonist, has also been shown to improve anxiety (some with generalised anxiety disorder) in alcoholism and also to improve drinking behaviour and reduce craving (Kranzler *et al*, 1994). The impact of SSRIs in treating comorbid alcohol misuse and anxiety is not clear.

When considering the use of SSRIs, it is important to recognise that subgroups of alcoholism do exist, in particular types 1 and 2 (Cloninger *et al*, 1981). In treating alcoholism either with or without a comorbid depressive disorder, SSRIs in type B (akin to type 2) alcoholism may not only result in no improvement but may actually reduce the impact of psychological treatment such as CBT (Kranzler *et al*, 1996). Thus, it should be borne in mind that for some people, SSRIs are not the drug of choice.

The use of benzodiazepines in an alcohol-dependent population is controversial (excluding use for alcohol withdrawal) and should not be undertaken without expert advice and monitoring. When abstinent, people with alcohol dependence may be at higher risk of benzodiazepine misuse and dependence because of the greater rewarding effects of these drugs (Ciraulo & Nace, 2000). Despite the level of concern, there is evidence to suggest that a history of alcohol misuse or dependence does not necessarily result in greater use of benzodiazepines, particularly for those who are less severely dependent. Therefore, their use should not be automatically excluded if the patient is misusing alcohol. Patients who are severely dependent or have antisocial personality disorder or polysubstance misuse are most at risk of misusing benzodiazepines. For some people, maintenance benzodiazepines can be indicated to maximise abstinence and minimise morbidity.

Although not specifically investigated in comorbid alcoholism and anxiety disorders, acamprosate may be useful. Most studies show that acamprosate as an adjunct to psychosocial treatment doubles the rate of abstinence, but clearly many patients are not helped. One study has suggested that patients who drink to overcome withdrawal or anxiety derived the greatest benefit (Lesch & Walter, 1996).

Conclusion

Successful treatment of an anxiety disorder can result in improved drinking behaviour. However, many patients will continue to drink alcohol, thus impairing their chance of recovery. In comorbid anxiety and alcohol misuse, drinking should be tackled first, but the anxiety disorder should be kept in mind and treatment for this should begin sooner rather than later. The picture is less clear for illicit drug misuse, with little data to guide management. Randomised controlled trials are needed to evaluate the efficacy of both psychological and pharmacological treatments, both singularly and together, in treating anxiety disorders complicated by substance misuse.

References

Argyropoulos, S. V., Sandford, J. J. & Nutt, D. J. (2000) The psychobiology of anxiolytic drugs. Part 2: Pharmacological treatments of anxiety. *Pharmacology and Therapeutics*, **88**, 213–227.

Baldwin, D. S., Anderson, I. M., Nutt, D. J., *et al* (2005) Evidence-based guidelines for the pharmacological treatment of anxiety disorders: recommendations from the British Association for Psychopharmacology. *Journal of Psychopharmacology*, **19**, 567–596.

Ballenger, J. C. (1993) Panic disorder: efficacy of current treatments. *Psychopharmacology Bulletin*, **29**, 477–486.

British Medical Association & Royal Pharmaceutical Society of Great Britain (2007) *British National Formulary* (March issue). BMJ Publishing Group and RPS Publishing.

Brooner, R. K., King, V. L., Kidorf, M., *et al* (1997) Psychiatric and substance use comorbidity among treatment-seeking opioid abusers. *Archives of General Psychiatry*, **54**, 71–80.

Brown, S. A., Irwin, M. & Schuckit, M. A. (1991) Changes in anxiety among abstinent male alcoholics. *Journal of Studies on Alcohol*, **52**, 55–61.

Carlson, J. G., Chemtob, C. M., Rusnak, K., *et al* (1998) Eye movement desensitization and reprocessing [EMDR] treatment for combat-related posttraumatic stress disorder. *Journal of Traumatic Stress*, **11**, 3–24.

Ciraulo, A. D & Nace, E. P. (2000) Benzodiazepine treatment of anxiety or insomnia in substance abuse patients. *American Journal of Addiction*, **9**, 276–284.

Cloninger, C. R., Bohman, M. & Sigvardsson, S. (1981) Inheritance of alcohol abuse. Cross-fostering analysis of adopted men. *Archives of General Psychiatry*, **38**, 861–868.

Coplan, J. D., Liebowitz, M. R., Gorman, J. M., *et al* (1992) Noradrenergic function in panic disorder. Effects of intravenous clonidine pre-treatment on lactate induced panic. *Biological Psychiatry*, **31**, 135–146.

Davidson, J. R., Potts, N., Richichi, E., *et al* (1993) Treatment of social phobia with clonazepam and placebo. *Journal of Clinical Psychopharmacology*, **13**, 423–428.

Devilly, G. J. & Spence, S. H. (1999) The relative efficacy and treatment distress of EMDR and a cognitive behavioural treatment protocol in the amelioration of post traumatic stress disorder. *Journal of Anxiety Disorders*, **13**, 131–157.

George, D. T., Zerby, A., Noble, S., *et al* (1988) Panic attacks and alcohol withdrawal: can subjects differentiate the symptoms? *Biological Psychiatry*, **24**, 240–243.

George, D. T., Nutt, D. J., Dwyer, B. A., *et al* (1990) Alcoholism and panic disorder: is the comorbidity more than coincidence? *Acta Psychiatrica Scandinavica*, **81**, 97–107.

George, D. T., Benkelfat, C., Rawlings, R. R., *et al* (1997) Behavioural and neuroendocrine responses to m-chlorophenylpiperazine in subtypes of alcoholics and in healthy comparison subjects. *American Journal of Psychiatry*, **154**, 81–87.

Heinz, A., Mann, K., Weinberger, D. R., et al (2001) Serotonergic dysfunction, negative mood states, and response to alcohol. *Alcoholism, Clinical and Experimental Research*, **25**, 487–495.

Himle, J. A., Abelson, J. L., Haghightgou, H., et al (1999) Effect of alcohol on social phobic anxiety. *American Journal of Psychiatry*, **156**, 1237–1243.

Keaney, K., Strang, J., Gossop, M., et al (2001) A double-blind randomized placebo-controlled trial of lofexidine in alcohol withdrawal: lofexidine is not a useful adjunct to chlordiazepoxide. *Alcohol and Alcoholism*, **36**, 426–430.

Kessler, R. C., McGonagle, K. A., Zhao, S., et al (1994) Lifetime and 12-month prevalence of DSM–III–R psychiatric disorders in the United States. *Archives of General Psychiatry*, **51**, 8–19.

Kessler, R. C., Crum, R. M., Warner, L. A., et al (1997) Lifetime co-occurrence of DSM–III–R alcohol abuse and dependence with other psychiatric disorders in the National Comorbidity Survey. *Archives of General Psychiatry*, **54**, 313–321.

Kranzler, H. R., Burleson, J. A., Del Boca, F. K., et al (1994) Buspirone treatment of anxious alcoholics. *Archives of General Psychiatry*, **51**, 720–734.

Kranzler, H. R., Burleson, J. A., Brown, J., et al (1996) Fluoxetine treatment seems to reduce the beneficial effects of cognitive–behavioural therapy in type B alcoholics. *Alcoholism, Clinical and Experimental Research*, **20**, 1534–1541.

Krausz, M., Degkwitz, P., Kühne, A., et al (1998) Comorbidity of opiate dependence and mental disorders. *Addictive Behaviors*, **23**, 767–783.

Kushner, M. G., Sher, K. J. & Beitman, B. D. (1990) The relation between alcohol problems and anxiety disorders. *American Journal of Psychiatry*, **147**, 685–695.

Lesch, O. & Walter, H. (1996) Subtypes of alcoholism and their role in therapy. *Alcohol and Alcoholism*, **31** (suppl. 1), 63–67.

Lingford-Hughes, A. R., Acton, P. D., Gacinovic, S., et al (1998) Reduced levels of the GABA-benzodiazepine receptor in alcohol dependency in the absence of grey matter atrophy. *British Journal of Psychiatry*, **173**, 116–122.

Lingford-Hughes, A. R., Welch, S. & Nutt, D. J. (2004) Evidence-based guidelines for the pharmacological management of substance misuse, addiction and comorbidity: recommendations from the British Association for Psychopharmacology. *Journal of Psychopharmacology*, **18**, 293–335.

Malizia, A. L., Cunningham, V. J, Bell, C. J., et al (1998) Decreased brain GABA A-benzodiazepine receptor binding in panic disorder. *Archives of General Psychiatry*, **55**, 715–720.

Merikangas, K. R., Mehta, R. L., Molnar, B. E., et al (1998) Comorbidity of substance use disorders with mood and anxiety disorders: results of the international consortium in psychiatric epidemiology. *Addictive Behaviors*, **23**, 893–907.

National Institute for Clinical Excellence (2004) *Management of Anxiety (Panic Disorder, with or without Agoraphobia, and Generalised Anxiety Disorder) in Adults in Primary, Secondary and Community Care. Clinical Guideline 22.* National Institute for Health and Clinical Excellence. http://www.nice.org.uk/guidance/CG22/niceguidance/pdf/English

Nutt, D. J. (1999) Alcohol and the brain. Pharmacological insights for psychiatrists. *British Journal of Psychiatry*, **175**, 114–119.

Nutt, D. J. & Cowen, P. J. (1987) Diazepam alters brain 5HT function in man: implications for the acute and chronic effects of benzodiazepines. *Psychological Medicine*, **17**, 601–607.

Pitman, R. K., Orr, S. P., Altman, B., et al (1996) Emotional processing during eye movement desensitization and reprocessing [EMDR] therapy of Vietnam veterans with post-traumatic stress disorder. *Comprehensive Psychiatry*, **37**, 419–429.

Potokar, J., Coupland, N., Wilson, S., et al (1999) Assessment of GABA A benzodiazepine receptor (GBzR) sensitivity in patients on benzodiazepines. *Psychopharmacology*, **146**, 180–184.

Quitkin, F. M., Rifkin, A., Kaplan, J., et al (1972) Phobic anxiety syndrome complicated by drug dependence and addiction. A treatable form of drug abuse. *Archives of General Psychiatry*, **27**, 159–162.

Randall, C. L., Thomas, S. E. & Thevos, A. K. (2000) Gender comparison in alcoholics with concurrent social phobia: implications for alcoholism treatment. *American Journal of Addiction*, **9**, 202–215.

Randall, C. L., Thomas, S. E. & Thevos, A. K. (2001) Concurrent alcoholism and social anxiety disorder: a first step toward developing effective treatments. *Alcoholism, Clinical and Experimental Research*, **25**, 210–220.

Regier, D. A., Farmer, M. E., Rae, D. S., *et al* (1990) Comorbidity of mental disorders with alcohol and other drug abuse. *JAMA*, **264**, 2511–2518.

Rothbaum, B. O. (1997) A controlled study of eye movement desensitization and reprocessing in the treatment of posttraumatic stress disordered sexual assault victims. *Bulletin of the Menninger Clinic*, **61**, 317–334.

Roy-Byrne, P. P., Lewis, N., Villacres, E., *et al* (1989) Preliminary evidence of benzodiazepine subsensitivity in panic disorder. *Biological Psychiatry*, **26**, 744–748.

Rudolph, U., Crestani, F. & Mohler, H. (2001) GABAA receptor subtypes: dissecting out their pharmacological functions. *Trends in Pharmacological Sciences*, **22**, 188–194.

Saunders, J. B., Aasland, O. G., Babor, T. F., *et al* (1993) Development of the Alcohol Use Disorders Identification Test (AUDIT): WHO Collaborative Project on Early Detection of Persons with Harmful Alcohol Consumption – II. *Addiction*, **88**, 791–804.

Schneier, F. R., Goetz, D., Campeas, R., *et al* (1998) Placebo-controlled trial of moclobemide in social phobia. *British Journal of Psychiatry*, **172**, 70–77.

Scott, J., Gilvarry, E. & Farrell, M. (1998) Managing anxiety and depression in alcohol and drug dependence. *Addictive Behaviors*, **23**, 919–931.

Versiani, M., Nardi, A. E., Mundim, F. D., *et al* (1992) Pharmacotherapy of social phobia. A controlled study with moclobemide and phenelzine. *British Journal of Psychiatry*, **161**, 353–360.

World Health Organization (1992) *The ICD–10 Classification of Mental and Behavioural Disorders. Clinical Descriptions and Diagnostic Guidelines*. WHO.

CHAPTER 16

An overview of psychological interventions for addictive behaviours

Adam Huxley and Alex Copello

Summary The efficacy of psychological interventions for the treatment of addiction problems has received considerable attention in the research literature as well as within the policy and service arenas. Psychological interventions can be used on their own or as an adjunct to pharmacological treatments. In UK drug treatment services attempts have been made to disseminate interventions based on psychological models of understanding addictive behaviours. There is an encouraging evidence base for the effectiveness of psychological interventions for a wide variety of addictive behaviours. Evidence-based psychological treatments include cognitive–behavioural and motivational treatments, contingency management, 12-step approaches and family and social interventions. Although the literature suggests that such treatments lead to improved outcomes when compared with no treatment at all, the evidence favouring one type of psychological intervention over another is less clear. Further research comparing the effectiveness of a broad range of psychological interventions delivered as brief or longer-term treatments needs to be undertaken with particular emphasis on pragmatic trials delivered in routine clinical settings and cost-effectiveness analyses. Other factors such as therapist characteristics and service variables are important in determining treatment effectiveness and need to be the focus of further research studies.

Psychological approaches to the treatment of drug and alcohol problems vary depending on the specific theoretical model on which they are based (e.g. cognitive, behavioural or social). Most psychological approaches, however, make use of the interaction between a therapist and a client (or client and family and/or other members of the social network) in order to raise awareness of and elicit changes in the client's behaviour (e.g. drug or alcohol use) as well as related factors, including thoughts and emotions.

Psychological interventions for clients misusing drugs or alcohol can be said to fall within two broad categories: (i) those that aim to help the individual make changes in their substance misuse behaviour, through reduction, stabilisation or abstinence; and (ii) those that aim to address co-occurring psychological difficulties such as anxiety, low mood, trauma, obsessive–compulsive problems and personality disorder (Wanigaratne *et al*, 2005). In practice, these psychological adjustment difficulties might be important in the origin and/or maintenance of an individual's substance-using behaviour and so to some extent these may need to be addressed even when the main focus of treatment is attempting to change that behaviour.

This chapter will focus on the first type of intervention, i.e. psychological interventions that aim to help people make changes in drug-using behaviour. The treatments described are based on processes hypothesised to influence substance use behaviour such as motivational factors, cognitive processes, skill development and social interactions.

Over recent years, there has been an increase in the development and evaluation of psychological interventions in the treatment of drug and alcohol problems. A comprehensive review of the evidence base for such interventions is beyond the scope of this chapter, and we focus on a description of the key clinical components of the various psychological treatments. Where relevant, recent key research studies are highlighted for each intervention type. For a more detailed analysis of the effectiveness of psychological interventions for addictive behaviours the reader is referred to reviews (e.g. Amato *et al*, 2004; Mayet *et al*, 2004; Wanigaratne *et al*, 2005) and to the National Institute for Health and Clinical Excellence's recently published guidelines on psychosocial interventions for drug problems in the UK (National Collaborating Centre for Mental Health, 2007). For a review of the effectiveness of psychological interventions for other psychological difficulties the reader is referred to Roth & Fonagy (2004).

Effectiveness of psychological interventions

The evidence for the effectiveness of psychological interventions is substantial across many diagnostic groups and settings (Department of Health, 2004). The research literature has shown that psychological interventions that target substance misusing behaviour lead to positive outcomes in treatment, most commonly indicated by either a reduction in, or abstinence from, the substance of choice. Further indication that psychological interventions promote improvements in clients' lives can be seen from the evidence of demonstrable changes in global functioning (quality of intimate relationships, physical health, employment and criminal behaviour, among others) and improvements in engagement and retention in treatment over time.

Wanigaratne *et al* (2005) have summarised the findings from the research on psychological treatments and put forward a variety of conclusions (Box 16.1).

The remainder of this chapter will concentrate on the psychological interventions that have been the focus of most research evaluation. For ease of reference we group the most rigorously evaluated psychological interventions into five categories: cognitive–behavioural approaches, motivational approaches, contingency-management-based interventions,

---

Box 16.1 Key components of psychological interventions for addiction

- There is a good evidence base for the efficacy of psychological treatments for substance misuse
- Making use of treatments that combine substitute prescribing and psychological interventions is more effective than either in isolation
- Psychological treatments are effective for substances where there are no substitute prescribing treatments
- Motivational interviewing and relapse prevention are effective across a range of substances
- The majority of the research suggests that no one form of psychological treatment is superior to another, although any form of psychological treatment leads to better outcomes than no treatment at all

(Wanigaratne *et al*, 2005)

12-step treatments, and family and social interventions. These categories are not perfectly delineated and there is some overlap, with some interventions focusing on common factors, for example the salient role of cognitions in both cognitive–behavioural therapy (CBT) and motivational approaches. However, they are useful for organising and reviewing existing treatments, and we outline key principles and strategies for each treatment type, with relevant recent studies.

Cognitive–behavioural approaches

Cognitive–behavioural therapy is based on the notion that thoughts and feelings govern our information processing system (i.e. how we view the world and make sense of it) and influence behaviour. In relation to substance misuse, the main goal of CBT is to reduce the level of substance use and associated harm. The basic premise of CBT as applied to substance misuse is that clients' thoughts and beliefs are central to the development and maintenance of addiction problems. For example, a client who believes that using drugs will help make them less anxious when meeting others is likely to continue using these drugs in social situations unless the belief is challenged or changed. The role of the therapist is to work collaboratively with the client in order to identify key patterns of thinking and behaviour that are involved in the maintenance of continued substance use and help the client to identify and develop skills to deal more adaptively with problems or difficult situations.

A key component of CBT is the development of a formulation that identifies factors and developmental processes that are involved in the origin and maintenance of the problem behaviour. This work may involve the identification of particular cycles, patterns or core beliefs that are implicated in the maintenance of the addictive behaviour. Cognitive–behavioural therapy is highly structured and collaborative, and sessions may include reviewing practice exercises (homework), debriefing on problems that have occurred between sessions, skills training and planning for the next session. Key strategies in CBT involve challenging faulty cognitions through alternative beliefs and the implementation of behavioural experiments.

Cognitive–behavioural therapy has good short-term outcomes among individuals misusing benzodiazepines (Vorma *et al*, 2002) and stimulants (Rosenblum *et al*, 1999; Baker *et al*, 2005). It has also shown good outcomes among pathological gamblers (Ladouceur *et al*, 2002), is reported to be more cost-effective than other treatments for those misusing opiates (Avants *et al*, 1999) and to reduce drug use by female opiate users (Pollack *et al*, 2002). Miller & Wilbourne's (2002) meta-analysis showed that a number of the top ten treatments for alcohol use disorders included interventions that had elements of CBT. Project MATCH found CBT as effective as motivational enhancement therapy and 12-step facilitation therapy (Project MATCH Research Group, 1997). A form of CBT called cognitive–behavioural integrated treatment (C–BIT) has been developed as an intervention for people with severe mental health problems who use substances and initial results show some promise (Graham *et al*, 2004, 2006).

Relapse prevention

Relapse prevention therapy is one of the most widely used cognitive–behavioural approaches to the treatment of addictive behaviours. It specifically addresses the nature of the relapse process and suggests coping strategies that are helpful when attempting to maintain positive change (Marlatt & Gordon, 1985). Relapse prevention is based on the idea that the likelihood of someone relapsing into previous problematic levels of substance use after a period of successful change or reduction is mostly determined by cognitive and behavioural processes as opposed to biological ones. Immediate determinants (e.g. high-risk situations, coping skills, outcome expectancies and the abstinence violation effect) and covert antecedents (e.g. lifestyle factors and urges and cravings) can both contribute to relapse. The original relapse prevention model (Marlatt & Gordon, 1985) and subsequent adaptations (e.g. Wanigaratne *et al*, 1990) outline a series of events and associated processes that may lead an individual from a high-risk situation to a lapse, a full-blown relapse or a successful outcome. The relapse prevention model incorporates numerous specific and global intervention strategies that allow therapist and client to address each step of the relapse process (Fig 16.1). Specific interventions include identifying high-risk situations for each client and enhancing the client's skills for coping with those situations, increasing the client's self-efficacy, managing lapses and restructuring the client's perceptions of the relapse process. Global strategies comprise balancing the client's lifestyle and helping him or her

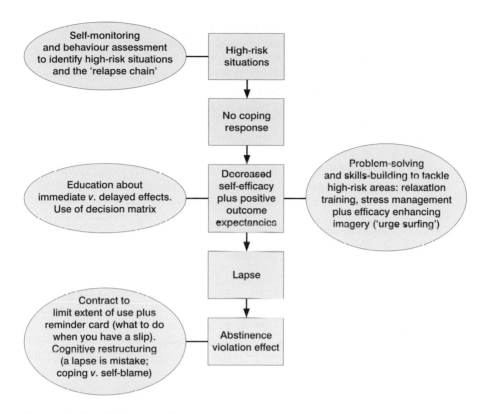

Fig. 16.1 Specific intervention strategies in the relapse prevention model (adapted from Dimeff & Marlatt, 1995: p. 181).

develop 'positive addictions', using stimulus-control and urge-management techniques, and developing 'relapse road maps'.

There is evidence of the effectiveness of relapse prevention with users of stimulants (McKay *et al*, 2002), cannabis (Stephens *et al*, 2000), alcohol (Irvin *et al*, 1999) and opiates (Abbot *et al*, 1998).

Motivational approaches

Motivational interviewing

Motivational interviewing was first described by Miller & Rollnick (1991) as a directive, client-centred counselling style for eliciting behavioural change by helping clients to explore and resolve ambivalence. In contrast to non-directive counselling, motivational interviewing is more focused and goal-directed. The examination and resolution of ambivalence is its central purpose, and the counsellor is intentionally directive in pursuing this goal. The spirit of motivational interviewing is centred on a collaborative relationship between therapist and client in which the therapist uses techniques such as reflection, summarising, open-ended questions and affirmations.

A significant amount of research details the efficacy of motivational interviewing as a brief intervention for substance misusing behaviours (Burke *et al*, 2003) as well as across other behavioural domains (Dunn *et al*, 2001). There is evidence of its efficacy for alcohol use problems (Miller & Wilbourne, 2002; Burke *et al*, 2003) as well as cannabis (Stephens *et al*, 2000), opiates (Saunders *et al*, 1995), stimulants (Stotts *et al*, 2001) and gambling (Hodgins *et al*, 2001) problems. Hettema *et al*'s (2005) meta-analysis of research on the effectiveness of motivational interviewing concluded that it generally increases treatment retention and adherence and that the effects emerge relatively quickly, although they tend to be highly variable across sites and providers.

Motivational enhancement therapy

Motivational enhancement therapy is a brief (3–5 sessions) structured clinical intervention derived from motivational interviewing. It is a style of counselling designed to engage ambivalent or resistant individuals in the treatment process and its focus is the resolution of ambivalence as a way of evoking intrinsic motivation to change (Miller *et al*, 1995a). Within an integrated treatment programme, the task of the motivational enhancement therapist is to prepare unmotivated clients for a course of treatment by encouraging 'change talk' and decreasing resistance to the notion of reducing their use of alcohol or drugs. Heather *et al*'s (1996) study showed that motivational enhancement therapy is more effective than behaviour-change skills training among problem drinkers. Motivational enhancement therapy has been shown to be as effective as other psychosocial approaches in two large randomised trials: Project MATCH (Project MATCH Research Group, 1997) and the United Kingdom Alcohol Treatment Trial (UKATT Research Team, 2005). For a further more detailed description of motivational approaches the reader is referred to chapter 17 in this volume.

Contingency-management-based interventions

The community reinforcement approach

The community reinforcement approach as described by Meyers & Smith (1995) is a broad-spectrum behavioural treatment for substance use problems that was developed to utilise social, recreational, familial and vocational reinforcers to aid clients in the recovery process. The community reinforcement approach acknowledges the powerful role of environmental contingencies in encouraging or discouraging substance use, and thus attempts to rearrange these contingencies such that non-using behaviour is more rewarding than using. The overall aim is to use the community to reward non-using behaviour so that the clients make healthy lifestyle changes. The community reinforcement approach is based on positive reinforcement instead of confrontation.

The approach has been developed to help clients work towards their specific goals by making use of functional analysis, a process that allows therapist and client to examine the triggers (thoughts, feelings and behaviours) leading to substance use and the immediate and long-term consequences of this behaviour. Community reinforcement works to replace clients' maladaptive behaviours with new coping strategies. 'Sobriety sampling' is a technique that teaches the client to abstain from alcohol for a mutually agreed limited period. Communication skills training is an important component of the approach's behavioural skills training. It helps clients increase positive interchanges in their intimate relationships. Clients also are taught problem-solving to develop more appropriate strategies for coping with their stressful environments than resorting to substance use.

The community reinforcement approach has been reported to be significantly more effective than drug counselling among stimulant users (Higgins et al, 1993) and more effective than standard treatment among clients using opiates (Gruber et al, 2000). There is also evidence of the effectiveness of community reinforcement combined with an incentive (vouchers) among cocaine users (Higgins et al, 1995; Roozen et al, 2004) and opiate users (Bickel et al, 1997). The community reinforcement approach and its components have been identified in several meta-analytic reviews of treatment for serious alcohol problems as having among the highest levels of treatment efficacy (Holder et al, 1991; Miller et al, 1995b; Finney & Monahan, 1986; Miller & Wilbourne, 2002).

Contingency management

Contingency management views substance addiction as a form of operant conditioning, i.e. drug use is controlled and shaped by its consequences. Reinforcers can therefore change behaviour if they are of sufficient magnitude and incompatible with substance use. A number of reinforcers have been used in contingency management programmes. The most common include vouchers that are given contingent on evidence of non-using behaviour such as urine test results. These vouchers can be exchanged for goods and services, including leisure activities. Some programmes, particularly in the USA where this approach has been implemented and researched, have provided privileges as reinforcers for change, for example 'take home' sorts of methadone or decreased level of supervised consumption.

Contingency management approaches have a strong evidence base, including a number of rigorously designed and conducted trials in the USA. A recent systematic review by Prendergast et al (2006) showed that such techniques can be particularly effective for the treatment of opiate and cocaine problems. The magnitude of the treatment effect was found to decline over time, although it was found that contingency management can establish and maintain abstinence for clients in order to encourage further engagement with psychosocial services. Although rarely used at present in UK practice, contingency management holds promise as an evidence-based approach to be used more widely in addiction services in the future.

Twelve-step approaches

Twelve-step approaches have their origins in self-help organisations such as Alcoholics Anonymous (AA) and Narcotics Anonymous (NA) (the Twelve Steps of NA are shown in chapter 1, Box 1.2). Addictive behaviours are viewed as a relapsing 'illness' and complete abstinence is the only treatment goal. Addiction is seen as the inability to control one's use of any mood-altering substance or behaviour despite awareness of its damaging consequences. Twelve-step approaches vary considerably but are based on the notion of working through a series of steps, on an individual or group basis, in order to facilitate recovery from addictive behaviours. The steps include admitting to a substance-related addiction, self-disclosure and self-appraisal, making amends where possible and supporting others in similar situations. Working through the steps, having one-to-one guidance and support from a senior member (a 'sponsor' who is also engaged in the programme) and participating in group meetings that can give rise to therapeutic processes similar to those found in psychotherapy groups (Emrick et al, 1977) are all integral components of 12-step approaches. Acceptance of the need for 'surrender' and abstinence from alcohol or other drugs are goals of the therapy. An important part of the therapeutic process is regular active participation in meetings and a willingness to accept a higher power as the locus of change in one's life.

Data concerning the effectiveness of 12-step treatments have been difficult to gather. Cook (1988) reviewed studies and found some indication of treatment efficacy but these studies were limited by the lack of a control group. Crits-Cristoph et al (1999) found that 12-step counselling led to better outcomes than other treatments for stimulant use. In Project MATCH, 12-step facilitation therapy was shown to be as effective as motivational enhancement therapy and cognitive–behavioural coping skills (Project MATCH Research Group, 1997). Emrick et al's (1993) meta-analysis of 107 studies on AA suggests a positive relationship between AA affiliation and psychological health.

Family and social interventions

An increasing range of family interventions are available to work with people with substance misuse problems, although implementation in routine addiction services remains limited (Copello & Orford, 2002). Two recent reviews of family interventions (Copello et al, 2005, 2006a) concluded that there is a growing evidence base to support family-focused interventions for substance misuse, with improved outcomes for both the misuser and affected family members. Such interventions can be categorised into three types:

- those aimed at involving the family in engaging the misuser in treatment
- those focused on treating the misuser after problems have developed
- those focused on affected family members in their own right.

A comprehensive review of these interventions is beyond the scope of this chapter, but three of the most commonly used are briefly described below.

Community reinforcement and family training

Community reinforcement and family training (CRAFT; Meyers et al, 1996) is an outgrowth of the community reinforcement approach. CRAFT was developed from a long tradition of work focusing on the influence of familial, social and vocational factors on people with drinking problems, in terms of reinforcing abstinence and assisting substance-related behavioural change. When Sisson & Azrin (1986) used this behavioural approach to give community reinforcement counselling to 12 family members of alcohol misusers, it improved the latter's treatment-seeking and reduced their drinking.

CRAFT has adapted a number of intervention strategies to work directly with 'concerned significant others' of treatment-resistant substance users, and has positive treatment outcomes with both alcohol and drug-misusing populations. The CRAFT process explores the interactions between the concerned significant other and the substance user in an attempt to increase rewarding interactions for non-using behaviour, as well as developing strategies to reduce levels of stress in the concerned significant other.

Behavioural couples therapy

Behavioural couples therapy (Fals-Stewart et al, 2004) has been subjected to a programme of well-designed studies. Behavioural couples therapy includes two main components:

- assessing and enhancing positive behavioural interactions between the substance user and partner
- improving communication skills.

It has mostly been evaluated on people with alcohol problems, and specific components for this application are shown in Box 16.2.

Reviews of efficacy indicate that, compared with individual approaches, behavioural couples therapy leads to reduced drinking and improved marital functioning (Fals-Stewart et al, 2004). Walitzer & Dermen (2004) found behavioural couples therapy also to be effective when the goal was one of moderation rather than abstinence: clients whose partners were included in treatment experienced fewer heavy drinking days and more abstinent/light drinking days in the year following treatment than clients who received individual treatment without the partner being involved.

> **Box 16.2** Specific components of behavioural couples therapy for alcohol misuse
>
> - Cognitive-behavioural strategies to help the drinker stop drinking and acquire coping skills to respond to both drinking-specific and general life problems
> - Strategies that teach family members to support the drinker's efforts to change, reduce protection for drinking-related consequences, develop better skills to cope with negative affect, and talk about alcohol-related topics
> - Strategies to improve the couple's relationship by increasing positive exchanges and improving communication and problem-solving skills
> - Behavioural contracts between intimate partners to support the use of medication
>
> (O'Farrell & Fals-Stewart, 1999)

Social behaviour and network therapy

Social behaviour and network therapy is a synthesis that incorporates a number of strategies used in other evidence-based family and social-network-based treatment approaches (Copello *et al*, 2002). It is based on the premise that to give the best chance of a good outcome, people with serious drinking and/or drug problems need to develop a social network that promotes and supports behavioural change. As part of the treatment the therapist attempts to engage members of this network in sessions with the misuser and network members where possible, and uses strategies based on communication, interactions between the user and the network members, and relapse management techniques. The aim is to develop positive support for change in the substance-misusing behaviour.

The UKATT trial (UKATT Research Team, 2005) involved a large randomised comparison of social behaviour and network therapy and motivational enhancement therapy in a range of treatment services in the UK. Results showed both therapies to be equally effective and cost-effective. In addition, a feasibility study of social behaviour and network therapy for drug misuse has shown promising outcomes in terms of reduced drug use and high levels of acceptance of the therapy by both clients and therapists in routine drug services (Copello *et al*, 2006*b*).

The evidence for counselling

The counselling approaches offered within most substance misuse services vary in nature, frequency, theoretical model and application. Most counselling approaches share some similarity in the interactional style used with clients, which is usually person-centred, non-directive and humanistic. Because of the variation of these approaches and the limited data from controlled studies it is difficult to ascertain the extent of the evidence for general counselling approaches for addiction. There are studies that show greater improvements in opiate-dependent clients who have had counselling than in those receiving methadone treatment only (Woody *et al*, 1983; McLellan *et al*, 1993). There is also evidence of some effectiveness of general alcohol counselling (Finney & Monahan, 1986), although Holder *et al* (1991) found it to be less effective than CBT and 12-step approaches. Kletter (2003) showed that cocaine use was reduced during court-enforced counselling, and Gossop *et al* (2006) found that drug-focused counselling was associated with less frequent heroin and cocaine use among clients attending methadone treatment when compared with no counselling at all. In the latter study, drug- or alcohol-focused 'counselling' was defined as spending 'quite a lot' or 'a great deal' of time discussing drug or alcohol problems, and non-counselling was defined as spending only 'a little' time discussing these issues. The lack of clarity in relation to the content and structure of the various and varied 'counselling' interventions makes it difficult to establish with any degree of certainty the efficacy or effectiveness of these approaches.

Other psychological interventions

Almost every therapeutic approach has been used at some time to treat addictive behaviour. As Orford (2001: p. 280) notes, psychological treatments for addiction have been particularly diverse and different forms of therapy have been in vogue for different types of behaviour at different times, almost always backed up by impressive rationale. Yet the research evidence base for some approaches is less clear.

Smith *et al* (2006) conclude that there is little evidence that therapeutic communities offer significant benefits in comparison with other residential treatments, or that one type of therapeutic community is better than another. There is some evidence to suggest the usefulness of other psychological interventions such as cue exposure treatments (Monti *et al*, 1993). Cue exposure is a technique that considers tolerance, withdrawal and cravings for drugs or alcohol as conditioned states that are amenable to change or extinction. Some evidence has been put forward for aversion therapy for stimulant users (Frawley & Smith 1992) and assertiveness training for alcohol misuse (Chaney 1989). Other therapeutic techniques being applied in addiction treatment settings include neuro-linguistic programming (Lewis, 1994) and other talking therapies. The evidence for these approaches is limited and caution must be exercised when considering approaches that claim to be deliverable with minimal training and support. Psychodynamic perspectives in addiction have also been considered (Potik *et al*, 2007).

Other important factors

With few exceptions, most of the published research has come from studies in the USA and there is a paucity of UK data comparing the efficacy of psychological treatments for substance misuse. Drummond *et al*'s (2004) study shows that US research may not be comparable when applied to UK treatment services, and Curran & Drummond (2005) suggest that further research is required on the effectiveness of psychological treatments delivered in differing clinical contexts by a wide variety of professionals in 'typical' rather then 'ideal' settings.

Research suggests that other factors often contribute to the efficacy of psychological interventions. There is evidence to suggest that therapists who are empathic and authoritative (Truax & Carkhoff, 1967), non-judgemental (Stanton & Standish, 1997) and who display a high level of interpersonal skill (Najavits & Weiss, 1994) have better outcomes with substance-misusing clients. Other factors, such as speed of uptake, length and intensity of treatment (Raistrick & Tober, 2004), have been found to influence treatment outcomes and hence need to be considered in future research.

Conclusion

Research indicates that a number of psychological interventions are efficacious in reducing substance use or maintaining abstinence, either as the sole intervention or as an adjunct to pharmacological treatment. These interventions are more likely to be effective when they are administered in a structured way by therapists who have had the appropriate training and receive regular supervision and support. Key skills include reflective practice, case formulation and an awareness of the complexities associated with someone who presents with addictive behaviours.

Future research on psychological interventions needs to consider the efficacy of such approaches as well as their cost-effectiveness. Psychological interventions have an important place among the range of treatments available for substance misuse. The ever-increasing evidence base of their efficacy means that they should no longer be considered optional adjuncts to pharmacological treatments. The recently published NICE guidelines for psychosocial interventions (National Collaborating Centre for Mental Health, 2007) should assist in the identification and implementation of effective psychosocial treatments across provider settings.

References

Abbott, P. J., Weller, S. B., Delaney, H. D., *et al* (1998) Community reinforcement approach in the treatment of opiate addicts. *American Journal of Drug and Alcohol Abuse*, 24, 17–30.

Amato, L., Davoli, M., Ferri, M., *et al* (2004) Effectiveness of interventions on opiate withdrawal treatment: an overview of systematic reviews. *Drug and Alcohol Dependence*, 73, 219–226.

Avants, S. K., Margolin, A., Sindelar, J. L., et al (1999) Day treatment versus enhanced standard methadone services for opioid dependent patients. A comparison of clinical efficacy and cost. *American Journal of Psychiatry*, **156**, 27–33.

Baker, A., Lee, N. K., Claire, M., et al (2005) Brief cognitive behavioural interventions for regular amphetamine users. A step in the right direction. *Addiction*, **100**, 367–378.

Bickel, H. K., Amass, L., Higgins, S., et al (1997) Effects of adding behavioral treatment to opioid detoxification with buprenorphine. *Journal of Counseling and Clinical Psychology*, **65**, 803–810.

Burke, B. L., Arkowitz, H. & Menchola, M. (2003) The efficacy of motivational interviewing: a meta-analysis of controlled clinical trials. *Journal of Consulting and Clinical Psychology*, **71**, 843 861.

Chaney, E. F. (1989) Social skills training. In *Handbook of Alcoholism Treatment Approaches: Effective Alternatives* (eds R. K. Hester & W. R. Miller), pp. 206–221. Pergamon Press.

Cook, C. H. (1988) The Minnesota Model in the management of drug and alcohol dependency: miracle, method or myth? *British Journal of Addiction*, **83**, 625–634.

Copello, A. & Orford, J. (2002) Addiction and the family: is it time for services to take notice of the evidence? *Addiction*, **97**, 1361–1363.

Copello, A., Orford, J., Hodgson, R., et al (2002) Social behaviour and network therapy: basic principles and early experiences. *Addictive Behaviours*, **27**, 345–366.

Copello, A., Velleman, R. & Templeton, L. (2005) Family interventions in the treatment of alcohol and drug problems. *Drug and Alcohol Review*, **24**, 369–385.

Copello, A., Templeton, L. & Velleman, R. (2006a) Family intervention for drug and alcohol misuse. Is there a best practice? *Current Opinion in Psychiatry*, **19**, 271–276.

Copello, A., Williamson, E., Orford, J., et al (2006b) Implementing and evaluating social behaviour and network therapy in drug treatment practice in the UK: a feasibility study, *Addictive Behaviours*, **31**, 802–810.

Crits-Cristoph, P., Siqueland, L., Blaine, J., et al (1999) Psychosocial treatment for cocaine dependence. National Institute for Drug Abuse Collaborative Cocaine Treatment Study. *Archives of General Psychiatry*, **56**, 493–502.

Curran, H. V. & Drummond, C. (2005) *Psychological Treatments for Substance Misuse and Dependence* (Foresight Brain Science, Addiction and Drugs Project). Department of Trade and Industry.

Department of Health (2004) *Organising and Delivering Psychological Therapies. July 2004.* Department of Health.

Dimeff, L. A. & Marlatt, G. A. (1995) Relapse prevention. In *Handbook of Alcoholism Treatment Approaches: Effective Alternatives* (2nd edn) (eds R. K. Hester & W. R. Miller). Allyn & Bacon.

Drummond, D. C., Kouimtsidis, C., Reynolds, M., et al (2004) *The Effectiveness and Cost-effectiveness of Cognitive Behaviour Therapy for Opiate Misusers in Methadone Maintenance Treatment: A Multicentre Randomised Controlled Trial (UKCBTMM [UK CBT in Methadone Maintenance Treatment Project]). Final Report to the Department of Health Research and Development Directorate.* Department of Health.

Dunn, E. C., Deroo, L. & Rivara, F. P. (2001) The use of brief interventions adapted from motivational interviewing across behavioural domains: a systematic review. *Addiction*, **96**, 1725–1742.

Emrick, C. D., Lassen, C. L. & Edwards, M. T. (1977) *Non-Professional Peers as Therapeutic Agents.* Pergamon Press.

Emrick, C. D., Tonigan, J. S., Montgomery, H., et al (1993) Alcoholics Anonymous: what is currently known? In *Research on Alcoholics Anonymous: Opportunities and Alternatives* (eds B. S. McCrady & W. R. Miller), pp. 41–76. Rutgers University Center of Alcohol Studies.

Fals-Stewart, W., O'Farrell, T. & Birchler, G. (2004) Behavioural couples therapy for substance abuse. Rationale, methods and findings. *Science and Practice Perspectives*, **2**, 30–41.

Finney, J. W. & Monahan, S. C. (1986) The cost effectiveness of treatment of alcoholism: a second approximation. *Journal of Studies on Alcohol*, **47**, 122–134.

Frawley, P. & Smith, J. (1992) One-year follow up after multi-modal in-patient treatment for cocaine and methamphetamine dependencies. *Journal of Substance Abuse Treatment*, **9**, 271–286.

Gossop, M., Stewart, D. & Marsden, J. (2006) Effectiveness of drug and alcohol counselling during methadone treatment: content, frequency and duration of counselling and association with substance use outcomes. *Addiction*, **101**, 404–412.

Graham, H., Copello, A., Birchwood, M., *et al* (2004) *Cognitive–Behavioural Integrated Treatment*. John Wiley & Sons.

Graham, H., Copello, A., Birchwood, M., *et al* (2006) A preliminary evaluation of integrated treatment for co-existing substance use and severe mental health problems: impact on teams and service users. *Journal of Mental Health*, **15**, 577–591.

Gruber, K., Chutuape, M. A. & Stitzer, M. L. (2000) Reinforcement-based intensive outpatient treatment for inner city opiate abusers. A short-term evaluation. *Drug and Alcohol Dependence*, **57**, 211–223.

Heather, N., Rollnick, S., Bell, A., *et al* (1996) Effects of brief counselling among male heavy drinkers identified on general hospital wards. *Drug and Alcohol Review*, **15**, 29–38.

Hettema, J., Steele, J. & Miller, W. (2005) Motivational interviewing. *Annual Review of Clinical Psychology*, **1**, 91–111.

Higgins, S. T., Budney, A. J., Bickel, W. K., *et al* (1993) Achieving cocaine abstinence with a behavioral approach. *American Journal of Psychiatry*, **150**, 763–769.

Higgins, S. T., Budney, A. J., Bickel, H. K., *et al* (1995) Outpatient behavioural treatment for cocaine dependence: one-year outcome. *Experimental and Clinical Psychopharmacology*, **3**, 205–212.

Hodgins, D. C., Currie, S. R. & el-Guebaly, N. (2001) Motivational enhancement and self-help treatments for problem gambling. *Journal of Consulting and Clinical Psychology*, **69**, 50–57.

Holder, H., Longabaugh, R., Miller, W. R., *et al* (1991) The cost effectiveness of treatment for alcoholism: a first approximation. *Journal of Studies on Alcohol*, **52**, 517–540.

Irvin, J. E., Bowers, C. A., Dunn, M. E., *et al* (1999) Efficacy of relapse prevention: a meta-analytic review. *Journal of Consulting and Clinical Psychology*, **67**, 563–570.

Kletter, E. (2003) Counselling as an intervention for cocaine-abusing methadone maintenance patients. *Journal of Psychoactive Drugs*, **35**, 271–277.

Ladouceur, R., Sylvain, C., Boutin, C., *et al* (2002) Cognitive treatment of pathological gambling. *Journal of Nervous and Mental Disease*, **189**, 774–780.

Lewis, B. (1994) *Sobriety Demystified: Getting Clean and Sober with NLP and CBT*. Kelsey & Company Publishing.

Marlatt, G. A., & Gordon, J. R. (1985) *Relapse Prevention: Maintenance Strategies in the Treatment of Addictive Behaviours*. Guilford Press.

Mayet, S., Farrell, M., Ferri, M., *et al* (2004) Psychosocial treatment for opiate abuse and dependence. *Cochrane Database of Systematic Reviews*, issue 4. Wiley InterScience.

McKay, J. R., Pettinati, H. M., Morrison, R., *et al* (2002) Relation of depression diagnoses to 2-year outcomes in cocaine-dependent patients in a randomised continuing care study. *Psychology of Addictive Behaviours*, **16**, 225–235.

McLellan, A. T., Arndt, I., Metzger, D. S., *et al* (1993) The effects of psychosocial services in substance abuse treatment. *JAMA*, **269**, 1953–1959.

Meyers, R. J. & Smith, J. E. (1995) *Clinical Guide to Alcohol Treatment: The Community Reinforcement Approach*. Guilford Press.

Meyers, R. J., Dominguez, T. P. & Smith, J. E. (1996) Community reinforcement training with concerned others. In *Sourcebook of Psychological Treatment Manual for Adult Disorders* (eds V. B. Van Hasselt & M. Hersen), pp. 257–294. Plenum Press.

Miller, W. R., & Rollnick, S. (1991) *Motivational Interviewing*. Guilford Press.

Miller, W., & Wilbourne, P. L. (2002) Mesa Grande: a methodological analysis of clinical trials of treatment for alcohol use disorders. *Addiction*, **97**, 265–277.

Miller, W. R., Zweben, A., DiClemente, C. C., *et al* (1995a) *Motivational Enhancement Therapy Manual: A Clinical Research Guide for Therapists Treating Individuals with Alcohol Abuse and*

Dependence (Project MATCH Monograph Series, vol. 2). National Institute on Alcohol Abuse and Alcoholism.

Miller, W. R., Brown, J. M., Simpson, T. L., *et al* (1995b) What works? Methodological analysis of the alcohol treatment outcome literature. In In *Handbook of Alcoholism Treatment Approaches: Effective Alternatives* (2nd edn) (eds R. K. Hester & W. R. Miller), pp. 278–291. Allyn and Bacon.

Monti, P. M., Rohsenow, D. J., Rubonis, A.V., Niaura, *et al* (1993) Cue exposure with coping skills treatment for male alcoholics: a preliminary investigation. *Journal of Consulting and Clinical Psychology*, **61**, 1011–1019.

Najavits, L. M. & Weiss, R. D. (1994) Variations in therapist effectiveness in the treatment of patients with substance use disorders: an empirical review. *Addiction*, **89**, 679–688.

National Collaborating Centre for Mental Health (2007) *Drug Misuse: Psychosocial Interventions* (NICE Clinical Guideline 51). NICE.

O'Farrell, T. J. & Fals-Stewart, W. (1999) Treatment models and methods: family models. In *Addictions: A Comprehensive Guidebook* (eds B. S. McCrady & E. E. Epstein), pp. 287–305. Oxford University Press.

Orford, J. (2001) *Excessive Appetites: A Psychological View of Addictions* (2nd edn). John Wiley & Sons.

Pollack, M. H., Penara, S. A., Bolton, E., *et al* (2002) A novel cognitive behavioural approach for treatment resistant drug dependence. *Journal of Substance Abuse Treatment*, **23**, 335–342.

Potik, P., Adelson, M. & Schreiber, S. (2007) Drug addiction from a psychodynamic perspective: methadone maintenance treatment (MMT) as transitional phenomena. *Psychology and Psychotherapy: Theory and Research*, **80**, 311–325.

Prendergast, M., Podus, D., Finney, J., *et al* (2006) Contingency management for treatment of substance use disorders: a meta analysis. *Addiction*, **101**, 1546–1560.

Project MATCH Research Group (1997) Matching alcoholism treatments to clients heterogeneity: Project MATCH post treatment drinking outcomes. *Journal of Studies in Alcohol*, **58**, 6–29.

Raistrick, D. & Tober, G. (2004) Psychosocial interventions. *Psychiatry*, **3**, 36–39.

Roozen, H., Boulogne, J., Tulder, M., *et al* (2004) A systematic review of the effectiveness of the community reinforcement approach in alcohol, cocaine and opioid addiction. *Drug and Alcohol Dependence*, **74**, 1–13.

Rosenblum, A., Magura, S., Palij, M., *et al* (1999) Enhanced treatment outcomes for cocaine-using methadone patients. *Drug and Alcohol Dependence*, **54**, 207–218.

Roth, T. & Fonagy, P. (2004) *What Works for Whom? A Critical Review of Psychotherapy Research* (2nd edn). Guilford Press.

Saunders, B., Wilkinson, C. & Phillips, M. (1995) The impact of brief motivational intervention with opiate users attending a methadone programme. *Addiction*, **90**, 415–424.

Sisson, R. W. & Azrin, N. H. (1986) Family member involvement to initiate and promote treatment of problem drinkers. *Journal of Behavior Therapy and Experimental Psychiatry*, **17**, 15–21.

Smith, L. A., Gates, S. & Foxcroft, D. (2006) Therapeutic communities for substance related disorder. *Cochrane Database of Systematic Reviews*, issue 1. Wiley InterScience.

Stanton, M. D. & Standish, W. R. (1997) Outcome, attrition and family-couples treatment for drug abuse: a meta-analysis and review of the controlled, comparative studies. *Psychological Bulletin*, **122**, 170–191.

Stephens, R. S., Roffman, R. A. & Curtin, L. (2000) Comparison of extended versus brief treatments for marijuana use. *Journal of Consulting and Clinical Psychology*, **68**, 898–908.

Stotts, A. L., Schmitz, J. M., Rhoades, H. M., *et al* (2001) Motivational interviewing with cocaine-dependent patients: a pilot study. *Journal of Consulting and Clinical Psychology*, **69**, 858–862.

Truax, D. B. & Carkhuff, R. R. (1967) *Toward Effective Counselling and Psychotherapy*. Aldine Publishing.

UKATT Research Team (2005) Effectiveness of treatment for alcohol problems: findings of the randomised UK alcohol treatment trial. *BMJ*, **331**, 541–544.

Vorma, H., Naukkarinen, H., Sarna, S., *et al* (2002) Treatment of out-patients with complicated benzodiazepine dependence: comparison of two approaches. *Addiction*, **97**, 851–859.

Walitzer, K. S. & Dermen, K. H. (2004) Alcohol-focused spouse involvement and behavioural couples therapy: evaluation of enhancements to drinking reduction treatment for male problem drinkers. *Journal of Consulting and Clinical Psychology*, **72**, 944–955.

Wanigaratne, S., Pullin, J., Wallace, W., *et al* (1990) *Relapse Prevention for Addictive Behaviours: A Manual for Therapists*. Blackwell Publishing.

Wanigaratne, S., Davies, P., Pryce, K., *et al* (2005) *The Effectiveness of Psychological Therapies on Drug Misusing Clients*. National Treatment Agency for Substance Misuse.

Woody, G. E., Luborsky, L., McLellan, A. T., *et al* (1983) Psychotherapy for opiate addicts: does it help? *Archives of General Psychiatry*, **40**, 639–645.

CHAPTER 17

Motivational interviewing

Janet Treasure

Summary   Motivational interviewing is a style of patient-centred counselling developed to facilitate change in health-related behaviours. The core principle of the approach is negotiation rather than conflict. In this chapter I review the historical development of motivational interviewing and give some of the theoretical underpinnings of the approach. I summarise the available evidence on its usefulness and discuss practical details of its implementation, using vignettes to illustrate particular techniques.

Motivational interviewing was conceived when Bill Miller, a psychologist from the USA, sat with colleagues from Norway and described what sort of therapeutic approach worked for people with alcohol problems. The process of discovery may have been like the technique itself: a gradual process of listening, reflecting to check understanding, and clarification. Once the form was crystallised it was subjected to a detailed academic analysis. Questions concerning what, how, when, why and for whom have been studied. The approach has been fitted with various theoretical models relating to interpersonal processes and behaviour change. The resultant technique was described in a textbook co-written with Steve Rollnick, a South African psychologist working in Wales (Miller & Rollnick, 1991). International training has meant that the approach has been widely disseminated and evaluated in a variety of settings.

What is motivational interviewing?

Motivational interviewing is a directive, patient-centred counselling style that aims to help patients explore and resolve their ambivalence about behaviour change. It combines elements of style (warmth and empathy) with technique (e.g. focused reflective listening and the development of discrepancy). A core tenet of the technique is that the patient's motivation to change is enhanced if there is a gentle process of negotiation in which the patient, not the practitioner, articulates the benefits and costs involved. A strong principle of this approach is that conflict is unhelpful and that a collaborative relationship between therapist and patient, in which they tackle

---

Box 17.1   The four central principles of motivational interviewing

1   Express empathy by using reflective listening to convey understanding of the patient's point of view and underlying drives

2   Develop the discrepancy between the patient's most deeply held values and their current behaviour (i.e. tease out ways in which current unhealthy behaviours conflict with the wish to 'be good' – or to be viewed to be good)

3   Sidestep resistance by responding with empathy and understanding rather than confrontation

4   Support self-efficacy by building the patient's confidence that change is possible

---

the problem together, is essential. The four central principles of motivational interviewing are shown in Box 17.1.

Rollnick & Miller (1995) defined specific behaviours, which could be taught to therapists, that they felt lead to a better therapeutic alliance and better outcome. These are summarised in Box 17.2.

The first four items in Box 17.2 explore the reasons that sustain the behaviour and aim to help the patient shift the decisional balance of pros and cons into the direction of change. The last two items cover the interpersonal aspects of the relationship. The therapist provides warmth and optimism and takes a subordinate, non-powerful position, which emphasises the patient's autonomy and right to choose whether to accept and make use of the therapist's knowledge and skills.

Instead of trying to fix the patient's health problem by forceful instruction, therapists need to use warmth and respect to persuade the patient to want

---

Box 17.2   The skills of a good motivational therapist

- Understand the other person's frame of reference
- Filter the patient's thoughts so that statements encouraging change are amplified and statements that reflect the status quo are dampened down
- Elicit from the patient statements that encourage change, such as expressions of problem recognition, concern, desire, intention to change and ability to change
- Match the processes used in the theory to the stage of change; ensure that they do not jump ahead of the patient
- Express acceptance and affirmation
- Affirm the patient's freedom of choice and self-direction

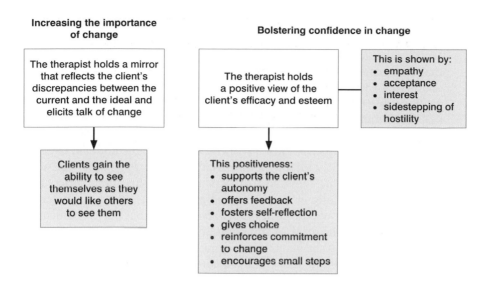

Increasing the importance of change

The therapist holds a mirror that reflects the client's discrepancies between the current and the ideal and elicits talk of change

Clients gain the ability to see themselves as they would like others to see them

Bolstering confidence in change

The therapist holds a positive view of the client's efficacy and esteem

This is shown by:
- empathy
- acceptance
- interest
- sidestepping of hostility

This positiveness:
- supports the client's autonomy
- offers feedback
- fosters self-reflection
- gives choice
- reinforces commitment to change
- encourages small steps

Fig. 17.1   How motivational therapy works.

to change. The process of motivational intervention is outlined in Fig. 17.1. Its aim is twofold: to increase the importance of change and to bolster the patient's confidence that change can happen. Motivational therapists have to be able to suppress any propensity they might have to show the 'righting reflex', i.e. to try to solve problems and set things right (this is not easy because health professionals are drawn into the field because they want actively to help others). Motivational therapists have to be flexible and able to have an appropriate balance between acceptance and drive for change.

Motivational interviewing helps change patterns of behaviour that have become habitual. It works in small doses to produce a large effect. It seems to work by reducing behaviours in the patient that interfere with therapy. Patient attributes regarded as markers of a poor prognosis, such as anger and low motivation, are less serious obstacles with motivational interviewing.

The evidence base

Miller and his group at the Center on Alcoholism, Substance Abuse, and Addictions (CASAA) in Albuquerque demonstrated that the style of the therapist's interaction is a critical component in facilitating change (for a review of this literature see Miller, 1995a). Therapists' expectations of change in their patients influenced patients' adherence and outcomes. The rate of patient resistance varied as a response to the therapeutic style: confrontation produced high levels of resistance, whereas a patient-centred approach reduced opposition.

Miller developed a short intervention (the Drinker's Check-Up) which operationalised some of the factors found to be useful in increasing motivation. Motivational feedback using this instrument was compared with feedback that used a standard confrontation-based approach. The outcome, in terms of drinking 1 year later, was poorer in the group of patients who were given confrontational feedback (Miller *et al*, 1993). In a further study it was found that if the motivational feedback of the Drinker's Check-Up was given as an initial intervention prior to admission to an in-patient clinic, outcome was improved (abstinence rates 3 months after discharge doubled to 57%, compared with 29% without the intervention). The therapists (unaware of group assignment) reported that patients given this intervention had participated more fully in treatment and appeared to be more motivated (Bien *et al*, 1993; Brown & Miller, 1993). The approach has been modified for pregnant women who drink. A similar intervention, developed for polydrug misuse, was found to be efficacious in pilot studies. However, this was not replicated in a later full study. The explanation for this was evident from analysis of the transcripts of the sessions. The need to complete the process of commitment to change within one session interfered with development of the patients' motivation, and some therapists were moving ahead of the patient in an attempt to complete the protocol (Miller *et al*, 2003).

Project MATCH: alcohol misuse

Motivational interviewing has been developed into a manualised four-session therapeutic intervention called motivational enhancement therapy for alcohol (Miller *et al*, 1994). This was used for the motivational inter-viewing intervention in Project MATCH (Box 17.3), the largest clinical trial ever conducted for alcoholism treatment methods. In this collaborative study, involving nine clinical sites in the USA, 1726 patients were randomly assigned to one of three interventions: 12 sessions of 12-step facilitation therapy, or 4 sessions of motivational enhancement therapy, or 12 sessions of cognitive–behavioural skills training. Five sites treated out-patients, and four gave intensive hospital in-patient treatment. Overall, the three treatment modalities yielded substantial and equivalent outcomes for up to a year following treatment (Project MATCH Research Group, 1998).

The primary aim of Project MATCH was to examine whether it is helpful to match patients to specific interventions. Over the 3-year follow-up period it was found that patients with higher state-trait anger responded best to motivational enhancement therapy (Project MATCH Research Group, 1997). It was concluded that motivational interviewing is a cost-effective technique to facilitate change in patients who might be resistant to treatment.

Other problem behaviours

Motivational enhancement therapy manuals are also available for cannabis and polydrug misuse (Miller, 1995*b*) and bulimia nervosa (Treasure & Schmidt, 1997).

Box 17.3   Information sources and manuals

- The standard text on motivational interviewing is *Motivational Interviewing: Preparing People for Change* (Miller & Rollnick, 2002). This is part of the growing 'Applications of Motivational Interviewing Series', edited by Stephen Rollnick and William Miller (Guilford Press).

- The Motivational Interviewing website gives information about the approach, training courses, research, abstracts, videos and so on (http://www.motivationalinterview.org)

- The Motivational Interviewing Skill Code (MISC) (http://casaa.unm.edu/download/misc.pdf) and the Motivational Interviewing Treatment Integrity (MITI) code (http://casaa.unm.edu/download/miti.pdf) are assessment instruments that may be used to maintain quality assurance in motivational interviewing

- Manuals for motivational enhancement therapy in alcohol and drug misuse (Miller *et al*, 1994; Miller, 1995*b*) and bulimia nervosa (Treasure & Schmidt, 1997)

- The Project MATCH website is at http://www.commed.uchc.edu/match/default.htm. Manuals of the treatment procedures used in the project are available from http://www.commed.uchc.edu/match/pubs/monograph.htm

---

Motivational interviewing has been found to be effective for various forms of behaviour change (for full details the systematic reviews of Dunn *et al* (2001) and Burke *et al* (2003) are recommended). Adaptations of motivational interviewing have been found to be useful for people whose problems involve alcohol, drugs, diabetes, dual diagnosis and bulimia. Mixed results have been found for its efficacy in smoking. Moderate treatment effect sizes of between 0.25 and 0.57 have been found for adaptations of motivational interviewing.

A detailed, regularly updated bibliography on the application of motivational interviewing for various clinical conditions can be found at http://www.motivationalinterview.org. Reviews have been published of the use of motivational interviewing in general (Hettema *et al*, 2005; Rubak *et al*, 2005; Knight *et al*, 2006), for alcohol problems (Vasilaki *et al*, 2006) and for adolescent substance use problems (Tait & Hulse, 2003). It is now being applied more widely in medicine and psychiatry to address poor treatment adherence in conditions such as hypertension (Shroeder *et al*, 2004), psychosis (Healey *et al*, 1998), eating disorders (Treasure & Schmidt, 1997; Wilson & Schlam, 2004) and comorbidity with drug and alcohol misuse (Barrowclough *et al*, 2001). It can also be used to improve the general health of patients with psychiatric disorders by focusing on maladaptive elements of their lifestyle, for example smoking, weight gain and inadequate exercise (e.g. VanWormer & Boucher, 2004).

What is effective implementation?

The process of change within motivational interviewing interventions has been studied in order to highlight the key strategies needed for their implementation. Miller *et al* (1993) found that a low level of resistance within the session predicts change. Resistance often arises in the presence of confrontation, and if the therapist behaves in a way that minimises resistance, change follows. An increase in the rate of 'self-motivational statements' (utterances by the patient that express interest in and/or intent to change) is positively associated with behaviour change.

Therapists differ in their adherence to the principles of motivational interviewing. Within Project MATCH, in which there was intensive training and monitoring to ensure equitable delivery between therapists, therapist effects on outcome persisted even after controlling for the effects of other variables. Empathy is a strong predictor of therapist efficacy. Other elements, which are more difficult to put into practice, include communicating belief in the patient's abilities and judgement, i.e. hope, respect, possibilities, freedom to change and faith in the person. The role of the therapist is to respect the patient and to hold an optimistic concept of the patient's potential for goodness (high self-esteem and self-efficacy) and to help the patient work within this framework. The therapist needs to be able to shift flexibly between acceptance and change.

Training courses in motivational interviewing are mostly relatively short (2–3 days). Miller & Mount (2001) evaluated the effectiveness of a 2–3 day training workshop in motivational interviewing for counsellors by studying samples of practice before and after the course. They found statistically significant changes in counsellors' behaviour consistent with the principles of motivational interviewing, but these changes were not large enough to make a difference for patients. Thus, continued practice, supervision and monitoring are needed in addition to 3-day training to attain and maintain standards.

The Albuquerque group led by Miller is developing instruments to measure therapist adherence to motivational interviewing principles. Two of these are now available: the Motivational Interviewing Skill Code (MISC) and the Motivational Interviewing Treatment Integrity (MITI) code (Box 17.3).

Theory

Although motivational interviewing started from a basis of clinical empiricism, several theoretical models (e.g. the transtheoretical model of change, which is described below, and dissonance theory) have been borrowed to provide an academic framework.

Models of health behaviour change

The basic principle that underpins most models of health behaviour change is that people hold a range of representations about their problematic symptoms and behaviours. For example, at one extreme are individuals who are stoical or in denial and neglect themselves or their symptoms. At the other are those who display abnormal illness behaviour and readily adopt the sick role. Most models of health behaviour change include the idea that there are at least two components to readiness to change. These are importance/conviction and confidence/self-efficacy (Keller & Kemp-White, 1997; Rollnick *et al*, 1999), encapsulated in the adage 'ready, willing and able'. 'Importance' relates to why change is needed. The concept includes the personal values and expectations that will accrue from change. 'Confidence' relates to the person's belief that they have the ability to master behaviour change. Motivational interviewing works on both of these dimensions by helping the patient to articulate why it is important for them to change and by increasing self-efficacy so that they have confidence to do so.

The transtheoretical model of change

Often there is confusion between, and fusion of, motivational interviewing and the transtheoretical model of change developed by Prochaska and co-workers (Prochaska & Norcross, 1994; Prochaska & Velicer, 1997).

The transtheoretical model of change breaks down the concept of readiness to change into stages, from not even thinking about it to maintaining change once it is made (Box 17.4). One of the implications of this model is that for each stage certain helping behaviours are particularly constructive.

Motivational interviewing and the transtheoretical model of change developed separately but synchronously. Motivational interviewing has no theoretical backbone, and the transtheoretical model filled some of this vacuum. Motivational interviewing is the type of process that is useful for people who are in the early stages of change. DiClemente, who worked with the Rhode Island group developing the transtheoretical model, was a co-author of the manual on motivational enhancement therapy used for project MATCH (Miller *et al*, 1994).

Box 17.4   The stages of change in the transtheoretical model

1   Precontemplation, not even ready to think about change seriously
2   Contemplation, ready to think about change
3   Determination, preparing to make plans for change
4   Action, implementing change
5   Maintenance, ensuring that the change in behaviour becomes habitual

---

Resistance to behaviour change

Two forms of resistance can impede behaviour change. The first relates to the 'problem' that is being considered and the second to the patient–therapist relationship. As regards the 'problem', there may be a conflict between the individual's conceptualisation of their behaviour and that of the family or society. Thus, individuals with, for example, anorexia nervosa or drug and alcohol misuse may not see any need to change their behaviour and will have been coerced into treatment by family and friends or statutory agencies. Human beings are inherently intolerant of lack of choice and can become motivated to do the opposite of what is requested: so-called 'reactance'. The propensity to this response lies on a behavioural dimension, with the poles ranging from oppositional to compliant.

The other source of resistance, the patient–therapist relationship, often relates to the patient's representations of helping/parental/authoritarian relationships or values about individual rights.

Individuals who are prone to both types of resistance are those with high levels of anger, aggressiveness and impulsivity and those with a need for control and with high levels of avoidance.

The effect of resistance in therapy has been reviewed in several studies by Beutler and colleagues (Beutler *et al*, 2002). Resistance, which is marked by anger or defensiveness, is associated with a poor outcome to therapy.

Motivational interviewing has an explicit focus on resistance in therapy. Indeed, in Project MATCH motivational interviewing was most effective in people who were angry. Within motivational interviewing there are special techniques to work with resistance. These are variations on reflective listening such as 'amplified' reflection, in which the patient's resistance and 'negative change' position is overstated. This works on the assumption that the oppositional tendency of the patient will lead to a withdrawal back to the middle ground. Another approach is to use a 'double-sided' reflection, which highlights the patient's ambivalence. The emphasis is on the individual's autonomy in the matter of change.

Motivational strategies in practice

The following examples of patient–therapist dialogue illustrate the use of some of the motivational techniques mentioned above. The patient is a young woman who attends an eating disorders clinic and is subsequently admitted to hospital to receive specialist treatment for severe weight loss.

Eliciting concerns – statements that affirm the need to change

The following open question is linked to a starting sentence setting the scene by acknowledging the ambivalence or resistance that is common in people with anorexia nervosa attending a clinic.

Therapist: Usually when people come to this clinic the driving force behind it has been other people such as their family or doctor. Please would you tell me how you got to come here today?

Patient: Well, my mother has been worried about me and kept nagging at me to do something.

Therapist: Your mother is concerned about your health. [A simple reflection.]

Patient: Yes, she says I'm too thin. She keeps crying and says that my heart might stop.

Therapist: Have you noticed any health difficulties that suggest that there might be some grounds for her concerns? For example, can you tell me about your periods? [This sentence sets the scene for eliciting concerns by encouraging the young woman to take an external perspective, in order to sidestep her resistance. The therapist opens up the conversation, focusing on the domains in which there are common difficulties in anorexia nervosa.]

Sidestepping resistance

It is important to try not to join in with a patient's anger and not to confront the patient. Instead, the therapist should reflect back the emotion of the outburst and take a low power position.

Patient: I'm just going to leave here and lose weight again!

Therapist: You're angry that after all the work you've done as an in-patient things don't feel much different. I'm sorry that the team haven't been able to help you to be able to recognise the need to nurture yourself. I'm sorry that we've been unable to help enough. [In this statement the therapist reflects the anger that underlies the patient's statement and expands on the meaning behind it, which is that the in-patient team has failed to live up to expectations.]

Reflecting ambivalence – the use of double-sided reflections

The therapist sidesteps a confrontational response to the following statement by making a double-sided reflection that highlights the patient's ambivalence about change.

Patient: I am not prepared to let my weight go above 35 kg.

Therapist: You're terrified about what will happen if you start to attend to your nutritional needs [empathy with the fear of change] and you know that there are clear signs that your body is suffering when your weight is below 40 kg – for example your blood glucose runs at a dangerously low level and your bones are continuing to dissolve.

Conclusion

Motivational interviewing has many applications within psychiatry, as it is particularly helpful for use in settings where there is resistance to change. The principles are simple but practice is less easy, and stringent quality control is needed to ensure that therapists adhere to the spirit of the process.

However, once the overall skill is integrated, honed and maintained it can be adapted to many situations. Practitioners following the implications of the transtheoretical model of change are flexible in their use of interventions. They might use a style of practice based on motivational interviewing for patients who are undecided about change (in precontemplation and contemplation) and later shift to a style of therapy informed more by cognitive–behavioural techniques when the person is committed to change. This is where the art and judgement of therapy come into play. People do not simply switch into a stable motivational state. A sensitive and empathic therapist will know when to back off from a skills-based approach into a more motivational stance. Unfortunately, time-limited and manualised therapies do not lend themselves to such an approach. There always needs to be room for flexibility to adjust for individual differences in the readiness to change.

References

Barrowclough, C., Haddock, G., Tarrier, N., *et al* (2001) Randomized controlled trial of motivational interviewing, cognitive behavior therapy, and family intervention for patients with comorbid schizophrenia and substance use disorders. *American Journal of Psychiatry*, **158**, 1706–1713.

Beutler, L. E., Moleiro, C. & Talebi, H. (2002) Resistance in psychotherapy: what conclusions are supported by research. *Journal of Clinical Psychology*, **58**, 207–217.

Bien, T. H., Miller, W. R. & Tonigan, J. S. (1993) Brief interventions for alcohol problems: a review. *Addiction*, **88**, 315–335.

Brown, K. L. & Miller, W. R. (1993) Impact of motivational interviewing on participation and outcome in residential alcoholism treatment. *Psychology of Addictive Behaviours*, **7**, 238–245.

Burke, B. L., Arkowitz, H. & Menchola, M. (2003) The efficacy of motivational interviewing: a meta-analysis of controlled clinical trials. *Journal of Consulting and Clinical Psychology*, **71**, 843–861.

Dunn, C., Deroo, L. & Rivara, F. P. (2001) The use of brief interventions adapted from motivational interviewing across behavioral domains: a systematic review. *Addiction*, **96**, 1725–1742.

Healey, A., Knapp, M., Astin, J., *et al* (1998) Cost-effectiveness evaluation of compliance therapy for people with psychosis. *British Journal of Psychiatry*, **172**, 420–424.

Hettema, J., Steele, J., & Miller, W. R. (2005) Motivational interviewing. *Annual Review of Clinical Psychology*, **1**, 91–111.

Keller, V. F. & Kemp-White, M. (1997) Choices and changes: a new model for influencing patient health behavior. *Journal of Clinical Outcome Management*, **4**, 33–36.

Knight, K. M., McGowan, L., Dickens, C., *et al* (2006) A systematic review of motivational interviewing in physical health care settings. *British Journal of Health Psychology*, **11**, 319–332.

Miller, W. (1995*a*) Increasing motivation for change. In *Handbook of Alcoholism Treatment Approaches. Effective Alternatives* (eds R. K. Hester & W. R. Miller), pp. 89–104. Allyn & Bacon.

Miller W. R. (1995*b*) *Motivational Enhancement Therapy with Drug Abusers.* University of Albuquerque Department of Psychology and CASAA. http://motivationalinterview. org/clinical/METDrugAbuse.PDF.

Miller, W. R. & Mount, K. A. (2001) A small study of training in motivational interviewing. Does one workshop change clinician and patient behavior? *Behavioural and Cognitive Psychotherapy*, **29**, 457–471.

Miller, W. & Rollnick, S. (1991) *Motivational Interviewing: Preparing People to Change Addictive Behaviour*. Guilford Press.

Miller, W. R. & Rollnick, S. (2002) *Motivational Interviewing: Preparing People for Change*. Guilford Press.

Miller, W. R., Benefield, R. G. & Tonigan, J. S. (1993) Enhancing motivation for change in problem drinking: a controlled comparison of two therapist styles. *Journal of Consulting and Clinical Psychology*, **61**, 455–461.

Miller, W. R., Zweben, A., DiClemente, C. C., *et al* (1994) *Motivational Enhancement Therapy Manual: A Clinical Research Guide for Therapists Treating Individuals with Alcohol Abuse and Dependence* (Project MATCH Monograph Series vol. 2). National Institute of Alcohol Abuse and Alcoholism.

Miller, W. R., Yahne, C. E. & Tonigan, J. S. (2003) Motivational interviewing in drug abuse services: a randomized trial. *Journal of Consulting Clinical Psychology*, **71**, 754–763.

Prochaska, J. O. & Norcross, J. (1994) *Systems of Psychotherapy: A Transtheoretical Analysis*. Brooks/Cole Publishing.

Prochaska, J. O. & Velicer, W. F. (1997) The transtheoretical model of health behavior change. *American Journal of Health Promotion*, **12**, 38–48.

Project MATCH Research Group (1997) Project MATCH secondary a priori hypotheses. *Addiction*, **92**, 1671–1698.

Project MATCH Research Group (1998) Matching alcoholism treatments to patient heterogeneity: Project MATCH three-year drinking outcomes. *Alcohol Clinical Experimental Research*, **22**, 1300–1311.

Rollnick, S. & Miller, W. R. (1995) What is motivational interviewing? *Behavioural and Cognitive Psychotherapy*, **23**, 325–335.

Rollnick, S., Mason, P. & Butler, C. (1999) *Health Behaviour Change*. Churchill Livingstone.

Rubak, S., Sandboek, A., Lauritzen, T., *et al* (2005) Motivational interviewing: a systematic review and meta-analysis. *British Journal of General Practice*, **55**, 305–312.

Schroeder, K., Fahey, T. & Ebrahim, S. (2004) How can we improve adherence to blood pressure-lowering medication in ambulatory care? Systematic review of randomized controlled trials. *Archives of Internal Medicine*, **164**, 722–732.

Tait, R. J. & Hulse, G. K. (2003) A systematic review of the effectiveness of brief interventions with substance using adolescents by type of drug. *Drug and Alcohol Dependence*, **22**, 337–346.

Treasure, J. L. & Schmidt, U. H. (1997) *A Clinician's Guide to Management of Bulimia Nervosa (Motivational Enhancement Therapy for Bulimia Nervosa)*. Psychology Press.

VanWormer, J. J. & Boucher, J. L. (2004) Motivational interviewing and diet modification: a review of the evidence. *Diabetes Educator*, **30**, 404–419.

Vasilaki, E. I., Hosier, S. G. & Cox, W. M. (2006) The efficacy of motivational interviewing as a brief intervention for excessive drinking: a meta-analytic review. *Alcohol and Alcoholism*, **41**, 328–335.

Wilson, G. T. & Schlam, T. R. (2004) The transtheoretical model and motivational interviewing in the treatment of eating and weight disorders. *Clinical Psychology Review*, **24**, 361–378.

CHAPTER 18

Substance misuse in adolescents

Harith Swadi and Sangeeta Ambegaokar

Summary   The increasing prevalence of substance misuse among adolescents means that child and adolescent mental health clinicians now have to seriously consider providing specialist assessment and treatment to young people with such disorders. This chapter outlines the differences between adolescent and adult substance misuse and why clinical approaches need to be different. It also proposes an assessment scheme that focuses on a contextual approach to understanding the drivers behind substance use in young people. Finally the possible screening treatment and intervention approaches are outlined. Two appendices provide a short screening instrument and the components of a semi-structured assessment.

There is increasing evidence that substance misuse among British adolescents is escalating (Miller & Plant, 1996; Sutherland & Willner, 1998). In 1992 the prevalence of drug use among adolescents aged 12–17 years referred to mental health services in England was 13.1% (16.3% among boys and 9.3% among girls) (Swadi, 1992). In more recent data from the USA, prevalence of substance use disorders in mental health treatment settings ranged from 19% to 87% (Deas-Nesmith *et al*, 1998; Aarons *et al*, 2001).

In the UK there has been historical emphasis on prevention rather than treatment for substance misuse by adolescents. However, there is increasing evidence that universal prevention strategies are relatively ineffective and limited to mild effects on drinking behaviour in adolescence (Spoth *et al*, 1998), although targeted selective prevention may be more effective (Tobler *et al*, 2000; Gottfredson & Wilson, 2003; Stewart *et al*, 2005). There has now been a significant increase in the provision of services for young people with substance misuse issues in the UK involving the development of a number of treatment models (Didlock & Cheshire, 2005).

Why treat adolescents?

Some have viewed substance use in adolescence as a normative behaviour during that period of development, given the fact that alcohol use and experimentation with drugs are so widespread among adolescents (Miller & Plant, 1996; Johnston *et al*, 1998). With that in mind, a potential point of contention is whether or not we should concern ourselves with treatment. Is it not possible that adolescents may just grow out of the habit of using psychoactive substances? There are several reasons supporting early and possibly vigorous intervention:

- while it is true that most adolescents using psychoactive substances will eventually grow out of it, some will not – they will become substance-dependent adults (Crome *et al*, 1998)
- substance misuse has an epidemic character through peer influence
- misuse is associated with significant comorbidity and psychosocial and health risks (Zeitlin, 1999)
- clinical experience suggests that substance misuse is possibly more likely to be treated successfully in adolescence than in adulthood
- the preventive value of treating adolescent substance misusers can be realised through a reduction in the demand for adult substance misuse services and the associated reduction in HIV and AIDS morbidity.

Substance misuse in adolescents is, on the whole, significantly dissimilar to that in adults. The aetiological factors, the patterns of use, the context of use and the therapeutic approaches can all be different:

- In adults attending substance misuse clinics, drug use is primarily a need to counter the effects of not taking drugs (i.e. the effects of the withdrawal syndrome). Adolescents take drugs because they provide them with something that they perceive as positive. Dependence is unusual among adolescents.
- In adolescents multiple drug use is the rule rather than the exception (Martin *et al*, 1996) and the idea of a favourite substance is uncommon. Adolescents are less likely to be involved in substances carrying higher prison tariffs and rarely inject. They are more involved in binges and are usually affected by the consequences of acute intoxication rather than chronic use.
- Motivation towards treatment is more likely to be an adult characteristic. Adults are particularly motivated by severe adverse consequences. Adolescents are usually reluctant patients and help-seeking behaviour is seldom their characteristic. They have usually experienced fewer adverse consequences and are less motivated to change. Although they may be motivated to resolve substance-related problems, they commonly have little motivation to abstain (Brown, 1999).
- Developmental differences make it necessary to take different approaches. Adolescents are still in the process of shaping their values and attitudes, and have different coping strategies from adults. For example, experience in handling stress, dealing with interpersonal conflict and negotiating change are more likely to be adult characteristics. Many adolescents have great difficulties in relationships and with personal and social skills – issues that almost always have to be addressed. Choice and decision-making are skills that have not yet fully developed in adolescents.

- Adult substance misusers often present to services at the later stages of the addiction process – usually physical and/or psychological dependence. Adolescents are usually at an earlier stage in the process. Therefore, detoxification is rarely needed in adolescents but rehabilitation is often needed because substance misuse seriously affects the development of many basic life skills – education, social relationships, employment skills, etc.

In conclusion, the needs of adolescent substance users are different from those of adults. Furthermore, they present to services with a complex pattern of psychological, personal and social problems and needs, including delinquent behaviour, homelessness, family problems, and educational and vocational needs.

First point of contact

The agencies most likely to first encounter (and so refer) adolescents who use drugs are social services, courts, schools and primary health workers. A proportion of individuals are referred to child mental health services for reasons other than substance misuse (usually behavioural problems). Substance misuse tends to emerge as a significant problem later in the assessment process. Unlike adults, adolescents rarely refer themselves for treatment. At the first point of contact, it is essential to determine whether substance use is problematic or not. This will in turn determine the need for further detailed and/or specialist assessment. The use of a screening instrument can be very useful in this respect. The Substance Misuse in Adolescence Questionnaire (SMAQ; Swadi, 1997) is a short questionnaire (nine yes/no items) which helps child welfare workers to identify adolescents who need a detailed multidisciplinary assessment (see Appendix 18.1). Psychometric evaluation in a British population of substance-misusing adolescents suggested that a total of five or more 'yes' answers is a strong indication for referral. Other, more detailed screening instruments have been used in the USA, but none has been validated in the UK (Meyers *et al*, 1999). They tend to be rather long and require some specialist training beyond that available to most agencies of first contact in the UK.

It is also important to determine whether the adolescent is in need of protection and/or crisis intervention, and whether there are any urgent legal issues that need to be addressed (Meyers *et al*, 1999).

Detailed assessment

If the screening process indicates that some kind of intervention or treatment is necessary, then the key to the latter lies in a comprehensive assessment of the individual (see Appendix 18.2 for a detailed assessment scheme). This will almost invariably be carried out by a number of professionals from different disciplines. The objective of the assessment is to determine the meaning and significance of the (substance-using) behaviour for the adolescent in the context of his or her family and environment. The type of intervention, its focus and its outcome depend to a large extent on the result of the assessment. The assessment also aims to identify the deficits that need to be addressed (such as social and life skills deficits, family communication problems and educational difficulties) and the assets that could be potentiated. An important issue is matching patients with treatment. The main factor in deciding this is the degree of handicap, the level of use and the adolescent's circumstances. For example, less affected adolescents, with a relatively short period of use and less severe or absent psychopathology, respond better to cognitive–behavioural approaches, whereas those with antisocial problems respond better to interactional therapy, particularly group therapy. Clinical experience suggests that those using substances socially often need less-intensive treatment – family intervention or individual counselling may suffice. The treatment process should have a well-defined and realistic goal and should address all the therapeutic needs of the individual, including substance misuse problems.

The assessment should also determine the most suitable treatment setting. The possibilities include out-patient, residential and day programmes. Unless the presentation is severe or chaotic, most individuals can be treated on an out-patient or day basis, with particular attention to educational needs. However, most will need input from different professionals with different skills and the support and collaboration of a number of agencies such as social services, voluntary organisations, education and health.

The main components of a comprehensive assessment are described below.

Pattern of use and its significance

Unlike adult addicts, who mainly use psychoactive substances just to feel 'normal', adolescents use such substances for many different reasons. It is essential to determine the context of use, as it has a crucial bearing on the intervention process. There are five different clinical contexts of adolescent involvement (Nowinski, 1990).

Exploratory or experimental

The primary motive in this type of substance misuse is curiosity and risk-taking. The mood-altering effects are secondary to the adventure of use. Use takes place mostly with others. The user may try more than one substance, but usually not more than a few times. The adolescent is experimenting with the 'mood swing' caused by psychoactive substances.

Social

The context here is strictly social, for example, parties, friends' houses, car parks, bicycle sheds. The primary motive is social acceptance. The peer group plays a large role. Substances are shared freely or sold at cost. The aim is to fit in with the crowd and to loosen up. The adolescent is usually still experimenting with the mood swing.

Emotional or instrumental

In this context, the adolescent learns to use substances purposefully to manipulate feelings, emotions and behaviour, i.e. to elicit or to inhibit certain behaviours and feelings. The adolescent is generally seeking the mood swing. There are two types of instrumental use.

Generative\hedonistic

The purpose is to seek pleasure and to have fun. Use is characterised by binges motivated by the desire to 'get high' and feel good. The purpose is to elicit pleasurable feelings or to explore new feelings or emotions.

Suppressive\compensatory

The purpose is to cope with stress and uncomfortable feelings, i.e. to suppress negative and distressing emotions. Mostly, use is solitary but it can also take place with the peer group.

Habitual

Typically, the frequency of use begins to show a characteristic of compulsiveness and preoccupation. Lifestyle and activities begin to converge around psychoactive substances. Former relationships, activities and friends begin to be replaced by new substance-related ones. Sleep and concentration difficulties begin to appear. Withdrawal symptoms appear occasionally, especially after periods of heavy sustained use. Craving may occur, tolerance may increase and the adolescent may begin to think about use most of the time. Behavioural problems increase and school performance becomes seriously affected. The adolescent is preoccupied with the mood swing.

Dependent or addictive

This is the stage at which physical and psychological addictions become the main feature. Tolerance, craving, withdrawal symptoms and the compulsion to use become prominent. The adolescent is completely preoccupied with use and life centres on the substance and the next 'fix'. The adolescent takes substances only to feel normal.

Adolescents in the first two categories of use (exploratory and social) tend to be primarily involved with lower-tariff substances such as volatile substances, cannabis and amphetamines, whereas those using habitually could be involved in a variety of substances, including opiates and crack cocaine.

Substance misuse has different consequences depending on the individual, the pattern of use and the environment. These consequences must be documented. Problematic substance use can be defined as that which has resulted in demonstrable or documented evidence of sustained adverse consequences, with evidence of continued use despite these consequences. This would be in areas related to education (e.g. being expelled or having left school prematurely), delinquency (e.g. being arrested or involved in theft), intra-familial relationships (e.g. running away from home or violence towards family members) and psychiatric symptomatology (e.g. severe conduct problems or depressive symptoms). Such consequences make treatment and/or intervention extremely desirable or even necessary.

Associated psychopathology (comorbidity)

Psychopathology is increasingly emerging as a very influential factor, in relation not only to initiation into substance use but also to response to intervention and outcome (Scourfield et al, 1996). Comorbidity is linked to earlier use of cannabis and alcohol, parental substance use, physical or sexual abuse, earlier relapse following treatment, a higher risk of suicide, violence and pregnancy, and poorer engagement in treatment (Riggs et al, 1995; Grella et al, 2001; Tomlinson et al, 2004).

Clinicians should be able to recognise and treat coexisting psycho-pathology. According to US data (Wilens et al, 2003) the most common disorders associated with young substance misusers are the disruptive behaviour disorders, which include conduct disorder, oppositional defiant disorder and attention-deficit hyperactivity disorder (ADHD). Treatment of ADHD with pharmacotherapy may halve the risk of later development of substance misuse. In addition, its treatment with psychostimulants in childhood has not been shown to increase the risk of developing later substance misuse problems.

The strong links with emotional problems are now also universally accepted. Studies have found that the prevalence of depressive disorders ranges from 24% to 50% in young substance misusers (Bukstein et al, 1992; Deykin et al, 1992). Consistently, reports indicate that affective symptoms predominate in females, whereas conduct problems are more common in males. It is very important to be aware of the existence of mood disorders among substance users, as they are easy to miss, particularly when associated with conduct problems and antisocial behaviour (Swadi, 1992). Substance misuse is also related to increased suicidal ideation and attempted suicide. Many adolescents who 'overdose' do so while under the influence of alcohol or other drugs. A major risk factor for completed suicide after parasuicide in adolescents is substance misuse (Hawton et al, 1993).

Young substance misusers also show higher rates of psychosomatic complaints, anxiety, relationship problems and social dysfunction. Adolescents with poor coping skills tend to use psychoactive substances to deal with stress (Labouvie, 1986) and as a means of emotional self-regulation. There is also an emerging link between eating disorders (both anorexia and bulimia) and substance misuse, particularly alcohol use (Lavik et al, 1991). A psychiatric assessment must include a good account of adverse life events, particularly victimisation and loss.

Another important point in the assessment is the need to ascertain the temporal relationship between existing psychopathology and substance misuse, although this can often be difficult to untangle. Particular care should be taken when assessing adolescents with coexisting affective problems and substance misuse. Psychiatric problems may be the result of substance misuse, particularly central nervous system depressants. On the other hand, many adolescents with psychopathology turn to psychoactive substances for psychological relief.

Functioning

The assessment of functioning should include an appraisal of the individual's motivation for treatment and their education, coping skills, social skills, self-perception and emotional adjustment. The primary objective is to determine strengths/assets and weaknesses/deficiencies. Building on assets and addressing deficiencies is an essential part of the intervention process.

Family assessment

This is almost a 'must', given the many different ways in which family factors play a role in adolescent substance misuse. Family background and parenting styles, including parental divorce, parental discord, family disruption, negative communication, inconsistent parental discipline and lack of closeness, have been identified as influential risk factors in adolescent drug use (Stoker & Swadi, 1990; Isohanni et al, 1991). Families of children who misuse drugs have been characterised as being those whose fathers are distant and disengaged and whose mothers are too involved (Kaufman & Kaufman, 1979; Stoker & Swadi, 1990). Families can also behave in a way that increases the risk of maintaining substance use. Commonly, clinicians refer to 'enabling behaviour' (Nowinski, 1990). This is a natural response by the family to stay intact and to survive. It motivates families to compensate for one dysfunctional member and to avoid issues that threaten family integrity. It may involve all family members – siblings may conspire to keep parents in the dark or parents may avoid the subject. Bailing out, minimising and avoiding are the most frequent enabling behaviours. The family assessment should focus on family dynamics, communication patterns, cohesion, affect and value transmission.

Treatment options

The need for treatment and its type and intensity depend on the stage of involvement and the degree of impairment or handicap caused by substance use. The treatment plan should address the personal and environmental needs of the adolescent, including any concurrent psychiatric illness, social skills and educational deficits, physical health and family problems. It should take the form of a multidisciplinary and inter-agency (usually involving social services and education) package that is agreed with the adolescent and the family.

Psychological treatments (see chapters 16 and 17)

Individual counselling

One approach in individual counselling is the use of brief intervention techniques. This began with the offering of simple advice in primary care settings, which led to significant reduction in substance use, particularly alcohol. Cognitive–behavioural therapy has also been found to have some benefit in the treatment of adolescent substance misuse (Waldron *et al*, 2001; Liddle, 2002). However, a more recent technique is motivational interviewing (Miller & Rollnick, 1991; chapter 17, this volume), based on the 'stages of change' model (Prochaska & DiClemente, 1982).

Motivational interviewing is becoming increasingly popular and has provided a new framework of understanding for therapeutic intervention. Intervention begins with identifying where the individual may currently be within the cycle of change. The objective is then to help them move from one stage to another by increasing their motivation to change behavioural patterns, including substance use. This approach is particularly useful with resistant clients (such as adolescents). Different stages require different techniques: Box 18.1 shows the stages and the therapist's main objectives at each stage, using the example of alcohol misuse.

In essence, people who are not sufficiently motivated to change, or who do not appear ready to use treatment to deal with their problem, are at higher risk for early relapse (DeLeon *et al*, 1997).

Motivational enhancement treatment has consistently been shown to be effective with substance-misusing adults (Burke *et al*, 2003). It has also been shown to be effective in combination with cognitive–behavioural therapy in the treatment of cannabis use in adolescents (Dennis *et al*, 2004).

Family work and therapy

Families can be helpful in the process of therapy, but they can also be obstacles. Families and family dynamics are influential as risk factors for initiation and progression (the process of moving from experimentation to chronic use). Nevertheless, most recovered addicts report that family systems were very helpful in their recovery. In particular, the family can help improve adherence to treatment that involves medication.

Family therapy can take the form of structural, strategic or behavioural work. It should be time limited and goal oriented, especially using goals identified by the family. Family tasks are very useful here. The therapist should keep the issue of drug use alive and avoid getting into other 'red herring' issues. If the family members wish to discuss other issues, they should be advised that they can do so after the current goal has been achieved. Parents' roles should be enhanced and they should be given a major advisory and decision-making capacity with regard to the treatment

Box 18.1   The therapist's role in motivational interviewing for alcohol misuse

Stage 1 Pre-contemplation
The individual is not thinking about stopping drinking – the therapist should raise doubt and increase the person's perception of the risks and problems involved in alcohol use

Stage 2 Contemplation
The individual is thinking about change: 'Maybe I should stop drinking' – tip the balance; evoke reasons for change; strengthen self-efficacy for change

Stage 3 Determination
The individual is determined to change: 'I must stop drinking' – help the individual to determine the best course of action for change

Stage 4 Action
The individual actually changes: 'I stopped drinking' – help to take steps towards maintaining change

Stage 5 Maintenance
The individual continues not to drink – help to identify and use strategies to prevent relapse

Stage 6 Relapse
The individual goes back to drinking – help to renew contemplation

process. Family therapy can reduce conflict among family members and help the adolescent replace friendships that encourage deviant behaviour with others that encourage social conformity (Knight & Simpson, 1996).

Multidimensional family therapy

A very effective and well-evaluated approach in family therapy, predominantly in the USA, is multidimensional family therapy. This is an out-patient, family-based, behaviourally or strategically oriented approach (Liddle, 1998). It views adolescent drug use in terms of a matrix of influences (individual, family, peer and community). Behavioural changes occur via multiple pathways, in differing contexts and through different mechanisms.

The therapy includes individual and family sessions (which may include people outside the family). The therapist helps to organise treatment by introducing several generic themes. These are different for the parents (e.g. feeling abused and without ways to influence their child) and the adolescent (e.g. feeling disconnected and angry with their parents). The therapist uses these themes of parent–child conflict as assessment tools and as a way to identify workable content in the sessions.

During individual sessions, the adolescent is helped to acquire communication skills and problem-solving skills to deal better with life stressors. Job skills and vocational training are also part of treatment. Sessions with the parents address parenting styles and belief systems. The parents are helped to examine their particular parenting style, to distinguish influence from control and to develop parenting approaches that allow them to have a positive influence on their child (Liddle *et al*, 1998).

Studies have shown that multidimensional family therapy leads to a significant reduction in substance use, and treatment gains seem to persist following treatment discharge. Psychiatric symptoms are much reduced during therapy and continue to improve following discharge (Liddle *et al*, 2001, 2004, 2005, 2006; Liddle & Dakof, 2002).

Group work (therapy)

This can focus on the substance misuse or on other issues. The latter can include social skills and relationships and can have an element of education and catharsis. Group therapy, particularly that which involves peer confrontation, seems to be effective for adolescents, at least in the short term (Wheeler & Malmquist, 1987). Some work focusing on the substance misuse has been based on the 12-step (Alcoholics Anonymous) model (Alford *et al*, 1991). The basic objective is self-help and relapse prevention. However, although this model can be beneficial for adults, for young people the concept of self-help has to be modified to take into account the process of adolescent development.

Group cognitive–behavioural therapy, particularly in combination with motivational enhancement treatment, has been found to be effective with adolescent substance misusers (Waldron *et al*, 2001; Kaminer *et al*, 2002). Psychodynamic approaches such as interpersonal group psychotherapy can also be helpful, particularly in improving self-regulation and bio-psychosocial functioning, which can in turn lead to a decrease in drug use and other problem behaviours (Brook *et al*, 2002; Flores, 2002).

Pharmacological treatments

Alcohol

By the time they are referred, adolescents are unlikely to have developed an alcohol dependence syndrome that requires detoxification (see chapter 7, this volume). However, if assessment confirms the presence of dependence, then detoxification along the conventional lines used for adults is indicated. Benzodiazepines are useful for this as they reduce withdrawal severity and the likelihood of delirium (for a detailed account see Lejoyeux *et al*, 1998, and chapter 7). The dosage and type of benzodiazepine and the duration of the detoxification regimen depend on the severity of the withdrawal syndrome and the motivation of the adolescent. Withdrawal scales may help to guide the process.

Opiates

Treatment of opiate dependence follows lines similar to those used for adults. It may be carried out on an out-patient or residential basis, depending on the severity of the dependence and the presence of a supportive environment in the community. However, there are at present few residential facilities for adolescents in the UK. Methadone and buprenorphine are currently available for the treatment of opiate dependence in adolescents, although buprenorphine is licensed only for use in those aged 16 and above. Few studies have investigated pharmacological treatment of opiate dependence in adolescents, but buprenorphine may be preferable for a number of reasons. Although its efficacy appears to be similar to that of methadone, it is less likely to be fatal if taken in excess, either on its own or when mixed with other drugs (Auriacombe *et al*, 2001). Furthermore, it is less likely to cause dependence, can be more easily reduced and stopped (Gowing *et al*, 2000) and is less sedating than methadone. However, methadone treatment may be more effective at retaining adolescent patients and reducing premature discharge from and subsequent return to treatment (Bell & Mutch, 2006).

Studies in adults suggest that drugs such as alpha-2 agonists (e.g. clonidine or lofexidine) and naltrexone may also be useful, although buprenorphine has been found to be significantly more efficacious than clonidine in opioid-dependent adolescents (Marsch *et al*, 2005). Symptomatic relief from signs of the withdrawal syndrome (such as diarrhoea and central nervous system arousal) may also be appropriate. The dose and duration of treatment with methadone or buprenorphine depend, as in alcohol dependence, on the severity of dependence and the individual's motivation. However, the aim should be stabilisation and rapid reduction if possible – long-term methadone maintenance is not usually advisable in young people.

Other substances

Detoxification programmes for dependence on drugs such as benzodiazepines and cocaine also follow the same lines as with adults. No pharmacological substitutes are available for these and the objective should be gradual reduction of use. Antidepressants such as desipramine and fluoxetine have been found to be helpful, particularly in adolescents with coexisting affective disorders (Kaminer, 1992; Riggs *et al*, 1997). However, it is important to note that only fluoxetine is currently recommended for use in the treatment of depression in patients under 18 years of age in the UK (National Institute for Health and Clinical Excellence, 2005).

External support network, education and employment

For adolescents in treatment, abstinence is a major change in lifestyle and needs support to be maintained. Once treatment is completed, if the individual is to function satisfactorily and 'stay off' drugs, it is important that they be able to return to an environment that will support this. The nature and degree of support must be explored as part of the continued review and assessment process. Such support will inevitably involve opportunities for adequate accommodation, education, training and employment. Often, it is also useful to provide psychological support on either a regular or an *ad hoc* basis. Most well-developed treatment programmes include an element of extended day or community follow-up and support.

'Staying off'

Staying off psychoactive substances can be difficult. It depends on external support resources to a significant degree, but much can be achieved by individuals themselves, with pharmacological and psychological support.

Pharmacological methods of relapse prevention have been used mostly for alcohol dependence and aim at dealing with and reducing craving, which is the main cause of short-term relapse. Acamprosate may be an effective and well-tolerated pharmacological adjunct to psychosocial treatment programmes in adolescent alcohol dependence (Niederhofer & Staffen, 2003). In addition, a small open-label trial of naltrexone in adolescent alcohol dependence suggested that naltrexone is safe and well-tolerated and may lead to a significant reduction in alcohol consumption and craving

---

Box 18.2 Points of good practice

- Some parents panic when they learn that their child is abusing drugs – it is wise not to join them. In many cases, all that is needed is simple counselling
- Families must always be involved. They have a great deal to offer, but their involvement does not necessarily have to follow the conventional lines of family therapy
- Substance misuse may be a symptom of a dysfunctional family system, no more – that system must be helped to become more functional
- Always look for psychopathology and deal with it vigorously. It may not come in the form of a full-blown syndrome, but it may, nevertheless, be very significant to the adolescent
- Substance misuse is not necessarily a 'conduct disorder'. It is likely that it is a manifestation of an emotional problem
- Sometimes it is wiser to view substance misuse as a behaviour that needs to be changed, rather than a disorder that has to be treated
- The motivation to change always comes from within. The strategy is to facilitate that process. Human beings do not change a behaviour unless they have to or wish to
- A good assessment is a sound investment
- Try to avoid treating adolescents within adult services. Some bad habits of adult misusers (like injecting) tend to rub off
- Multi-agency intervention is the rule rather than the exception

---

(Deas *et al*, 2005). However, larger, randomised controlled trials are needed. Naltrexone can also help prolong abstinence from opiate use in adults, particularly when combined with psychological and social relapse prevention strategies (Kirchmayer *et al*, 2000; Tucker & Ritter, 2000).

Cognitive–behavioural therapy is increasingly gaining credence in relapse prevention. This approach aims to help the individual to generate mechanisms for coping with situations that have high risk for relapse. Social pressure is the most important high-risk situation for adolescents. The indications are that abstinence is directly related to the individual's ability to develop coping strategies to deal with social pressure. The most successful strategies are those characterised by a cognitive–behavioural approach, such as avoiding high-risk situations, refusal and engaging in alternative activity (Myers & Brown, 1990).

Conclusion

Points of good practice in the treatment of adolescents with substance misuse problems are summarised in Box 18.2, but the key to a successful outcome lies in a comprehensive assessment. Its findings will heavily influence the intervention strategy. Intervention is mostly multidisciplinary, multi-agency and requires multiple skills. It also requires careful planning and effective communication between the agencies and professionals involved.

Appendix 18.1

The Substance Misuse in Adolescence Questionnaire (Swadi, 1997; reprinted with permission)

Answers with a 'yes' score 1 and answers with a 'no' score 0. A total score of 5 or more is a strong indication for further detailed assessment.

1   Are the effects of the drug more important to you than the adventure of use?
2   Do you have a favourite drug?
3   Do you ever use alone?
4   Do you use to suppress feeling sad, bored, lonely, confused or anxious?
5   Are you thinking a lot about drugs and drug use?
6   Do you plan your day to make sure you can use?
7   Do you need to use more to get high now than before?
8   Do you feel depressed, irritable or anxious if you do not use?
9   Do you crave for or 'miss' your favourite drug?

Appendix 18.2

Suggested assessment scheme

A suggested scheme (the questions to ask) for the assessment of adolescents who misuse psychoactive substances. Information will inevitably come from multiple sources, including parents, teachers, social workers and the assessor's own observations.

History data

1 Reasons for referral
2 Recent events
3 Personal history
4 Family structure and situation
5 Life events within past year

Patterns of use

1 Substance
2 Route
3 Type
4 Quantity
5 Weekly expense

(Make a list of and inquire about all possible substances, by name.)

Clinical contexts of substance misuse (the questions to ask)

1 Which is more important – the effects of the drug or the atmosphere of use?
2 What is remembered more – the effects of the drug or the atmosphere of use?
3 How often does the individual use?
4 Is use regular or occasional?
5 Most of the time, does the individual use alone or with others?
6 Where does most 'use' take place? Home, pub, school, etc.
7 Does the individual tend to use more often at social events such as parties?
8 Does use help the individual fit in with the crowd?
9 Does the individual use more often under the influence of friends?
10 When using with others, does it help the individual to relax and loosen up?
11 Does the individual participate in drinking or drug use games?
12 If the drug of choice is not available, would the individual use an alternative drug?
13 Does the individual use combinations of substances?
14 Does the individual use one substance to counter some effects of another?
15 Does the individual feel physically/psychologically normal the day after use?
16 Has use affected school work and behaviour?
17 Has use affected the individual's family relationships?
18 Does the individual use to make them feel a certain way, e.g. high, happy or relaxed?
19 Does the individual plan/seek to use to feel like that?
20 Does the individual ever use alone?
21 Does the individual use to feel less restrained, shy or inhibited?
22 Does the individual use to suppress feeling sad, bored, lonely, confused or anxious?
23 Does the individual plan/seek to use to feel like that?
24 How does the individual get on with their parents?
25 Has the individual made new friends since starting to use?
26 Do any of the new friends use? If yes, heavily or frequently, or harder drugs?
27 Has the individual lost any old friends?
28 Does the individual think a lot about use? Is the individual preoccupied with the idea of use?
29 Does the individual plan their day to make sure they can use?
30 Is the individual losing interest in usual activities or hobbies?
31 Does the individual need to use more to get high now than before, say a year ago?
32 Does the individual suffer from physical withdrawal symptoms?
33 If yes, what? How severe?
34 If yes, does the individual use to get over these symptoms?
35 Does the individual feel depressed, irritable or anxious if they do not use?
36 Does the individual use to get over these feelings?
37 Has the individual ever put limits or rules for use, e.g. only weekends or no mixing of substances?

38 How often does the individual break these limits?
39 Does the individual crave for or 'miss' their favourite substance?
40 If so, what does it feel like?
41 How many negative consequences has the individual had because of use?
    Physical:
    Social:
    Legal:
    Educational:
    Psychological:

Functional assessment

Attitude towards referral

1 Is the individual agreeable with the referral?
2 Does the individual think there is a problem? If yes, where do they think the problem lies? In him- or herself? In others? If no, why do they think they are here?
3 Does the individual think there is a problem with their use? If yes, who is it a problem for?
4 Where does the individual think the solution lies?

Education

1 What was the individual's attitude towards schooling earlier in life?
2 How did the individual do at school then? Grades?
3 Did the individual have any concentration problems then?
4 What is the individual's attitude towards schooling now?
5 How is the individual doing at school now? Grades?
6 Does the individual have any specific learning problems now?
7 Does the individual have any concentration problems now?
8 What does the individual see as their best subjects?
9 What does the individual see as their worst subjects?
10 Has their schoolwork declined?
11 At what grade did their schoolwork start to decline?
12 Does the individual have any academic aspirations? College?

Life skills

1 How does the individual communicate and relate to the interviewer?
2 Can the individual express him- or herself clearly?
3 Is the individual outgoing or shy?
4 How assertive or timid is the individual?
5 Is the individual passive or aggressive?
6 What does the individual do to relax?
7 What does the individual normally do to cope with stress?
8 What does the individual do recreationally and to have fun?
9 What interests and hobbies does the individual have?

Emotional adjustment

1 What emotions trigger use and how often?
2 What situations trigger these emotions?
3 Is the individual aware of the process/temporal link between triggers, emotions and use?
4 Has the individual tried to develop strategies to avoid setting this process off? If yes, what?

Self-esteem

1 Does the individual appear to take care of appearance, hair and clothes?
2 What does the individual believe they can do well?

254

3   What is the individual most proud of?
4   What is the individual least proud of?
5   What does the individual hope to achieve in life?
6   How does the individual see him- or herself in 5–10 years' time?
7   What does the individual not like most about him- or herself?
8   What does the individual think other people like about them?
9   What does the individual think other people dislike about them?
10 Does the individual feel guilty or ashamed about anything to do with him- or herself?

Psychiatric assessment

(Record any evidence of psychopathology.)

Physical health

Record the results of a full physical examination (and necessary investigations).

References

Aarons, G. A., Brown, S. A., Hough, R. I., *et al* (2001) Prevalence of adolescent substance use disorders across five sectors of care. *Journal of the American Academy of Child and Adolescent Psychiatry*, **40**, 419–426.

Alford, G., Koehler, R. & Leonard, J. (1991) Alcoholics Anonymous–Narcotics Anonymous model of in-patient treatment of chemically dependent adolescents: a 2-year outcome study. *Journal of Studies on Alcohol*, **52**, 118–126.

Auriacombe, M., Franques, P. & Tignol, J. (2001) Deaths attributable to methadone vs buprenorphine in France. *Journal of the American Medical Association*, **285**, 45.

Bell, J. & Mutch, C. (2006) Treatment retention in adolescent patients treated with methadone or buprenorphine: a file review. *Drug and Alcohol Review*, **25**, 167–171.

Brook, J. S, Finch, S., Whiteman, M, *et al* (2002) Drug use and neurobehavioural, respiratory and cognitive problems: precursors and mediators. *Journal of Adolescent Health*, **30**, 433–441.

Brown, S. A. (1999) Treatment of adolescent alcohol problems: research review and appraisal. In *NIAA Extramural Scientific Advisory Board: Treatment* (eds Extramural Scientific Advisory Board), pp. 1–26. National Institute on Alcohol Abuse and Alcoholism.

Bukstein, O., Glancy, L. J. & Kaminer, Y. (1992) Patterns of affective comorbidity in a clinical population of dually diagnosed substance abusers. *Journal of the American Academy of Child and Adolescent Substance Misuse*, **31**, 1041–1045.

Burke, B. L., Arkowitz, H. & Menchola, M. (2003) The efficacy of motivational interviewing: a meta-analysis of controlled clinical trials. *Journal of Consulting and Clinical Psychology*, **71**, 843–861.

Crome, I., Christian, J. & Green C. (1998) Tip of the national iceberg? Profile of adolescent patients prescribed methadone in an innovative community drug service. *Drugs: Education, Prevention and Policy*, **5**, 195–197.

Dcas, D., May, M. P., Randall, C., *et al* (2005) Naltrexone treatment of adolescent alcoholics: an open-label pilot study. *Journal of Child and Adolescent Psychopharmacology*, **15**, 723–728.

Deas-Nesmith, D., Campbell, S. & Brady, K.T. (1998) Substance use disorders in adolescent inpatient psychiatric population. *Journal of the National Medical Association*, **90**, 233–238.

DeLeon, G., Melnick, G. & Kressel, D. (1997) Motivation and readiness for therapeutic community treatment among cocaine and other drug abusers. *American Journal of Drug and Alcohol Abuse*, **23**, 169–189.

*Dennis, M. L., Godley, S. H., Diamond, G., *et al* (2004) The Cannabis Youth Treatment (CYT) study: main findings from two randomized trials. *Journal of Substance Abuse Treatment*, **27**, 197–213.

Deykin, E. Y., Buka, S. L. & Zeena, T. H. (1992) Depressive illness among chemically dependent adolescents. *American Journal of Psychiatry*, **149**, 1341–1347.

*Didlock, N. & Cheshire, R. (2005) *Developing The Evidence Base: Young People with Substance Misuse Problems*. Turning Point/Addaction.

Flores, P. J. (2002) The interpersonal approach. In *The Group Therapy of Substance Abuse* (eds D. W. Brook & H. I. Spitz), pp. 19–36. Haworth Press.

Gottfredson, D. C. & Wilson, D. B. (2003) Characteristics of effective school-based substance abuse prevention. *Prevention Science*, **4**, 27–38.

Gowing, L., Ali, R. & White, J. (2000) Buprenorphine for the management of opioid withdrawal. *Cochrane Library*, issue 3. Update Software.

Grella, C. E., Hser, Y., Joshi, V., *et al* (2001) Drug treatment outcomes for adolescents with comorbid mental and substance use disorders. *Journal of Nervous and Mental Disease*, **189**, 384–392.

Hawton, K., Fagg, J., Platt, S., *et al* (1993) Factors associated with suicide after parasuicide in young people. *BMJ*, **306**, 1641–1644.

Isohanni, M., Moilanen, I. & Rantakallio, P. (1991) Determinants of teenage smoking, with special reference to non-standard family background. *British Journal of Addiction*, **86**, 391–398.

Johnston, L., O'Malley, P. & Bachman, J. (1998) *National Survey Results from Monitoring the Future Study, 1975–1997, Secondary School Students*. Vol. I. National Institute on Drug Abuse.

Kaminer, Y. (1992) Desipramine facilitation of cocaine abstinence in an adolescent. *Journal of the American Academy of Child and Adolescent Psychiatry*, **31**, 312–317.

Kaminer, Y., Burleson, J. & Goldberger, R. (2002) Psychotherapies for adolescent substance abusers: short- and long-term outcomes. *Journal of Nervous and Mental Disease*, **190**, 737–745.

*Kaufman, E. & Kaufman, P. (1979) *Family Therapy of Drug and Alcohol Abuse*. Gardner Press.

Kirchmayer, U., Davoli, M. & Verster, A. (2000) Naltrexone maintenance treatment for opioid dependence. *Cochrane Library*, issue 3. Update Software.

Knight, D. K. & Simpson, D. D. (1996) Influences of family and friends on client progress during drug abuse treatment. *Journal of Substance Abuse Treatment*, **8**, 417–429.

Labouvie, E. (1986) Alcohol and marijuana use in relation to adolescent stress. *International Journal of the Addictions*, **21**, 333–345.

Lavik, N., Clausen, S. & Pedersen, W. (1991) Eating behaviour, drug use, psychopathology and parental bonding in adolescents in Norway. *Acta Psychiatrica Scandinavica*, **84**, 387–390.

*Lejoyeux, M., Solomon, J. & Adès, J. (1998) Benzodiazepine treatment for alcohol-dependent patients. *Alcohol and Alcoholism*, **33**, 563–575.

Liddle, H. A. (1998) *Multidimensional Family Therapy Treatment Manual*. Center for Treatment Research on Adolescent Drug Abuse (University of Miami School of Medicine).

Liddle, H. A. (2002) Advances in family-based therapy for adolescent substance abuse: findings from the multidimensional family therapy research program. In *Research Monograph No. 182: Problems of Drug Dependence 2001* (ed. L. S. Harris), pp. 113–115. National Institute on Drug Abuse.

Liddle, H. A. & Dakof, G. A. (2002) Abstract. A randomized controlled trial of intensive outpatient, family based therapy vs. residential drug treatment for co-morbid adolescent drug abusers. *Drug and Alcohol Dependence*, **66** (suppl. 1), S103 (#385).

*Liddle, H. A., Rowe, C. L., Dakof, G. A., *et al* (1998) Translating parenting research into clinical interventions. *Clinical Child Psychology and Psychiatry*, **3**, 419–442.

Liddle, H. A., Dakof, G. A., Parker, K., *et al* (2001) Multidimensional Family Therapy for adolescent substance abuse. Results of a randomized clinical trial. *American Journal of Drug and Alcohol Abuse*, **27**, 651–687.

Liddle, H. A., Rowe, C. L., Dakof, G. A., *et al* (2004) Early intervention for adolescent substance abuse. Pre-treatment to post treatment outcomes of a randomized controlled trial comparing multidimensional family therapy and peer group treatment. *Journal of Psychoactive Drugs*, **36**, 49–63.

Liddle, H. A., Rodriguez, R. A., Dakof, G. A., *et al* (2005) Multidimensional Family Therapy: a science-based treatment for adolescent drug abuse. In *Handbook of Clinical Family Therapy* (ed J. Lebow), pp. 128–163. John Wiley & Sons.

Liddle, H. A., Rodriguez, R. A. & Marvel, F. A. (2006) Multidimensional Family Therapy (MDFT): an effective treatment for adolescent substance abuse. In *Proceedings of the 2005 International Conference on Tackling Drug Abuse* (ed. D. Shek), pp. 228–240. Hong Kong University Press.

Marsch, L. A., Bickel, W. K., Badger, G. J., *et al* (2005) Comparison of pharmacological treatments for opioid-dependent adolescents: a randomised controlled trial. *Archives of General Psychiatry*, **62**, 1157–1164.

Martin, C. S., Kaczynski, N. A., Maisto, S. A., *et al* (1996) Polydrug use in adolescent drinkers with and without DSM–IV alcohol abuse and dependence. *Alcoholism: Clinical and Experimental Research*, **20**, 1099–1108.

*Meyers, K., Hagan, T., Zanis, D., *et al* (1999) Critical issues in adolescent substance use assessment. *Drug and Alcohol Dependence*, **55**, 235–246.

Miller, P. & Plant, M. (1996) Drinking, smoking and illicit drug use among 15 and 16 year olds in the United Kingdom. *BMJ*, **313**, 394–397.

*Miller, W. & Rollnick, S. (1991) *Motivational Interviewing: Preparing People to Change Addictive Behaviour*. Guilford Press.

Myers, M. & Brown, S. (1990) Coping responses and relapse among adolescent substance abusers. *Journal of Substance Abuse*, **2**, 177–189.

National Institute for Health and Clinical Excellence (2005) *Depression in Children and Young People: Identification and Management in Primary, Community and Secondary Care* (Clinical guideline CG28). NICE.

Niederhofer, H. & Staffen, W. (2003) Acamprosate and its efficacy in treating alcohol dependent adolescents. *European Child and Adolescent Psychiatry*, **12**, 144–148.

*Nowinski, J. (1990) *Substance Abuse in Adolescents and Young Adults: A Guide to Treatment*. Norton.

*Prochaska, J. & DiClemente, C. (1982) Transtheoretical therapy. Toward a more integrative model of change. *Psychotherapy: Theory, Research and Practice*, **19**, 276–288.

Riggs, P., Baker, S., Mikulich, S. K., *et al* (1995) Depression in substance-dependent delinquents, *Journal of the American Academy of Child and Adolescent Psychiatry*, **34**, 764–771.

Riggs, P., Mikulich, S., Coffman, L., *et al* (1997) Fluoxetine in drug-dependent delinquents with major depression: an open trial. *Child and Adolescent Psychopharmacology*, **7**, 87–95.

Scourfield, J., Stevens, D. E. & Merikangas, K. R. (1996) Substance abuse, comorbidity, and sensation seeking: gender differences. *Comprehensive Psychiatry*, **37**, 384–392.

Spoth, R., Redmond, C. & Shin, C. (1998) Direct and indirect latent-variable parenting outcomes of two universal family-focused preventive interventions: extending a public health-oriented research base. *Journal of Consulting and Clinical Psychology*, **66**, 385–399.

Stewart, S. H., Conrod, P. J., Marlatt, G. M., *et al* (2005) New developments in prevention and early intervention for alcohol abuse in youth. *Alcoholism: Clinical and Experimental Research*, **29**, 278–286.

Stoker, A. & Swadi, H. (1990) Perceived family relationships in drug abusing adolescents. *Drug and Alcohol Dependence*, **25**, 293–297.

Sutherland, I. & Willner, P. (1998) Patterns of alcohol, cigarette and illicit drug use in English adolescents. *Addiction*, **93**, 1199–1208.

Swadi, H. (1992) Psychiatric symptoms in drug abusing adolescents. *Drug and Alcohol Dependence*, **31**, 77–83.

*Swadi, H. (1997) Substance Misuse in Adolescence Questionnaire (SMAQ): a pilot study of a screening instrument for problematic use of drugs and volatile substances in adolescents. *Child Psychology and Psychiatry Review*, **2**, 63–69.

Tobler, N. S., Roona, M. R., Ochshorn, P., *et al* (2000) School-based adolescent drug prevention programs: 1998 meta-analysis. *Journal of Primary Prevention*, **20**, 275–336.

Tomlinson, K. L., Brown, S. A. & Abrantes, A. M. (2004) Psychiatric comorbidity and substance use treatment outcomes of adolescents. *Psychology of Addictive Behaviours*, **18**, 160–169.

Tucker, T. & Ritter, A. (2000). Naltrexone in the treatment of heroin dependence: a literature review. *Drug and Alcohol Review*, **19**, 73–82.

Waldron, H. B., Slesnick, N., Brody, J. L., *et al* (2001) Treatment outcomes for adolescent substance abuse at 4 and 7 month assessments. *Journal of Consulting and Clinical Psychology*, **69**, 802–813.

Wheeler, K. & Malmquist, J. (1987) Treatment approaches in adolescent chemical dependency. *Pediatric Clinics of North America*, **34**, 437–448.

*Wilens, T., Faraone, S., Biederman, J., *et al* (2003) Does the stimulant pharmacotherapy of ADHD beget later substance misuse? A meta-analysis of the literature. *Pediatrics*, **111**, 179–185.

*Zeitlin, H. (1999) Psychiatric comorbidity with substance misuse in children and teenagers. *Drug and Alcohol Dependence*, **55**, 225–234.

*Publications of particular interest.

CHAPTER 19

Management of drug misuse in pregnancy

Ed Day and Sanju George

Summary   Use of both licit and illicit drugs can lead to a range of medical, psychiatric and social problems, and the situation becomes further complicated if the user is pregnant. Prescribed and non-prescribed substances can affect a pregnancy, and substances are seldom used in isolation. This chapter focuses on the use of illicit drugs (including prescribed drugs used illicitly) during pregnancy and describes some of the issues in managing such cases. The impact of substance use on the foetus, the mother and the new-born child is considered, and the importance of multidisciplinary working in this area is highlighted. Space precludes a detailed account of the issues surrounding the use of legal substances such as alcohol and tobacco during pregnancy, but they also have a significant impact in this group (see chapters 6 and 8).

It is difficult accurately to estimate the prevalence of high-risk drug use during pregnancy for a variety of reasons: feelings of shame, denial and stigma experienced by the drug user, lack of awareness among professionals in antenatal services, the presence of comorbid psychiatric disorders, and sociocultural barriers that prevent a thorough assessment. However, we know that about one-third of drug users in treatment in the UK are female, and over 90% of these women are of childbearing age (15–39 years). A number of large surveys of drug use in different populations conducted in the USA provide a further insight. For example, the National Pregnancy and Health Survey gathered self-report data from a sample of 2613 women whose babies were delivered in 52 urban and rural hospitals during 1992 (National Institute of Drug Abuse, 1996). Over 5% of those who gave birth during the study period had used illicit drugs while they were pregnant, with 2.9% using cannabis and 1.1% using cocaine at some point in their pregnancy (compared with 20% smoking tobacco and 18.5% drinking alcohol). A further report combined 2 years of US National Household Survey data (1994 and 1995) for women and girls 15–44 years old and found that 9.3% reported current use of illicit drugs, with 2.3% doing so while pregnant. The problem is therefore a significant one, particularly as it has implications for both mother and child.

Effects of drug use on the mother

Dependence on heroin or other drugs can lead to neglect in many areas of the user's life. The need to obtain a steady supply of the drug is both time-consuming and expensive, and so neglect of medical, nutritional and social well-being is common. Injected drug use leads to an increased risk of acquiring blood-borne viruses such as HIV and hepatitis, as well as abscesses and endocarditis. Maternal infection, neglect and malnourishment are partly responsible for the observed low birth weights, high incidence of preterm birth and poor nutritional status of neonates born to drug users (Fischer, 2000). Women may become involved in crime such as prostitution, robbery and burglary in an attempt to finance their drug habit.

Parenting issues

Parental drug use during and after pregnancy can have a serious impact on the emotional, cognitive and behavioural development of children. It has been estimated that 200 000–300 000 children in England and Wales have one or both parents with a serious drug problem (Advisory Council on the Misuse of Drugs, 2003). After the birth, parental drug use may present the child with a range of difficulties that can affect emotional, behavioural, cognitive and psychological development (Box 19.1).

Drug use does not necessarily lead to problems in child care or the neglect or abuse of children, and substance misuse treatment services have long played an important role in supporting mothers. However, it is important to consider the impact of parents' substance misuse on the welfare of children in their care: some of the risks posed are shown in Box 19.2.

Effects of drug use on the child

As a general principle, exposure to substances in the first trimester of pregnancy affects foetal organogenesis, whereas use in the second and third trimesters mainly results in growth and functional abnormalities or

---

Box 19.1 Potential difficulties faced by the children of drug users

- Physical and emotional abuse or neglect
- Inadequate parenting or supervision
- Separation
- Poverty
- Poor education
- Exposure to criminal behaviour
- Social isolation

Box 19.2   Potential impact of parental drug use on children's welfare

- Impaired judgement, coordination and consciousness can affect a parent's ability to care for and supervise young children
- Drug-induced disinhibition can lead to aggressive behaviour, including domestic violence
- Withdrawal from certain drugs can cause irritability and mood disturbance
- Unemployment, poverty and criminality may impair family functioning
- Drug use can become a higher priority for the parent than buying basic essentials for the family
- Reduced parental vigilance may leave children vulnerable to abuse by visitors to the home
- The presence in the home of drugs and/or injecting equipment puts children at risk

(National Treatment Agency for Substance Misuse, 2002; Advisory Council on the Misuse of Drugs, 2003; Department for Education and Skills, 2003)

---

impairments in the newborn. Persistent drug use close to term can result in preterm labour, sudden infant death syndrome (SIDS) and neonatal abstinence syndromes.

Shorter-term effects

It is often difficult to establish direct causal effects of substances. The foetus is potentially at risk of harm from the direct effects of drugs, infection and poor maternal health and nutrition. These effects may be compounded by lack of adequate antenatal care.

Opioids

Dependent heroin use during pregnancy is associated with a reduction of foetal growth, resulting in low birth weight, prematurity, and foetal and neonatal death (Hulse *et al*, 1997, 1998; Dunlop *et al*, 2003). The specific effects of opioids on the neonate are confounded by harm associated with the mother's lifestyle (intoxication–withdrawal cycle, drug contaminants, infections, poverty), the difficulty specifying and quantifying drugs taken and the influence of other factors, for example the almost universal incidence of cigarette-smoking among opioid users (Ward *et al*, 1998).

The clinical signs of opioid neonatal abstinence syndrome (Box 19.3) occur in 48–94% of infants exposed to opioids *in utero*, with signs of withdrawal from methadone being more common than from heroin (Osborn *et al*, 2004). The onset, duration and severity vary and are mainly influenced by the type of drug used, the severity of maternal drug dependence, the timing of the last drug intake and foetal metabolic factors. Onset usually occurs within

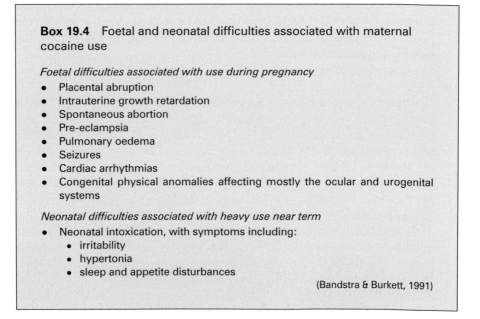

Box 19.3 Characteristics of opioid neonatal abstinence syndrome

- Gastrointestinal disturbances
- Irritability
- Hyperactivity
- Feeding and sleeping disturbances
- Autonomic hyperactivity
- Seizures (these are rare, occurring in less than 5%)

(Osborn *et al*, 2004)

24–72 h of birth, but it can be delayed by up to 7–10 days. Methadone tends to produce withdrawal symptoms of later onset, longer duration and greater severity (Coghlan *et al*, 1999). Neonatal opioid withdrawal may result in sleep–wake abnormalities, feeding difficulties and weight loss, which can disrupt the mother–infant relationship (Osborn *et al*, 2004).

Cocaine and amphetamines

Cocaine is available as a powder that can be snorted or injected and as 'crack', a 'free base' form that is suitable for smoking and has a more immediate and intense high. However it is used, cocaine is a potent vasoconstrictor and can

Box 19.4 Foetal and neonatal difficulties associated with maternal cocaine use

Foetal difficulties associated with use during pregnancy
- Placental abruption
- Intrauterine growth retardation
- Spontaneous abortion
- Pre-eclampsia
- Pulmonary oedema
- Seizures
- Cardiac arrhythmias
- Congenital physical anomalies affecting mostly the ocular and urogenital systems

Neonatal difficulties associated with heavy use near term
- Neonatal intoxication, with symptoms including:
  - irritability
  - hypertonia
  - sleep and appetite disturbances

(Bandstra & Burkett, 1991)

reduce blood flow and oxygen supply to the foetus. Maternal cocaine use during pregnancy has been associated with numerous foetal and neonatal problems (Box 19.4). However, cocaine and amphetamines appear to have low specific teratogenicity, and as yet a 'foetal cocaine syndrome' has not been conclusively demonstrated (Plessinger & Woods, 1993).

Benzodiazepines

Benzodiazepines also have low teratogenic potential, although high-dosage use during pregnancy has been associated with abnormalities such as cleft lip and cleft palate. Continued maternal use near term can result in 'floppy baby syndrome', characterised by lethargy, irritability, reduced muscle tone and respiratory depression in the newborn, and a neonatal abstinence syndrome (Sanchis et al, 1991).

Blood-borne viral infections

Intravenous drug users who share needles or injecting paraphernalia are at particular risk of contracting blood-borne viral infections such as HIV, hepatitis B and hepatitis C. Pregnant women who are infected can transmit the infection to their babies (vertical transmission) during pregnancy, during the process of birth or through breastfeeding. Early detection and prompt initiation of treatment and other protective interventions can reduce the risk of mother-to-baby transmission.

Many HIV-infected children die in the first few years of life, whereas hepatitis B or C infection can result in babies becoming chronic 'carriers' or can lead to chronic liver disease, cirrhosis and death. Therefore routine antenatal screening for such infections is recommended, provided that informed consent is obtained and adequate pre- and post-test counselling is provided. If the mother is infected, all possible measures should be taken to prevent mother-to-baby transmission, and appropriate immunisation and treatment should be instituted at the earliest opportunity to prevent long-term sequelae for the mother and the child.

Longer-term effects

Knowledge about longer-term effects of drugs on children is limited and contradictory. Some studies report a range of behavioural and learning difficulties, whereas others show few or none, especially if the research controls for other life conditions and health problems. Children of opioid-dependent mothers show high levels of irritability, hyperactivity, and feeding and sleep disturbances in the first few weeks of life that may render them liable to difficulties with attachment behaviour (Householder et al, 1982). Furthermore, these behavioural and psychological problems appear to continue throughout early and middle childhood. However, it is difficult to draw firm conclusions because huge methodological difficulties affect research in this area and longitudinal studies are needed (Householder et al, 1982; Johnson & Leff, 1999). It is also important to remember that developmental problems may result primarily from severe environmental deprivation and the fact that one or both parents are using drugs: *in utero* heroin exposure, for example, may be less important than the home environment (Ornoy *et al*, 1996).

Maternal drug use may continue to have an impact on the child's cognitive, educational, emotional and behavioural development throughout early life. Studies of pre-school children with drug-using parents have noted high rates of inattention, hyperactivity and aggression (Ornoy *et al*, 1996), as well as lower school attendance and reduced concentration when compared with controls (Hogan & Higgins, 2001). Kandel's research on parents of primary school children noted an association between parental drug use in the past year and more punitive forms of parental disciplining and less supervision of the child (Kandel, 1990). In early adolescence, having drug-using parents is associated with increased risk of offending and bullying behaviour, and adolescent children of drug-using parents are also more likely to play truant from school, repeat a year or even be suspended from school (Kolar *et al*, 1994). There is also a strong correlation between parents' and adolescents' use of illicit substances: adolescents who use drugs are likely to have one or more parents who are users (Fergusson & Lynskey, 1998; Johnson & Leff, 1999).

Formulating a management plan

The medical and social problems associated with drug use make it especially important that drug-using women do not become pregnant unless they want to. Treatment services should aim to help users to maximise their health before becoming pregnant, and attempts to improve lifestyle and diet are helpful (Hepburn, 2002). When heroin-using women do become pregnant it is often unexpected, as menstrual problems such as amenorrhoea are common in this population. Early signs and symptoms of pregnancy such as nausea, headaches and fatigue may become lost among withdrawal-related effects. This may lead drug-using women to present late for treatment, and many factors can dissuade them from seeking professional help. One such factor is the fear of being seen as irresponsible or inadequate carers, which often results in poor self-esteem, guilt, depression and denial of drug use (Klee *et al*, 2002).

The basic principles underlying good treatment of substance misuse problems in general (see chapter 1) apply to pregnant women, with special emphasis on the health of the unborn child. Drug use is only one of a number of interacting physical, psychological, social and environmental factors that influence the course and outcome of any pregnancy. It is wrong to assume that drug use by itself makes a woman incapable of caring for a baby in a healthy, supportive environment. Unfortunately, practice varies widely in different locations, and approaches to antenatal care and addiction treatment often conflict.

Box 19.5   Assessment factors specific to pregnant women

- Past obstetric and gynaecological history
- Screening for sexually transmitted diseases and blood-borne viral infections such as HIV and hepatitis B and C
- Feelings about the pregnancy and the baby
- Plans for the baby's future
- Feelings of guilt or self-blame
- Fears that the baby will be taken into care
- Existing needs and available resources

Assessment

A comprehensive assessment forms the cornerstone of a good care plan. It is often best provided as the first step in a well-integrated care package by a multidisciplinary team in a shared specialised clinic. The specialist drug service needs to work in conjunction with the general practitioner, midwife, obstetrician, paediatrician and social worker in organising and providing care for drug-dependent women throughout the antenatal, intranatal and postnatal periods. The pregnant drug user (and possibly her partner) needs to be actively involved in all phases of planning and decision-making. Assessment of drug use should include the type and quantity of drug used, route of administration, injecting behaviour, degree of dependence, previous treatment history and motivation to change. Good practice guidelines for assessment of drug use are outlined elsewhere (Department of Health, 1999), and these should be supplemented by a more detailed history of factors relevant to the pregnancy (Box 19.5). The assessment process must consider the risk to the physical and mental health of the mother during pregnancy, the risk of teratogenicity or the development of a neonatal abstinence syndrome, and ongoing child care and parenting issues. It should ultimately lead to a plan involving well-coordinated, multidisciplinary care with realistic and practical treatment goals.

Neonatal abstinence syndrome

Drug-using women should be prepared for the possibility that their newborn child will experience withdrawal symptoms (neonatal abstinence syndrome). Such preparation may help to allay their fears and engage them in treatment. They may be advised to stay in hospital for at least 3 days after delivery, to allow monitoring of the child for a neonatal abstinence syndrome. Mild to moderate symptoms can be managed by purely supportive measures (Box 19.6) and no specific pharmacological intervention is required. After discharge from hospital, the midwife should provide support at home in the

> **Box 19.6** Supportive measures for a neonate with a neonatal abstinence syndrome
>
> - Keep the baby in a quiet, dimly lit room
> - Ensure close, gentle interaction with the mother
> - Provide small, frequent feeds
> - Ensure close monitoring by nursing and medical staff

form of daily visits. Parents are taught before leaving hospital to seek medical advice should any withdrawal symptoms emerge.

More severe withdrawal symptoms may necessitate a longer stay in hospital with a period of observation and treatment by specialist staff. There is no evidence that well-managed neonatal abstinence syndrome is associated with long-term health problems (Dunlop *et al*, 2003). However, there is debate as to what constitutes optimum management, and a survey of 213 maternity units in England and Wales showed that only 65 had formulated policies for the drug treatment of neonatal opioid withdrawal (Morrison & Siney, 1996). Furthermore, there was wide variation in practice surrounding the monitoring and treatment of neonatal opioid withdrawal, with eight different rating scales and nine different drugs used for treatment. There is a danger that if a baby is being monitored specifically for withdrawal the appearance of signs is automatically attributed to maternal substance misuse, when other conditions such as mild cerebral irritation caused by foetal hypoxia or instrumentally assisted delivery can produce a similar picture. The American Academy of Pediatrics recommends tincture of opium as the preferred drug for opioid withdrawal symptoms in infants with confirmed drug exposure (American Academy of Pediatrics, 1998; Box 19.7). However, many infants with neonatal abstinence syndrome have been exposed to multiple substances *in utero*, and further research is required to determine the best treatment option in such cases (Johnson *et al*, 2003).

Pharmacological management

Opioid dependence

Methadone

There is a significant body of evidence to suggest that methadone maintenance treatment during pregnancy, when combined with a comprehensive psychosocial treatment programme, can reduce the incidence of obstetric and foetal complications as well as neonatal morbidity and mortality (Finnegan, 1991; Ward *et al*, 1998). Methadone maintenance enables stabilisation of the

---

Box 19.7 Indications for drug therapy in neonates with confirmed *in utero* exposure to opioids

- Seizures
- Poor feeding
- Diarrhoea and vomiting, resulting in excessive weight loss and dehydration
- Inability to sleep
- Fever unrelated to infection

(American Academy of Pediatrics, 1998)

---

mother's drug use and lifestyle, and can also facilitate access to comprehensive antenatal and postnatal care. Furthermore, by reducing or eliminating illicit drug use it can help to stabilise the *in utero* environment, while not increasing the risk of congenital abnormalities in the foetus. Research evidence has consistently shown that methadone maintenance during pregnancy produces superior outcomes compared with not being in treatment (Ward *et al*, 1998). Opioid-dependent women who receive methadone maintenance therapy during their pregnancy are more stable both physically and psychologically, and receive more prenatal care than women who are not in treatment (Fischer *et al*, 2000). Obstetric complications may be seen in any woman not receiving prenatal care, but the incidence of such problems in pregnant heroin users maintained on methadone is lower than that in those who continue to use heroin during pregnancy (Kaltenbach *et al*, 1998).

Use of street heroin presents the foetus with problems created by the cycle of withdrawal and intoxication produced by using a relatively short-acting drug. Both intoxication and withdrawal place stress on the foetus, and withdrawal in particular has been associated with foetal death (Ward *et al*, 1998). A further problem is the teratogenic nature of many of the adulterants added to illicit drugs to increase their bulk.

Many of the difficulties experienced by infants born to opioid-dependent mothers are due to premature birth and being small for gestational age (Finnegan, 1991). Infants born to methadone-maintained mothers are born later and are larger for gestational age than those born to opioid-dependent women who are not in treatment (Householder *et al*, 1982). In addition, pregnant women in methadone maintenance therapy attend for more antenatal care, and this can be an important predictor of outcome for both mother and foetus.

Most clinicians recommend that methadone maintenance therapy should be started as soon as possible after confirmation of pregnancy. If the woman is already on a methadone programme, maintenance should be continued. Detoxification from all drugs is unrealistic for most of this population, and often results in the mother experiencing an abstinence syndrome leading to foetal distress (Ward *et al*, 1998). The overall aim should therefore be to maintain the woman on methadone for the entire pregnancy, as withdrawal may lead to a risk of miscarriage in the first trimester or premature labour and foetal death *in utero* in the third trimester (Finnegan, 1991). However, many women express a strong desire to undertake a detoxification process, and there is some dispute as to how many are able to achieve this goal (Day *et al*, 2003; Luty *et al*, 2003). The metabolism of methadone is increased by pregnancy, and this may cause previously stable women to experience withdrawal symptoms in the final trimester. This can lead to an increased risk of relapse if not carefully managed. An alternative to increasing the daily methadone dose is to use a split dose in order to maintain steadier plasma levels (Wittman & Segal, 1991).

Buprenorphine

Buprenorphine shows considerable potential as a treatment for opioid-dependent pregnant women, and may be associated with a low incidence of neonatal abstinence syndrome (Fischer *et al*, 2000). However, as yet there is insufficient controlled research with adequate follow-up periods to demonstrate its safety during pregnancy and breastfeeding (Dunlop *et al*, 2003). Buprenorphine does not have a specific licence to be used in pregnancy, and methadone maintenance remains the treatment of choice for pregnant and breastfeeding women.

Cocaine dependence

Despite the wide range of pharmacological treatments for cocaine dependence (antipsychotics, antidepressants, dopamine agonists, anti-epileptics), no one drug has been found to be unequivocally effective. Furthermore, many of these treatments are not recommended in pregnancy, and should be initiated and monitored only by a specialist in a hospital setting. Withdrawal symptoms that emerge on abrupt cessation of cocaine during pregnancy may be reduced with short-term use of benzodiazepines or antipsychotics, but the use of dopaminergic drugs or desipramine in the longer term for managing craving and depressive symptoms is not recommended. Unlike the situation with opioids, there is no safe drug for substitute prescribing during pregnancy (Kaltenbach & Finnegan, 1998). Treatment is often a combination of symptomatic interventions during the withdrawal phase and psychosocial interventions, and there has been very little systematic research into the effectiveness of this approach in pregnant women. A similar approach should be adopted in managing the use of other psychostimulant drugs such as amphetamines and 3,4-methylenedioxymethamphetamine (MDMA, ecstasy), where the evidence base is also limited.

Benzodiazepine dependence

Sudden cessation of benzodiazepines can lead to maternal convulsions and so should be avoided (Hepburn, 2002). The primary aim in treating benzodiazepine dependence in pregnant women is usually to identify a mutually agreed and realistic goal, be it low-dose 'maintenance', gradual reduction or detoxification. For women using high doses of benzodiazepine alone, without any significant psychosocial or medical complications, gradual reduction and detoxification in the community are recommended. Women who are taking short- or medium-acting benzodiazepines (e.g. lorazepam, oxazepam) should be transferred to an equivalent dose of diazepam and the dose gradually reduced to zero. Women who are using high doses of benzodiazepine in combination with other drugs, or those who have complicating medical, psychiatric or psychosocial problems, are best managed in hospital. Once admitted for detoxification, the level of withdrawal symptoms and other problems should be objectively assessed. With long-acting benzodiazepines, symptoms of withdrawal may not be manifest for the first 5–7 days, and post-withdrawal problems such as sleep disturbance may take several weeks to resolve. Pharmacological treatment is best supplemented with individual supportive psychotherapy, anxiety management and other supportive measures.

Alcohol

It is worth noting that many drug-dependent pregnant women also misuse alcohol, and this should be assessed and managed appropriately (Mayo-Smith, 1997). Alcohol is an established human teratogen and there is no clear safe level of consumption during pregnancy. Consumption of less than 7 units per week is thought to cause no significant harm to the baby, but more regular use can adversely affect the developing foetal brain and result in a series of physical, neurological and behavioural abnormalities known as foetal alcohol syndrome (Jones & Smith, 1973). It is therefore recommended that pregnant women abstain from drinking alcohol.

Drug use and breastfeeding

Most substances of misuse are lipid soluble and hence are excreted in significant amounts in breast milk and easily cross the blood–brain barrier of the infant (O'Mara & Nahata, 2002). This exposes the newborn child to a range of adverse effects, including intoxication and withdrawal. Guidelines are slowly being developed about breastfeeding by women dependent on either legal or illegal drugs (Drug Misuse in Pregnancy Breastfeeding Project, 2003). Contraindications for breastfeeding are listed in Box 19.8. It is generally accepted that women who are well stabilised on reasonably low doses of prescribed drugs may breastfeed their babies, as the potential benefits far outweigh the risks. Breastfeeding is not thought to be a significant route of transmission of hepatitis B or C.

It is preferable to avoid breastfeeding a baby for 1–2 h after taking any street drug or medication, as this is the time of highest plasma drug concentration.

Box 19.8 Contraindications for breastfeeding

Breastfeeding is not advisable if the woman is:
- using multiple substances in large quantities
- using in a very inconsistent manner
- injecting drugs
- using cocaine, crack or large doses of amphetamines
- HIV positive

Mothers should be taught about signs and symptoms of intoxication and withdrawal in the baby and should seek medical advice if any doubts arise. Breastfeeding should not be abruptly discontinued, as this can precipitate withdrawal symptoms, and gradual weaning with slow introduction of alternative semi-solid foods should be instituted (Drug Misuse in Pregnancy Breastfeeding Project, 2003).

Psychosocial issues

There is a wide range of psychosocial approaches available for the treatment of drug dependence (see chapter 16), but no single approach has been found to be better than the others for use with pregnant drug users. Therefore the principles used to guide addiction treatment in general apply to this subgroup (Ghodse, 2002: pp. 211–241). However, the impact of drug use on parenting capacity and any risks to the children must also be assessed in order to guide the most appropriate intervention. Questions about child care and parenting issues are sensitive and can have important implications for drug-using parents. Although parents have the right to confidentiality in most circumstances, society has a duty to protect children, particularly as they often cannot advocate for themselves. The emphasis should be on working collaboratively with parents to maximise the care of children and protect them from harm (Department of Health et al, 1999). There is some evidence to suggest that deficiencies in parenting attitudes and skills may be prevalent among drug misusers, but that parenting training can lead to dramatic improvements in self-esteem, parenting knowledge and attitudes (Camp & Finkelstein, 1995).

In many cases, children's welfare can be safeguarded by appropriate health and social care without recourse to formal child protection measures (Department of Health et al, 1999), but more formal steps sometimes need to be taken. Section 17 of the Children Act 1989 obliges local authorities to make appropriate enquiries and take action to protect children if there is reasonable cause to suspect that they are likely to suffer 'significant harm'.

A child protection case conference may be convened to determine the facts and decide on further action. The child's name may be placed on the child protection register or proceedings may be instituted for a care or supervision order if the case warrants such intervention. Each local authority has an area child protection committee (ACPC) responsible for developing and promoting local child protection arrangements and effective multiagency working and information-sharing.

Outcome of treatment

Pregnancy is a temporary phase in a woman's life and her patterns of drug use, engagement with treatment services and eventual outcome will be only partially determined by what happens during this period. It is often hoped that pregnancy will act as a catalyst for change in a drug-using woman, although there is little evidence that this is true. The outcome of drug treatment in pregnancy can be viewed from the perspective of both the woman and the child. The successful delivery of a healthy baby is in itself a good outcome in the short term. However, few studies have focused on the long-term outcome of children born to drug-dependent women and the effectiveness of various maternal treatment interventions in preventing adverse consequences. A further problem is the lack of consensus about which outcome measures should be used in this subgroup of patients. Abstinence rates during pregnancy or soon after birth are commonly used, but this approach neglects long-term relapse rates and the impact on the child's development.

Most research on drug use during pregnancy has focused on opioid users in methadone treatment programmes, and overall it shows better birth outcomes and more regular antenatal care visits for women maintained on methadone than for those not in treatment (Edelin et al, 1988). Methadone maintenance has been shown to retain a higher proportion of pregnant women in treatment than briefer abstinence-focused interventions (Anderson et al, 1996). Furthermore, enhancing methadone maintenance therapy with more frequent antenatal care and relapse prevention groups can lead to further improvements in treatment engagement, fewer positive urine screen results and higher birth weights (Chang et al, 1992).

The treatment setting

Treatment may take place in residential or out-patient settings, although the capacity of the former is limited in the UK. There is some evidence that residential treatment programmes that include facilities to admit children alongside their parents have improved rates of retention in treatment and higher abstinence rates (Hughes et al, 1995), and that the more comprehensive a residential programme is, the better the outcome (Stevens & Arbiter, 1995). However, other work has found out-patient programmes to be as effective as residential ones for this group (Strantz & Welch, 1995). There is evidence that significant improvement in the health of pregnant opioid-dependent women and their babies occurs if they are monitored as out-patients by specialist obstetric units with expertise in managing substance use (Ward *et al*, 1998; Dunlop *et al*, 2003).

A range of service models have been developed in the UK in response to specific local needs, and many report positive results (Dawe *et al*, 1992; Morrison *et al*, 1995; Hepburn, 2002; Day *et al*, 2003).

Conclusion

Drug use in pregnancy is a potentially complex bio-psychosocial problem and is best managed through careful assessment leading to a care plan that is implemented by a multidisciplinary team. The predominantly negative attitudes towards drug-using pregnant women must be taken into consideration, as these will have an impact on whether an individual seeks help and subsequently enters a treatment programme. Medical management through maintenance prescribing can have a significant effect on both health and social outcomes, but the best results are obtained when working in conjunction with obstetric, neonatal and social services. Taking illicit drugs certainly does not preclude a woman from providing adequate child care, but there is a need to provide support in more than just the high-risk cases if poor long-term outcomes for the child are to be avoided (Advisory Council on the Misuse of Drugs, 2003).

References

Advisory Council on the Misuse of Drugs (2003) *Hidden Harm: Responding to the Needs of Children of Problem Drug Users*. Home Office.

American Academy of Pediatrics (1998) Neonatal drug withdrawal. *Pediatrics*, **101**, 1079–1088.

Anderson, F., Svikis, D., Lee, J., *et al* (1996) Methadone maintenance in the treatment of opiate dependant pregnant women. In *Problems of Drug Dependence 1995: Proceedings of the 57th Annual Scientific Meeting* (ed. L. S. Harris). National Institute of Drug Abuse.

Bandstra, E. S. & Burkett, G. (1991) Maternal–fetal and neonatal effects of *in utero* cocaine exposure. *Seminars in Perinatology*, **15**, 288–301.

Camp, J. M. & Finkelstein, N. (1995) *Fostering Effective Parenting Skills and Healthy Child Development within Residential Substance Abuse Treatment Settings*. Coalition on Addiction, Pregnancy and Parenting.

Chang, G., Carroll, K. M. & Behr, H. M. (1992) Improving treatment outcome in pregnant opiate-dependent women. *Journal of Substance Abuse Treatment*, **9**, 327–330.

Coghlan, D., Milner, M., Clarke, T., *et al* (1999) Neonatal abstinence syndrome. *Irish Medical Journal*, **92**, 232–236.

Dawe, S., Gerada, C. & Strang, J. (1992) Establishment of a liaison service for pregnant opiate-dependent women. *British Journal of Addiction*, **87**, 867–871.

Day, E., Porter, L., Clarke, A., *et al* (2003) Drug misuse in pregnancy: the impact of a specialist treatment service. *Psychiatric Bulletin*, **27**, 99–101.

Department for Education and Skills (2003) *Every Child Matters*. TSO (The Stationery Office).

Department of Health (1999) *Drug Misuse and Dependence – Guidelines on Clinical Management.* Department of Health.

Department of Health, Home Office & Department for Education and Employment (1999) *Working Together to Safeguard Children.* TSO (The Stationery Office).

Drug Misuse in Pregnancy Breastfeeding Project (2003) *Breastfeeding and Drug Misuse: An Information Guide For Mothers.* University of Plymouth.

Dunlop, A. J., Panjari, M., O'Sullivan, H., *et al* (2003) *Clinical Guidelines for the Use of Buprenorphine in Pregnancy.* Turning Point Alcohol and Drug Centre.

Edelin, K. C., Gurganious, L. & Golar, K. (1988) Methadone maintenance in pregnancy: consequences of care and outcome. *Obstetrics and Gynecology,* **71**, 399–404.

Fergusson, D. M. & Lynskey, M. T. (1998) Conduct problems in childhood and psychosocial outcomes in adolescence. A prospective study. *Journal of Emotional and Behavioral Disorders,* **6**, 6–12.

Finnegan, L. P. (1991) Treatment issues for opioid-dependent women during the perinatal period. *Journal of Psychoactive Drugs,* **23**, 191–201.

Fischer, G. (2000) Treatment of opioid dependence in pregnant women. *Addiction,* **95**, 1141–1144.

Fischer, G., Johnson, R. E., Eder, H., *et al* (2000) Treatment of opioid-dependent pregnant women with buprenorphine. *Addiction,* **95**, 239–244.

Ghodse, H. (2002) *Drugs and Addictive Behaviour: A Guide to Treatment* (3rd edn). Cambridge University Press.

Hepburn, M. (2002) Drug use and women's reproductive health. In *Working with Substance Misusers: A Guide to Theory and Practice* (eds T. Peterson & A. McBride). Routledge.

Hogan, D. & Higgins, L. (2001) *When Parents Use Drugs: Key Findings from a Study of Children in the Care of Drug-Using Parents.* Trinity College Dublin.

Householder, J., Hatcher, R., Burns, W., *et al* (1982) Infants born to narcotic-addicted mothers. *Psychological Bulletin,* **92**, 453–468.

Hughes, P. H., Coletti, S. D. & Neri, R. L. (1995) Retaining cocaine-abusing women in a therapeutic community: the effect of a child live-in program. *American Journal of Public Health,* **85**, 1149–1152.

Hulse, G. K., Milne, E., English, D. R., *et al* (1997) The relationship between maternal use of heroin and methadone and infant birth weight. *Addiction,* **92**, 1571–1579.

Hulse, G. K., Milne, E., English, D. R., *et al* (1998) Assessing the relationship between maternal opiate use and neonatal mortality. *Addiction,* **93**, 1033–1042.

Johnson, J. L. & Leff, M. (1999) Children of substance abusers: overview of research findings. *Pediatrics,* **103**, 1085–1099.

Johnson, K., Gerada, C. & Greenough, A. (2003) Treatment of neonatal abstinence syndrome. *Archives of Disease in Childhood: Fetal Neonatal Edition,* **88**, F2–F5.

Jones, K. L. & Smith, D. W. (1973) Recognition of the foetal alcohol syndrome in early infancy. *Lancet,* **ii**, 999–1001.

Kaltenbach, K. & Finnegan, L. (1998) Prevention and treatment issues for pregnant cocaine-dependent women and their infants. *Annals of the New York Academy of Sciences,* **846**, 329–334.

Kaltenbach, K., Berghella, V. & Finnegan, L. (1998) Opioid dependence during pregnancy. *Obstetrics and Gynecology Clinics of North America,* **25**, 139–151.

Kandel, D. (1990) Parenting styles, drug use and children's adjustment in families of young adults. *Journal of Marriage and the Family,* **52**, 183–196.

Klee, H., Jackson, M. & Lewis, S. (2002) *Drug Misuse and Motherhood.* Routledge.

Kolar, A. F., Brown, B. S., Haertzen, C. A., *et al* (1994) Children of substance abusers. The life experiences of children of opiate addicts in methadone maintenance. *American Journal of Drug and Alcohol Abuse,* **20**, 159–171.

Luty, J., Nikolaou, V. & Bearn, J. (2003) Is opiate detoxification unsafe in pregnancy? *Journal of Substance Abuse Treatment,* **24**, 363–367.

Mayo-Smith, M. F. (1997) Pharmacological treatment of alcohol withdrawal: a meta-analysis and evidence-based practice guideline. *JAMA,* **160**, 649–655.

Morrison, C. L. & Siney, C. (1996) A survey of the management of neonatal opiate withdrawal in England and Wales. *European Journal of Pediatrics*, **155**, 323–326.

Morrison, C. L., Siney, C., Ruben, S. M., *et al* (1995) Obstetric liaison in drug dependency. *Addiction Research*, **3**, 93–101.

National Institute of Drug Abuse (1996) *National Pregnancy and Health Survey: Drug Use among Women Delivering Livebirths 1992*. National Institute of Drug Abuse.

National Treatment Agency for Substance Misuse (2002) *Models of Care for the Treatment of Drug Misusers*. National Treatment Agency for Substance Misuse.

O'Mara, N. B. & Nahata, M. C. (2002) Drugs excreted in human breast milk. In *Problems in Pediatric Drug Therapy* (eds L. A. Pagliaro & A. M. Pagliaro). American Pharmaceutical Association.

Ornoy, A., Michailevskaya, V., Lukashov, I., *et al* (1996) The developmental outcome of children born to heroin-dependent mothers raised at home or adopted. *Child Abuse and Neglect*, **20**, 385–396.

Osborn, D. A., Cole, M. J. & Jeffrey, H. E. (2004) Opiate treatment for opiate withdrawal in newborn infants. *Cochrane Library*, issue 3. Update Software.

Plessinger, M. A. & Woods, J. R., Jr (1993) Maternal, placental and fetal pathophysiology of cocaine exposure during pregnancy. *Clinical Obstetrics and Gynecology*, **36**, 267–268.

Sanchis, A., Rosique, D. & Catala, J. (1991) Adverse effects of maternal lorazepam on neonates. *DICP, The Annals of Pharmacotherapy*, **25**, 1137–1138.

Stevens, S. J. & Arbiter, N. (1995) A therapeutic community for substance abusing pregnant women and women with children. Process and outcome. *Journal of Psychoactive Drugs*, **27**, 49–56.

Strantz, I. H. & Welch, S. P. (1995) Post partum women in outpatient drug abuse treatment: correlates of retention/completion. *Journal of Psychoactive Drugs*, **27**, 357–373.

Ward, J., Mattick, R. P. & Hall, W. (1998) Methadone maintenance during pregnancy. In *Methadone Maintenance Treatment and Other Opioid Replacement Therapies* (eds J. Ward, R. P. Mattick & W. Hall). Harwood Academic Publishers.

Wittman, B. K. & Segal, S. (1991) A comparison of the effects of single- and split-dose methadone administration on the fetus: ultrasound evaluation. *International Journal of the Addictions*, **26**, 213–218.

CHAPTER 20

Intoxication and legal defences

Quazi Haque and Ian Cumming

Summary Intoxication with alcohol and drugs is commonly associated with criminal offending. The relationship between intoxication and criminal culpability is complex and may be of psychiatric relevance, especially if a legal defence resting on mental condition is being considered. This chapter outlines the legal issues (such as they apply in England and Wales) of which psychiatrists should be aware when preparing medico-legal opinions about mentally disordered offenders.

Intoxication with alcohol or drugs is the obvious theme of certain charges such as drunk and disorderly conduct or drink-driving. In other offences, intoxication may be a factor that can affect or complicate the issue of criminal responsibility.

Approximately 50% of violent offences and property offences are committed after drugs or alcohol have been consumed, and although consumption may not be directly linked to the offence, there is often a strong association between the two.

Psychiatrists are frequently asked to comment on the effects of intoxication on mental responsibility. Although the legal defences of insanity and diminished responsibility are familiar to psychiatrists, the relationship between intoxication and criminal intent is a complex issue that can raise the possibility of defences against particular offences. This chapter will mainly consider the law in England and Wales. The major differences in the legislation of the other jurisdictions in the UK are given in Box 20.1.

The issues surrounding intoxication and legal defence appear to be addressed in a variety of ways, which might reflect the complexity of the legal arguments. The law has arisen as a 'compromise' between acknowledging the effects of alcohol and drugs on mental condition and maintaining criminal liability, for the benefit of society. These are areas into which psychiatrists often stray and may even introduce their own moral code. The legal issues that they should be aware of when considering such a venture are outlined below.

There is a generally held belief that many of the legal issues in this area are centred around a theme of intoxication. This is ill-founded and opinions

---

Box 20.1   Other UK jurisdictions

The law in Scotland attaches rather less importance to subjective *mens rea* than that in England and Wales. Most Scottish criminal charges allege no mental element at all but refer only to the proscribed harm. The *mens rea* terms such as recklessness and negligence are often interpreted with an objectivist slant. Liability for causing inadvertent harm while drunk departs little from normal principles. The distinction between offences of basic and specific intent has therefore not developed to the same extent as south of the border. For example, in *Brennan v HM Adv.* [1977], the accused stabbed his father to death after consuming between 20 and 25 pints of beer together with lysergic acid diethyamide (LSD). He was convicted of murder and his appeal was dismissed: voluntary intoxication was considered to be a continuing element of criminal recklessness which Scottish law needed to retain in the interests of its citizens.

Similar positions are held in Northern Ireland and the Republic of Ireland. Although the Beard rules (*DPP v Beard*, 1920) have never been overruled, voluntary intoxication does not provide the basis for a defence against criminal charges.

---

may be sought about the effects of alcohol and drugs without reliable indices of actual intake. The law is less concerned with more modest and minor consumption, although clinicians are often aware of individual variability and the hazards of estimating consumed quantity from the appearance and behaviour of the defendant at the time of the offence.

The law pays little attention to the claim of individuals that they had a drink in order to 'remove their inhibitions'. It is seen as irrelevant that the individual would not have committed the crime if he[1] had not had a drink: he is seen as being fully responsible at the time of the offence. The law is, however, applicable when the person is so intoxicated as to lack the state of mind required in relation to that crime (the *mens rea*) or to be in a state of automatism. It is not a matter as to whether the defendant was capable of forming *mens rea*. It is a question of whether *mens rea* was, in fact, formed.

Case law has been described for the following circumstances:

(a)   intent – specific and basic
(b)   intoxication – involuntary and voluntary
(c)   voluntary intoxication and offences of basic intent
(d)   partial intoxication
(e)   intoxication and mistake

---

1. To avoid repetitive use of his/her and he/she, throughout this chapter defendants and offenders are taken to be male. This does not imply that women are not also defendants and offenders.

(f) voluntary intoxicated beliefs
(g) intoxication and mental health defences of:
  • insanity
  • diminished responsibility
  • automatism.

Crimes of specific and basic intent

The essence of the law is that intoxication can provide a defence to crimes that are of specific intent, but not to those that are of basic intent. In crimes of specific intent, it must be proved that the defendant lacked the necessary *mens rea* at the time of the offence. It is for the prosecution to establish the actual intent of the defendant, taking into account the fact that he was intoxicated. In crimes of basic intent, the fact that intoxication was self-induced provides the necessary *mens rea*.

The original distinction between crimes of specific and of basic intent was based on common sense: the court did not want alcohol to allow a defendant to escape responsibility for his crimes. It did, however, wish to have flexibility so that in certain cases intoxication afforded, in effect, some mitigation. The allocation of crimes to the categories of basic or of specific intent is not based on any established legal test and has often arisen from previous court decisions (Smith & Hogan, 1996). In practice, the terms are difficult to define and are sometimes anomalous. They seem to escape definition; their purpose may be to reduce criminal liability while not allowing the defendant to escape all punishment, but the delineation of crimes into the two categories is less rigorous.

Examples of crimes that have been held to be of specific intent (Box 20.2) include murder (*R v Sheehan*, 1975), wounding or causing grievous bodily harm with intent (*R v Pordage*, 1975), theft (*Ruse v Read*, 1949), deception and handling stolen goods (*R v Durante*, 1972). Crimes that are held to require only a basic intent (Box 20.2) include manslaughter (*R v Lipman*, 1970), malicious wounding or inflicting grievous bodily harm under section 20 of the Offences Against the Person Act 1861 (*Bratty v A-G for Northern Ireland*, 1963), rape (*R v Fotheringham*, 1989) and various offences of assault.

Voluntary and involuntary intoxication

Voluntary intoxication

Voluntary intoxication refers to the knowing intake of alcohol and/or some other drug or intoxicating substance. The individual must be aware that the substance is, or may be, an intoxicant and have taken it in such a quantity that it impairs his awareness or understanding. The law presumes that intoxication is voluntary unless evidence is produced that allows the court or jury to conclude the possibility that it was involuntary.

Box 20.2 Offences requiring specific or basic intent

Specific intent	*Basic intent*
Murder	Manslaughter
Grievous bodily harm with intent	Malicious wounding
Theft	Rape
Deception	Grievous bodily harm under section 20
Handling stolen goods	False imprisonment

Voluntary intoxication is not, and never has been, a defence in itself. It is not a defence to plead that by taking alcohol one's judgement between right and wrong was impaired or that one was no longer able to resist an impulse. There are, however, three broad situations when voluntary intoxication may be forwarded as a defence or mitigating factor and thus be considered as a partial excuse to reduce the level of criminal liability. They are:

(a) when intoxication leads to the inability to form the specific intent requisite for a particular offence;

(b) where a statute expressly provides a false belief to be a defence against the particular offence;

(c) when mental conditions allow the defence of insanity or of diminished responsibility.

Involuntary intoxication

The most common cases of involuntary intoxication involve intoxication that is unknowingly induced by a third party. Intoxication can also be held as involuntary if it is caused by prescribed drugs taken within the required instructions of a doctor, or if caused by a drug, whether or not taken in excessive quantity, that is not normally liable to cause unpredictability or aggressiveness (for example, sedatives such as benzodiazepines).

Where a defendant is reduced to a state of intoxication through no fault of his own, he cannot be 'blamed' for his actions and will, accordingly, have a defence to any criminal charge. The defendant must, however, be so intoxicated that he did not form the requisite *mens rea*. If the *mens rea* is thought to be present, then the law approaches such cases in the same way as for voluntary intoxication, in that involuntary intoxication is not, in itself, a defence.

Thus, provided that the defendant acted voluntarily with the requisite *mens rea*, the fact that involuntary intoxication led him to commit an offence that he would not have committed when sober does not afford a defence

---

Box 20.3   A drugged intent is still an intent

D, who had paedophiliac homosexual tendencies, was in dispute with a couple who arranged for X to obtain damaging information that could be used against D. X invited a 15-year-old boy to his room and drugged him so that he fell asleep. While he was asleep, D visited X's room and performed indecent acts on the boy. These were video recorded by X. D was charged with indecent assault on the boy. His defence was that he had been involuntarily intoxicated at the time because X had laced his drink. He was convicted.

Judgment   The trial judge directed the jury to convict if they found that D had assaulted the boy pursuant to an intent resulting from the influence of intoxication secretly induced by X. Acquittal would arise only if he was so intoxicated, involuntarily, that he did not intend to commit the indecent assault (a basic intent offence). This ruling was held by the House of Lords on appeal.

R v Kingston [1994]

(although it may mitigate the punishment), and this is so even though he acted under an irresistible impulse because of intoxication (Box 20.3).

Voluntary intoxication and intent

Voluntary intoxication and crimes of specific intent

In case law, the meaning of specific intent has been clarified by Lord Birkenhead's decision of 1920 in the case of Beard who, when intoxicated with alcohol, suffocated a girl while raping her (*DPP v Beard*, 1920). From this case, 'insanity', whether produced by drunkenness or otherwise, is a defence against the criminal charge. An accused man could therefore be declared not guilty if intoxication rendered him incapable of forming the specific intent for that offence. According to the Beard rules:

'In a charge of murder based upon intention to kill or do grievous bodily harm, if the jury are satisfied that the accused was, by reason of his drunken condition, incapable of forming the intent to kill or do grievous bodily harm ... he cannot be convicted of murder. But nevertheless, unlawful homicide has been committed by the accused ... and that is manslaughter ... The law is plain beyond question that in cases falling short of insanity a condition of drunkenness at the time of committing an offence causing death can only, when it is available at all, have the effect of reducing the crime from murder to manslaughter.'

It has been argued that these rules are based on judicial policy to protect the public against the prospect of absolute acquittal. This view could be taken further to suggest that such a policy is imperfect; for example, rape is not a crime requiring specific intent and theft has, unlike murder, no charge of basic intent to fall back on. The law changed somewhat following the introduction of the Criminal Justice Act 1967. Section 8 of the Act no longer stipulates that incapacity is requisite in the proof of lack of specific intent. Also, under section 8, individuals are no longer presumed to intend the natural and probable consequences of their acts; rather, necessary intent is to be decided by the jury or magistrates on all the available evidence. Contradictory to the ruling in the Beard case, it is now established that the burden is on the prosecution to establish that, despite the evidence of intoxication, the accused had the necessary specific intent.

Voluntary intoxication and crimes of basic intent

For crimes that require only basic intent, intoxication is no defence. The case law is affirmed in *DPP v Majewski* [1976]. The accused had taken barbiturates, amphetamines and alcohol and subsequently assaulted a publican and three policemen. He was convicted of assault and his following appeal was dismissed.

The judgment from Majewski was that, if the offence charged is one of basic intent, the accused may be convicted of it if he was voluntarily intoxicated at the time of committing the offence, even though, because of intoxication, he did not have the *mens rea* normally required for the conviction of that offence, and despite the fact that he was in a state of automatism. Additionally, the House of Lords recognised in Majewski that, for a person charged with an offence of basic intent, the prosecution does not need to prove the *mens rea* required for that offence and the accused can be convicted simply on proof that he committed the offence (the *actus reus*).

This leads on to the complex concept of recklessness. Certain crimes, such as attempted murder, can only be committed intentionally; others may be committed recklessly. The distinction is important. A distinction must also exist between recklessness and negligence, so that the law can punish reckless wrongdoing, but, apart from certain crimes, it can exempt negligent wrongdoing from criminal liability.

The type of recklessness recognised by the majority of the House of Lords is termed Caldwell-type recklessness, following their Lordships' decision in *R v Caldwell* [1982]. An individual is Caldwell-type reckless with regard to a particular risk that attends his actions if the risk is obvious to an ordinary prudent person who has not given thought to the possibility of there being any such risk, or if the individual has recognised that there is some risk and has nevertheless persisted in his actions.

The effect of the ruling in Majewski that proof of *mens rea* is not required when an accused who is voluntarily intoxicated is charged with an offence of basic intent is reduced when Caldwell-type recklessness suffices for that offence. In *R v Caldwell*, Lord Diplock took the view that classification of offences into those of basic or specific intent was irrelevant where Caldwell-type recklessness sufficed for *mens rea*. The distinction between such offences is important, however, if the intoxicated person who is charged with an offence of basic intent has thought about a possible risk and wrongly concluded it to be negligible. In this case, a loophole in Caldwell-type recklessness (termed 'the lacuna') means that he could not be convicted of recklessness. Indeed, he would be acquitted unless convicted under the Majewski ruling on the basis that the *actus reus* of an offence of basic intent has been committed.

Drug-induced intoxication and intent

Theoretically, the same rules apply to intoxication with drugs. In *R v Lipman* [1969], the accused, in a state of intoxication caused primarily by lysergic acid diethylamide (LSD), asphyxiated a girl by forcing a bedsheet down her throat while believing that he was struggling with snakes. He was deemed to have been reckless, but his state of intoxication rendered him incapable of forming the specific intent for murder and he was therefore convicted of manslaughter.

Intoxication and rape

Rape is a crime of basic intent: the central theme of the charge of rape is one of consent. In the case of *R v Woods* [1981], the accused pleaded that he was so drunk that he had not realised that his victim had not provided consent. Section 1(2) of the Sexual Offences (Amendment) Act 1976 states that if a jury has to consider whether a man believed that a victim was consenting to sexual intercourse, it must have regard to the presence or absence of reasonable grounds for such a belief, in conjunction with any other relevant matters. The Court of Appeal held that intoxication was not a 'legally relevant matter' in this context and therefore the jury must examine the other evidence and disregard the evidence of his intoxication.

Partial intoxication

There is no legal distinction between being completely or partially intoxicated if a defence of intoxication is raised. The ruling from Majewski would therefore apply to partial intoxication in offences requiring a basic intent.

Intoxication and mistake

Intoxication has many effects, including the misinterpretation of the actions and words of others. In many cases, a defendant who committed a crime when drunk will claim that he made a mistake: therefore the necessary *mens rea* was lacking.

If a *sober* person kills another in the mistaken belief that the victim is coming towards him to stab him, he may be found not guilty of murder (provided that he used force that was reasonable on the basis of the facts as he believed them to have been) because he lacked an intent to kill unlawfully or cause grievous bodily harm. Where, however, the mistake arises by reason of voluntary intoxication, the Majewski principle applies, so that the defendant cannot rely on his mistake to acquit him of the crime.

Case law suggests that the Majewski ruling applies in this context even if the offence is one of specific intent. In *R v O'Grady* [1987], the defendant, when intoxicated, killed a man in the mistaken belief that he was being attacked. His appeal against his conviction for manslaughter, an offence of basic intent, was dismissed by the Court of Appeal. Lord Lane judged that a defence of mistake caused by voluntary intoxication would fail even in offences that required specific intent.

Dutch courage

On occasion, individuals use alcohol or drugs to make it easier for them to take certain actions, including criminal ones. The law has ruled that with such offences (including those of specific intent), one is liable, even if, because intoxicated, one lacks the appropriate mental element at the time of the offence. According to Lord Denning's interpretation of the Court of Appeal's decision in *A-G for Northern Ireland v. Gallagher* [1963]:

'... if a man, whilst sane and sober, forms an intention to kill and makes preparations for it, knowing it is the wrong thing to do, and then gets himself drunk so as to give himself Dutch courage to do the thing, and whilst drunk carries out his intention, he cannot rely on this self-induced drunkenness as a defence to a charge of murder, nor even as reducing it to manslaughter. He cannot say that he got himself into such a stupid state that he was incapable of an intent to kill. So, also, when he is a psychopath, he cannot by drinking rely on his self-induced defect of reason as a defence of insanity. The wickedness of his mind before he got drunk is enough to condemn him, coupled with the act which he intended to do and did do. A psychopath who goes out intending to kill, knowing it is wrong, and does kill, cannot escape the consequences of making himself drunk before doing it.'

Intoxicated belief as a defence

There is one type of case where an intoxicated belief can be used as a defence. In *Jaggard v Dickinson* [1980, 1981], the accused was allowed to appeal against conviction of intentional or reckless criminal damage to property. The accused, owing to voluntary intoxication, mistakenly but honestly believed that she was damaging the property of a friend and that the latter would have consented to her doing so. Section 5(3) of the Criminal Damage Act 1971 states that a belief of entitlement to consent to the destruction of property is a lawful excuse and it is immaterial whether such a belief is justified or not, if it is honestly held.

Intoxication and mental health defences

Insanity, diminished responsibility and automatism are mental condition defences within the criminal law of England and Wales. They are not specific to intoxication-related defences.

Insanity

Ever since their inception in 1843, the M'Naghten rules (Mackay, 1995) have been the standard test of criminal responsibility when applied to the defence of insanity. Mackay states that:

'To establish a defence on the ground of insanity, it must be clearly proved that, at the time of the committing of the act, the party accused was labouring under such a defect of reason, from disease of the mind, as not to know the nature and quality of the act he was doing; or if he did know it, that he did not know he was doing what was wrong. "Disease of the mind" is a wide-ranging concept which is capable of encompassing all forms of mental disorder which give rise to a "defect of reason". The courts tend to have a narrower interpretation of "knowledge" requirements of the rules, that is, "nature", "quality" and "wrong". The lack of knowledge of these elements when committing a criminal act is restricted to the lack of legal rather than moral knowledge. The courts therefore apply an extremely restricted approach to the rules which is cognitively, rather than morally, based.'

Therefore, intoxication can satisfy the legal definition of insanity only if the associated state of mind satisfies the strict legal interpretations of disease of the mind and defect of reason. Certain states, such as delirium tremens or drug-induced psychosis, may satisfy all of these criteria. It is also worth noting that if the defendant's state of mind results partly from drink or drugs and partly from a condition that is capable of forming the insanity defence in its own right (e.g. psychopathy), intoxication is usually disregarded as a defence unless it has induced the latter condition within the meaning of the M'Naghten rules.

Diminished responsibility

The defence of diminished responsibility, under section 2 of the Homicide Act 1957, is available for the charge of murder only. There are three components to the defence:

(a) that the accused was suffering from an abnormality of mind at the material time;
(b) that this arose from:
   • a condition of arrested or retarded development of mind
   • inherent causes
   • disease or injury
(c) that it substantially impaired his mental responsibility on such acts as will power, perception and judgement.

Box 20.4 The 'first drink of the day' test

The accused, an alcoholic, usually drank barley wine or Cinzano. On the day of the killing, she drank almost an entire bottle of vodka. That evening, she strangled her 11-year-old daughter after the child had said she had been sexually interfered with at home and wanted to live with her grandmother. The mother's blood alcohol level at the time of the killing was estimated to have been 300 mg per 100 ml, which can be fatal to non-alcoholics. The defendant's own evidence had suggested that she still had control over her drinking after the first drink, despite severe craving for alcohol. The jury convicted her of murder, having decided that she did not suffer from an abnormality of mind as a direct result of her alcoholism.

Her appeal was based on the medical evidence that she might have had a compulsion to drink, at least after the first drink of the day, and that the cumulative effects of such consumption had caused an intoxicated state at the time of the killing. Her counsel also argued the possibility that craving for drink and drugs could produce an abnormality of mind. The appeal was dismissed, the jury having been correctly told by the trial judge that if the taking of the first drink was not involuntary, then the whole of the drinking on the day in question was not involuntary. As for severe craving for drink leading to an abnormality of mind, such craving would need to lead to involuntary drinking and would thus be subject to the 'first drink of the day' test.

R v Tandy [1989]

Alcohol consumption can therefore find a defence of diminished responsibility if alcoholism has amounted to 'disease or injury'. A defence of diminished responsibility cannot, however, be based on an abnormality of mind brought about by voluntary intoxication, as this has not arisen from any inherent causes or been induced by disease or injury. The Court of Appeal has consistently ruled that the transient effects of alcohol on the brain do not amount to injury within the meaning of section 2(1) of the Homicide Act 1957.

For alcoholism to amount to disease or injury, the psychiatrist will have to consider whether cerebral damage has injured the brain to such an extent that there is a gross impairment of judgement and emotional responses. The appropriate physical investigations, such as neuroimaging, electro-encephalograms and psychometric testing, may be of value in supporting this defence.

If alcoholism has not led to extensive brain damage, a defence of diminished responsibility may still be available if drinking has become involuntary. Alcohol dependence could therefore theoretically support such a defence, but existing case law (see Box 20.4) imposes strict criteria. The legal test for such a loss of control, or inability to resist the impulse to drink, requires the first drink of the day to be completely involuntary. If the accused is able to resist the impulse to take the first drink, he does not suffer from a 'disease or injury' within section 2 of the Homicide Act, even if he finds the impulse to continue drinking irresistible. A defence of diminished responsibility cannot then apply.

One could argue that the judgment in *R v Tandy* [1989] could also apply to drug use alone for a defence of diminished responsibility, if the taking of drugs has been involuntary or has resulted in 'disease or injury to the mind' such as to substantially impair mental responsibility. At present there is no clear authority on this point (Mackay, 1999).

Automatism

A defence to a crime can be made if it was committed involuntarily. Where the involuntary act is beyond the control of the individual's mind, the situation is known as an automatism. In broad terms, there are two types of automatism: insane and non-insane. With automatism of the insane type, if the involuntary act can be shown to have occurred in the context of a 'defect of reason due to disease of the mind', the M'Naghten rules and special verdict apply. With automatism of the non-insane type, the accused may be acquitted. In general, therefore, if an act is performed in a state of automatism, criminal liability is negated.

In some cases, however, such action can be liable under Majewski if that automatic state is the result of voluntary intoxication and the offence is one of basic intent. The position is less clear if intoxication is one of a number of features alleged to have combined to produce an automatic state, for example automatism alleged to have been induced by head injury following intoxication. The current law (Law Commission, 1992) suggests that where causal factors are less easily separated, it would seem that the presence of intoxication, based on the Majewski ruling, excludes reliance on automatism.

Conclusion

The effect of alcohol on the individual is very complex and idiosyncratic. Psychiatrists making evaluations for the purposes of court reports face further hurdles in trying to untangle the legal arguments. A clinical evaluation that will be of use to the court will require a thorough history of the events, with a special focus on the defendant's account of the event and consumption of intoxicants in the period leading up to the offence. It is also essential to thoroughly tease out the history of alcohol and substance misuse. Clinical assessment may be complicated by amnesia, which is common in serious offences but is not in itself a defence in criminal proceedings (Taylor & Kopelman, 1984).

The principal problem when assessing the state of intoxication characterising an offender who has committed a criminal act is that many offenders lack one of the key premises for responsibility for a criminal act,

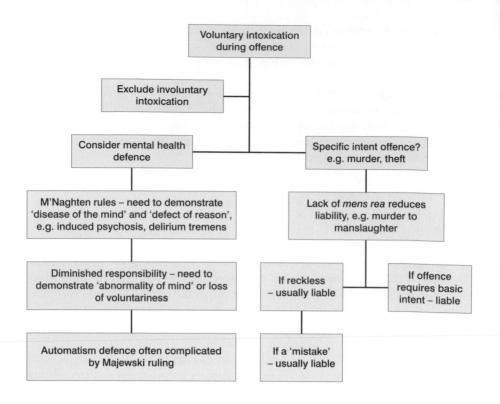

Fig. 20.1 Legal defences available to the intoxicated offender.

namely *mens rea*. The judgment of being legally guilty or culpable requires the conversion of legal and philosophical values into working jurisprudence. Case law provides practical guidance when considering issues of legal defences, but it is complex and subject to frequent reform (Fischer & Rehm, 1998; Gough, 2000). Although it is the court process that decides on culpability, it is not unusual for psychiatrists to be asked to comment on specific mental elements related to a criminal offence committed by an intoxicated defendant. Aside from the well-established mental condition defences of insanity and diminished responsibility, a working knowledge of the association between intoxication and intention is therefore helpful (Fig. 20.1).

References

Fischer, B. & Rehm, J. (1998) Intoxication, the law and criminal responsibility – a sparkling cocktail at times. *European Addiction Research*, 4, 89–101.

Gough, S. (2000) Surviving without Majewski? *Criminal Law Review*, (Sept.), pp. 719–733.

Law Commission (1992) *Intoxication and Criminal Liability*. Consultation Paper No. 127, TSO (The Stationery Office).

Mackay, R. D. (1995) *Mental Condition Defences in the Criminal Law*, pp. 180–214. Clarendon Press.

Mackay, R. D. (1999) Crim LR 105 at 121.

Smith, J. C. & Hogan, B. (1996) *Criminal Law* (8th edn), pp. 221–223. Butterworths.

Taylor, P. J. & Kopelman, M. D. (1984) Amnesia for criminal offences. *Psychological Medicine*, **14**, 581–588.

A-G for Northern Ireland v Gallagher [1963] AC 349.
Bratty v A-G for Northern Ireland [1963] AC 386, 410.
Brennan v HM Adv. [1977] Scots Law Times 151.
DPP v Beard [1920] AC 479 (64).
DPP v Majewski [1976] 2 All ER 142.
Jaggard v Dickinson [1981] QB 527, [1980] 3 All ER 716, DC.
R v Caldwell [1982] AC 341, [1981] 1 All ER 961.
R v Durante [1972] 1 WLR 1612.
R v Fotheringham [1989] 88 Cr App R 206.
R v Kingston [1994] 3 All ER 353, HL.
R v Lipman [1969] 3 All ER 410.
R v Lipman [1970] 1 QB 152, CA.
R v O'Grady [1987] QB 995, [1987] 3 All ER 420, CA.
R v Pordage [1975] Crim LR 575.
R v Sheehan [1975] 1 WLR 739.
R v Tandy [1989] 1 All ER 267, CA.
R v Woods [1981] 74 Cr App R 312, CA.
Ruse v Read [1949] 1 KB 377.

CHAPTER 21

Substance misuse and violence: the scope and limitations of forensic psychiatry's role

Peter Snowden

Summary Psychiatric disorder, substance misuse and violence often coexist in the work of a forensic psychiatrist, and forensic psychiatry should view the management of substance misuse problems as fundamental to practice. The causes are part of an interactional process involving the basic pharmacological effects of alcohol and drugs, the substance use context, environment, culture and personality factors such as predisposition to aggression. The prevalence of alcohol and drug use in prisoners is high, with 66% of prisoners reporting drug use in the month before being received into prison, and 39% whilst in prison. This is significant as individuals with comorbid mental health and substance misuse are more likely than those with only psychosis to report offending or aggression. The forensic psychiatrist may have a number of opportunities to identify offenders who misuse substances, and should be aware of the available treatment pathways and strategies.

For the past 30 years, forensic psychiatry has been concerned with violent offenders with psychosis and/or personality disorder. If dual diagnosis or comorbidity meant anything to a forensic psychiatrist, it would be the 'typical' forensic case – an individual with schizophrenia and a premorbid dissocial personality who had been arrested for a violent crime. In this chapter I use comorbidity to describe the co-occurrence of two or more conditions (here a psychiatric disorder and health problems arising from substance misuse) rather than dual diagnosis. In fact, many violent offenders have multiple diagnoses. Williams & Cohen (2000) argue that dual diagnosis suggests a closer relationship, perhaps including cause and effect, and is a subset of comorbidity.

Forensic psychiatrists have probably kept up with developments in criminal law as it relates to crimes associated with alcohol and drugs more than they have with the psychiatry of substance (alcohol and drug) misuse and its relationship to forensic psychiatry. Speciality training arguably encourages this narrow focus. This is unfortunate, as the Epidemiologic Catchment Area

> **Box 21.1** The role of the forensic psychiatrist
>
> *Identification* To identify and assess the degree of dependence and psycho-logical, physical and social problems associated with substance use, misuse and dependence
>
> *Decision-making* To make informed decisions on how to meet the needs of the patient, based on multidisciplinary expertise
>
> *Liaison* As necessary, to contact appropriate criminal justice system services
>
> *Referral* To contact other specialist services if the balance between the offender's risk to others and problems associated with the psychiatric disorder and substance misuse suggests that forensic services are not the most appropriate services to meet the individual's needs
>
> *Management* To manage jointly or take a lead in managing those whose risk to others is a major concern

(ECA) surveys (Regier *et al*, 1990) have shown that having a mental disorder doubles the risk of an alcohol misuse disorder and quadruples the risk of a drug-related disorder. The institutional ECA survey of psychiatric patients and prisoners shows even higher levels of comorbidity, with a lifetime prevalence of substance use disorders of 16.7% in the general population and 39% in patients of mental hospitals.

The role of the modern forensic psychiatrist

Forensic psychiatry should view the discipline of substance misuse as fundamental to practice. Practitioners should be able to make rational informed decisions when presented with offenders with a history of substance misuse, particularly when, in addition, there is a comorbid disorder (see Box 21.1).

Relationship of substance problems to violence and crime

Violence

Drugs and alcohol can produce effects that may lead to violence as part of an acute psychological disturbance or as a result of misuse, withdrawal and dependence. In general, alcohol is a major risk factor for violent offending, whereas illicit drug use is more likely to be associated with acquisitive offending and trafficking. Athanasiadis (1999) has reviewed the association between drugs, alcohol and violence, in a field of research limited by

---

Box 21.2   The relationship between drugs, alcohol and violence

Positive association

- Cocaine and 'crack'
- Amphetamines
- Anabolic androgenic steroids
- Alcohol
- Benzodiazepines
- Cannabis

No association

- Sole use of opiates
- Nicotine

---

methodological complexities inherent in the multifaceted nature of the problem. Not all drugs are associated with violence in populations without psychosis (Box 21.2).

There is a significant relationship between early development and onset of alcohol dependence and trait aggressiveness. The aetiology of violence is complex, and alcohol-induced aggression is not a uniform phenomenon. Three possible mechanisms have been proposed (Pihl & Lemarquand, 1998) to explain the association of alcohol and violence – potentiation, inhibition and disorganisation of behaviour. These might be mediated through serotonin pathways. Badawy (1998) suggests that in those with a susceptibility to aggression after alcohol consumption there is a marked depletion of brain serotonin, which may increase the likelihood of aggression in response to internal or external stimuli. Another approach has been to focus on executive cognitive functioning and it has been proposed that disruption of this system by alcohol is an underlying mechanism in alcohol-intoxicated aggression. Johns (1998) suggests that 'although the association between substance misuse and aggression is well recognised, the mechanisms are poorly understood'. Clearly, the causes are complex and are part of an interactional process involving the basic pharmacological effects of alcohol and drugs, the drinking (substance misuse) context and environment, culture and personal factors such as predisposition to aggression.

Crime

The prevalence of alcohol misuse in a survey of psychiatric morbidity of prisoners in England and Wales (Singleton et al, 1998) was 58% for male and 36% for female remand prisoners. For the sentenced population the results were 63% and 39% respectively. Only a minority denied any past drug use. Fifty per cent of the male and 33% of the female sentenced populations were

---

Box 21.3 Alcohol-related crime and harm to public order

The following points are taken from the Interim Analytical Report of the National Alcohol Harm Reduction Strategy (Prime Minister's Strategy Unit, 2002)

- Alcohol impairs cognitive skills, meaning that people may misread social cues, make bad judgements about risk, or respond inappropriately in social situations. In particular they are more likely to respond aggressively when they believe they are being provoked

- People arrested for breach of the peace, criminal damage, and assault (including sexual assault and domestic violence) are most likely to have been drinking

- The British Crime Survey (BCS) shows that in 2001/2, 47% of all victims of violence described their assailant as being under the influence of alcohol at the time

- BCS figures suggest that in 1999 there were an estimated 1.2 million incidents of alcohol-related violence. Over half of alcohol-related violence between strangers and acquaintances occurs in or around pubs, clubs or discos, with 70% of such incidents taking place on weekend evenings

- Over half of all incidents of alcohol-related violence between strangers and acquaintances resulted in some form of injury

- Alcohol plays a role in around a third of cases of violence between spouses and partners

- The total cost of alcohol-related crime in England and Wales is estimated to be up to £7.3 billion

---

using drugs in prison. A more recent study based on mandatory drug testing in prisons found that 39% of prisoners said that they had used drugs at least once while in their current prison, 25% had used in the past month and 16% had used in the week before interview (Singleton *et al*, 2005). In total, 66% of prisoners reported drug use in the month before being received into prison, and 25% reported that they had used while in prison.

An English special hospital study (Corbett *et al*, 1998) reviewed the case notes of patients admitted between 1972 and 1995. Patients with a history of substance misuse were significantly more likely to have taken illicit drugs at the time of the index offence than patients without such a history. Patients with personality disorder and a history of drug misuse were twice as likely to have taken alcohol at the time of a violent offence compared with controls.

While crime and drug misuse have been high on the political agenda, until recently there have been few initiatives to tackle the role played by alcohol in crime. The extent of the problem has been summarised in the Interim Analytical Report of the National Alcohol Harm Reduction Strategy (see Box 21.3). Box 21.4 summarises the risk factors for becoming a victim of alcohol-related stranger or acquaintance violence.

Box 21.4   Risk factors for becoming a victim of alcohol-related stranger or acquaintance violence

- Being a male 16–29 years old
- Being single
- Being unemployed
- Visiting a pub frequently
- Visiting a night club frequently
- Living in an urban or inner-city area
- Living in privately rented accommodation
- Drinking on average 3–4 times per week
- Drinking more than 10 units on a typical drinking day

Rasanen *et al* (1998) found in an unselected birth cohort study that men who misused alcohol and were diagnosed with schizophrenia were 25.2 times more likely to commit violent crime than well men. The risk for individuals with schizophrenia not dependent on alcohol was 3.6 times higher, and for individuals with other psychosis it was 7.7 times higher. This study also found that one-fifth of the men with schizophrenia were dependent on alcohol by the age of 27.

Other studies confirm that individuals with comorbidity are more likely than those with only psychosis to report offending or aggression. Steadman *et al* (1998) reported findings of the MacArthur Violence Risk Assessment Study, which compared violence by discharged psychiatric patients with that by others living in the same community. There was no difference between patients and controls, but substance misuse was associated with an increased risk of violence in both groups. For patients, the effect was more obvious, with a 1-year rate of violence of 18% for major mental disorder, increasing to 31% with comorbid substance misuse. The highest risk of violence (43%) occurred with a combination of substance misuse and personality or adjustment disorder. A significant risk of violent behaviour has also been reported in those with dual diagnosis complicated by non-adherence to medication. Thomson (1999) describes the synergistic effect between substance misuse and mental disorder in the causation of violence. Swartz *et al* (1998) postulate three explanations for this: substance misuse may impede medication adherence, non-adherence may lead to self-medication with illicit drugs, or non-adherence and substance misuse may both result from other factors such as personality traits and poor insight.

Of the 500 homicide court reports reviewed by Appleby *et al* (1999) in their Report on Safer Services (70% of the homicide cases identified), 39%

had a history of alcohol misuse and in 51% alcohol was thought to have contributed to the offence. For drug misuse the figures were 35% and 18%, respectively. The homicide group was further subdivided into those with a mental illness and a larger group of other individuals (i.e. those with a personality disorder) in contact with mental health services. Those with mental illness had a lower rate of drug misuse than those with no mental illness, but the same rate of alcohol misuse. Both alcohol and drugs were more likely to be implicated in homicide in those with no mental illness.

Forensic psychiatry's role: scope and limitations

Identification

Although the primary focus of forensic psychiatry treatment services (in-patient or community) is on the violent offender with mental disorder, a wider group of offenders is initially assessed. The forensic psychiatrist has a number of opportunities to identify offenders who misuse substances (whether or not the individual is violent) through contact with the probation service and prison healthcare service and through cases referred for assessment by the legal profession and the courts. Box 21.5 describes in general terms the purpose of any assessment by a psychiatrist of an individual who misuses drugs and alcohol. It is important to differentiate between recreational use, harmful use and a dependence syndrome. For a definite diagnosis of dependence in ICD–10, three or more of the following should have been experienced or exhibited some time during the previous year: a compulsion to take the substance, an impaired capacity to control use, a physiological withdrawal state, tolerance, preoccupation with substance use, and persistent use despite clear evidence of harmful effects (World Health Organization, 1992).

Brooke *et al* (1998), in a study based on self-report data, suggest that 23% of remand prisoners would like treatment for substance misuse. At

---

Box 21.5 The purpose of assessing drug and alcohol problems

- To differentiate recreational use, harmful use and dependence
- To distinguish between substance-related psychological symptoms and psychiatric syndromes
- To identify substance-related acute presentations
- To ensure adequate risk assessment
- To initiate appropriate and effective therapies safely
- To refer to specialist National Health Service, voluntary or statutory services

least half of such individuals have no history of contact with mental health services and a period in custody may be the first chance to offer treatment. Prison treatment programmes have been shown to be cost-effective, with significant reductions in recidivism rates. All offenders assessed by a forensic psychiatrist should be subjected to a full psychiatric history and mental state examination, with a focus on alcohol and substance misuse. The examination should include prescribed medication and non-adherence.

In England, the Drug Intervention Programme began in 2003 with three aims: to facilitate integration between criminal justice agencies and treatment providers, to deliver seamless treatment pathways across agencies, and to address drug-using offenders' needs across treatment journeys. The programme is based on the rationale that addressing the treatment needs of drug-using offenders will reduce their involvement in criminality. Its aim is to help adult drug-using offenders out of crime and into treatment by developing and integrating measures known as interventions (Home Office 2007). The key features are listed in Box 21.6.

The extension of the Drug Intervention Programme into prisons has been based on the development of the 'integrated drug treatment system' (IDTS) in prisons. The objective of the IDTS is to expand the quantity and quality of drug treatment within HM Prisons by:

- increasing the range of treatment options available to those in prison, notably substitute prescribing
- integrating clinical and psychological treatment in prison into one system that works to the standards of Models of Care (National Treatment Agency for Substance Misuse, 2006) and the Treatment Effectiveness Strategy (National Treatment Agency for Substance Misuse, 2005) and works to one care plan
- integrating prison and community treatment to prevent damaging interruptions either on reception into custody or on release back home.

The IDTS has to work closely with the Drug Intervention Programme in particular to ensure that offenders receive seamless support and are retained in treatment after release. The IDTS is being introduced throughout the prison estate in England and Wales in 2007 and will be evaluated as part of the overall integration of drug treatment within the criminal justice system.

Decision-making and liaison

If an individual gives a history suggestive of problem use, it must decided whether this is harmful to their physical, mental and social well-being and if so, whether there is evidence of dependence and comorbidity. Any psychiatrist working in prison, but particularly the forensic psychiatrist (because of the nature of the work), has a responsibility to encourage the development of appropriate treatment opportunities for offenders who misuse substances.

Box 21.6 Key elements of the Drug Interventions Programme

Criminal justice integrated teams (CJITs) facilitate delivery at a local level. Set up by the local drug action team (see chapter 2), CJITs case manage adult offenders and coordinate agencies and services. CJIT workers (previously known as arrest referral workers) are based in police custody suites and courts to provide a gateway into treatment and into the throughcare provided by CJITs. Their assessments of drug-misusing offenders are taken into consideration by judges and magistrates when they make bail and sentencing decisions.

Conditional cautioning targets offenders by attaching a condition of treatment to a police caution. The offender may be prosecuted if the condition is not met.

Drug testing on arrest was phased in during 2006 across 70 drug action team areas. Offenders who test positive for the use of heroin, cocaine or crack cocaine on arrest or charge are asked to undergo a required assessment of their drug misuse, and it is an offence to refuse the assessment. Information about an offender's drug misuse can provide an opportunity to identify their needs and offer support, even if they are never charged with the offence they were arrested for. If an offender is charged and goes to court, the information about their drug misuse is useful for informing bail and sentencing decisions.

Restriction on bail (RoB) reverses the presumption of court bail for defendants who have tested positive for heroin, cocaine or crack cocaine. It should be applied to any adult defendant attending court for a drugs offence, or an offence the court suspects was caused or contributed to by Class A drug misuse, unless the court believes there is no significant risk of the defendant reoffending. Restriction on bail makes the requirement to undergo an assessment of the defendant's drug misuse and/or any proposed follow-up treatment a condition of court bail. A failure to comply with this condition is treated in the same way as any other breach of bail.

Treatment-related community sentencing is predominantly carried out through drug rehabilitation requirements (DRRs) in community sentences. Drug rehabilitation requirements are the main delivery route for drug interventions within community sentences for adult offenders. The requirements involve treatment (either in the community or in a residential setting) and regular drug testing. The National Probation Service also has specific accredited programmes to tackle drug-related offending.

Counselling, assessment, referral, advice and throughcare (CARAT) services provide specialist advice and drug treatment to prisoners in order to reduce the harm caused by drugs and to secure access to treatment on release. CARAT workers take the lead role for the programme in prisons, and liaise closely with the local CJIT throughout an offender's sentence and particularly in the preparation of release plans at the end of a sentence to help offenders reintegrate into the community. CARAT teams also work closely with prison resettlement teams to help ensure that drug misusers' wider rehabilitative needs can be met.

(Adapted from Home Office, 2007)

The changes in the provision of healthcare in prison (HM Prison Service & NHS Executive, 1999), in conjunction with the Drug Interventions Programme (see above), have improved the provision of therapies and the quality of treatment, with less reliance on rapid detoxification as the only treatment strategy.

Referral

For violent offenders who misuse substances (without comorbidity), the clinical aspects of any inter-agency community strategy for risk management should involve interventions to reduce reliance on alcohol and drugs. The role of the forensic psychiatrist is limited to the referral of these individuals to the most appropriate service (NHS, independent probation or voluntary), and to encourage, with the Drug Interventions Programme and the probation service, a multi-agency risk-management approach. As a guide, where there is evidence of harmful substance use and/or dependence, specialist alcohol or substance misuse services should be involved and, if necessary (risk and the nature of the offence will dictate this), the probation service too. For non-dependent harmful use a decision will need to be made as to which is the most appropriate agency to undertake further work, and in most cases the probation service and voluntary sector should be considered.

Therapeutic work can always begin in prison at the point of assessment. All prisons have counselling, assessment, referral, advice and throughcare (CARAT) teams to provide specialist advice and drug treatment to prisoners (Box 21.6). They will facilitate the continuation of treatment when the individual is returned to the community. Advice to the court at the time of sentencing, and liaison with an offender's general practitioner (GP), the local mental health service, addiction service and probation are all routes to ensure that a treatment recommendation is put into practice. For those who do not have a GP, efforts should be made to identify one. No individual should be 'blacklisted' as a hopeless case. The health gains associated with success, or even partial success, are too great and therapeutic pessimism should be avoided.

Management of violent offenders with comorbidity

The forensic psychiatrist will be particularly involved in cases where there is a combination of a psychiatric disorder, substance misuse and violence. Such cases have become very much part of the core work of forensic psychiatrists in recent years (Marshall, 1998). The 'typical' forensic case could now be described as involving a violent offender with a personality disorder that pre-dates the development of a mental illness, complicated further by harmful substance misuse. The assessment of risk (Box 21.7) in these cases must consider the triangular relationship between the mental illness, violence and substance misuse. In some cases a period in a secure unit will be necessary, in order to improve the clinical risk assessment and to help with stabilisation and detoxification from drugs and/or alcohol. The risk assessment will then dictate the most appropriate and safest clinical risk management strategy. These are complex cases, and the risk assessment

---

Box 21.7 Factors to consider in risk assessment for violent offenders with a dual diagnosis

Index offence

- Nature and severity of index offence
- Past offending history

Substance misuse

- Alcohol history
- Drug history
- Nature and extent of harmful use/dependence
- Treatment adherence
- Insight and motivation for change
- Early identification of relapse of misuse

Mental illness

- Nature of the illness
- Treatment adherence
- Insight
- Early identification of relapse of illness

Relationship of violence to:

- use, misuse, withdrawal or chronic use of alcohol/drugs
- mental illness and alcohol/drug misuse

---

and management programme will have to be revisited on a regular basis and refined over time.

Offenders who pose a significant risk to others should be managed primarily by forensic services, who would be expected to address non-dependent harmful use (Box 21.8). Even in these cases specialist advice can be necessary, and in some cases other services could be involved in a secondary capacity. Those with dependence on or harmful misuse of substances will need at the very least an assessment by a specialist substance misuse service (Box 21.9). (Both case examples are fictitious.) In other cases a shared care approach may be more suitable, but the risk management plan will need to be clear about how the two clinical problems will be dealt with and whether other services are to be involved. Each individual will need an assessment such as that outlined in Box 21.7, and its outcome will dictate the most appropriate balance between forensic and other services.

High-risk individuals should be treated by forensic services as in-patients and then as community patients (Snowden *et al*, 1999). However, the limitations of such an approach must be recognised and addiction services have much to offer here. It would be unusual for a forensic team not to seek the advice of specialist addiction services in such cases. Where continuity of care is not such an issue and it is decided that the risks are better managed

Box 21.8   Case example 1

A 40-year-old man with a history of alcohol dependence kills his father, with whom he is living, in the setting of an acute psychotic episode and after a number of negative life events. Further investigation reveals that 9 years previously he had a grand mal fit and at around the same time he began to present with a paranoid psychosis. After admission to a medium secure unit, and a few days before a court date, he had his second grand mal fit. A computerised axial tomography scan showed clear generalised brain damage.

He was prescribed carbamazepine, primarily as an anticonvulsant, but the psychotic symptoms settled also. After much debate, and with his agreement, disulfiram was prescribed. Alongside other treatment interventions, a nurse specialist from an alcohol misuse service saw him for individual sessions. As he obtained greater leave privileges he was able to attend the specialist alcohol treatment service for group work and educational sessions. Now discharged, he is primarily supervised by the forensic community team, but he is also in regular contact with a community psychiatric nurse from the local community alcohol team.

Box 21.9   Case example 2

A male who developed schizophrenia in his 20s often presented to local adult mental health services after relapse. Non-adherence and associated cannabis misuse complicated his care. His use of cannabis became heavy and harmful, and relapses became more serious because he began to set fires when unwell. After causing a serious fire he was admitted to a medium secure unit. It took some considerable time to stabilise his mental state. The forensic team worked with him to reduce his cannabis habit and to show him the risks associated with cannabis use. He is now living in the community, and his illness is in remission. He cooperates with antipsychotic medication. However, he still finds it difficult to be totally abstinent from cannabis. Close supervision involving hostel staff, his brother and the multidisciplinary forensic team, with random urine testing, has managed, so far, to keep him safe in the community.

by a shared care approach, both forensic and local/addiction services can be involved. It is essential in such cases that responsibilities are clear, that the focus of each service is understood and that the planned response of health services to any potential increase in risk is known. Forensic mental health services cannot function and meet the needs of patients if too isolated from general adult and specialist addiction services. It is essential for service links to be strengthened. Effective community treatment of such patients requires careful attention to adherence to treatment, within an integrated substance misuse and mental health approach.

Service models for violent offenders with comorbidity

A number of prospective studies have shown that treatment outcomes such as symptom levels, hospitalisation rates and stability of social functioning are worse in dual diagnosis. Also, poorer adherence to treatment, more frequent violent behaviour and probably more severe clinical and social problems are found in dual diagnosis than in psychotic illness alone (Swanson *et al*, 1990). To make matters worse, the problems relating to the substance misuse can be as chronic as those associated with the mental illness.

Drake *et al* (1998) have reviewed treatment services for people with a dual diagnosis in the USA (see also chapters 12 and 13, this volume). By the 1980s many of these individuals were shunted from general services to specialist substance misuse services, and were often excluded from both systems. For violent offenders with dual diagnosis this could be catastrophic, and it led to the development of a single integrated service and clinical programme. Interventions for substance misuse and mental health were provided by the same clinical team.

Crome (1999) has reviewed the situation from a UK perspective in this underresearched field. The experience of services in the USA may not be appropriate for the UK, where various models could be considered (Box 21.10). Nevertheless, comprehensive out-patient programmes do appear to engage patients in services and may help them reduce substance misuse and attain remission. Service effectiveness appears to be associated with assertive outreach, case management and a longitudinal, stepwise, motivational approach to substance misuse and its treatment (see chapter 13).

Substance use and misuse in secure psychiatric units

The use of alcohol and drugs is an increasingly important issue in the management of in-patients, even in secure units. Many patients in medium secure units have leave and can therefore bring drugs into the unit. Visitors

---

Box 21.10 Strategies for managing substance misuse and dual diagnosis in the National Health Service

- Developing closer links between forensic and addiction services
- Facilitating at all levels (including consultant) joint discussions, cross-referrals, assessments and protocols
- Training and supervision in addiction techniques for all forensic teams
- Specialist dual-diagnosis keyworker liaison with community forensic teams

---

Box 21.11   Diagnosis of substance misuse in in-patients with psychosis

The individual

- Sudden unexplained exacerbation of psychosis
- Evidence of financial embarrassment
- Intoxication
- Deterioration of behaviour and violence
- Victim of assault or bullying

The patients

- Violence and bullying between patients
- Change in mental state and behaviour of a number of patients

The ward regime

- Problems following visits to the ward of specific visitors
- Problems after specific patients return from leave

---

to secure units are another source of illegal drugs and alcohol. Williams & Cohen (2000) have described the problems on psychiatric wards. There is as yet little information about the difficulties experienced in secure units. The Fallon Inquiry into events on the personality disorder unit at Ashworth High Security Hospital described a 'system which was lax enough to allow the importation of alcohol' (Fallon *et al*, 1999). There is a need to draw up policies and procedures in secure units to manage these issues, but it is difficult to manage the tension between therapy and security considerations. Measures to prevent and control drug misuse can have an oppressive effect, but drug misuse and its effects can frighten other patients and staff. This is because of violence, bullying, sexual misconduct, indebtedness and relapse (Poole & Brabbins, 1997). Box 21.11 provides a helpful framework for considering the clinical issues.

Conclusion

A series of powerful epidemiological studies (Johns, 1998) have quantified the increased risk of violent offending and the relative contributions of mental disorders and substance misuse. Substance misuse as a topic is central to the discipline of forensic psychiatry. The splitting of services for offender patients with mental disorder (particularly those with psychotic illnesses) and associated substance misuse problems and the separation of training schemes for doctors and other disciplines should be reviewed if we are to provide the best services for our patients.

References

Appleby, L., Shaw, J., Amos, T., et al (1999) *Safer Services: National Confidential Inquiry into Suicide and Homicide by People with Mental Illness*. Department of Health.

Athanasiadis, L. (1999) Drugs, alcohol and violence. *Current Opinion in Psychiatry*, **12**, 281–286.

Badawy, A. A. B. (1998) Alcohol, aggression and serotonin: metabolic aspects. *Alcohol and Alcoholism*, **33**, 66–72.

Brooke, D., Taylor, C., Gunn, J., et al (1998) Substance misusers in prison – a treatment opportunity? *Addiction*, **93**, 1851–1856.

Corbett, M., Duggan, C. & Larkin, E. (1998) Substance abuse and violence: a comparison of special hospital in-patients diagnosed with either schizophrenia or personality disorder. *Criminal Behaviour and Mental Health*, **8**, 311–321.

Crome, I. B. (1999) Substance misuse and psychiatric comorbidity: towards improved service provision. *Drugs: Education, Prevention and Policy*, **6**, 151–174.

Drake, R. E., Mercer-McFadden, C., Meuser, K. M., et al (1998) Review of integrated mental health and substance abuse treatment for patients with dual disorders. *Schizophrenia Bulletin*, **24**, 589–608.

Fallon, P., Bluglass, R., Edwards, B., et al (1999) *Report of the Committee of Inquiry into the Personality Disorder Unit, Ashworth Special Hospital*. Cm 4195. TSO (The Stationery Office).

HM Prison Service & NHS Executive (1999) *The Future Organisation of Prison Healthcare: Report by the Joint Prison Service and National Health Service Executive Working Group*. Department of Health.

Home Office (2007) *The Drug Interventions Programme*. Home Office. http://www.drugs.gov.uk/drug-interventions-programme

Johns, A. (1998) Substance misuse and offending. *Current Opinion in Psychiatry*, **11**, 669–673.

Marshall, J. (1998) Comordity of severe mental illness and substance misuse. *Journal of Forensic Psychiatry*, **9**, 9–12.

National Treatment Agency for Substance Misuse (2005) *Business Plan 2005/06: Towards Treatment Effectiveness*. NTA.

National Treatment Agency for Substance Misuse (2006) *Models of Care for the Treatment of Adult Drug Misusers: Update 2006*. NTA.

Pihl, R. O. & Lemarquand, D. (1998) Serotonin and aggression in the alcohol–aggression relationship. *Alcohol and Alcoholism*, **33**, 55–65.

Poole, R. & Brabbins, C. (1997) Substance misuse and psychosis. *British Journal of Hospital Medicine*, **58**, 447–450.

Prime Minister's Strategy Unit (2002) *Strategy Unit Alcohol Harm Reduction Project: Interim Analytical Report*. Cabinet Office. http://www.number-10.gov.uk/files/pdf/SU%20interim_report2.pdf

Rasanen, P., Tuhonen, J., Ishanni, M., et al (1998) Schizophrenia, alcohol abuse and violent behaviour: a 26 year follow-up study of an unselected birth cohort. *Schizophrenia Bulletin*, **24**, 437–441.

Regier, D. A., Farmer, M. E., Rae, D. S., et al (1990) Comorbidity of mental disorders with alcohol and other drug abuse. *Journal of the American Medical Association*, **264**, 2511–2518.

Singleton, N., Meltzer, H., Gatward, R., et al (1998) *Psychiatric Morbidity Among Prisoners in England and Wales*. HMSO.

Singleton, N., Pendry, E., Simpson, T., et al (2005) *The Impact and Effectiveness of Mandatory Drugs Tests in Prison*. Home Office.

Snowden, P., McKenna, J. & Jasper, A. (1999) Management of conditionally discharged patients and others who present similar risks in the community: integrated or parallel? *Journal of Forensic Psychiatry*, **10**, 583–596.

Steadman, H. J., Mulvey, E. P., Monahan, J., *et al* (1998) Violence by people discharged from acute psychiatric facilities and by others in the same neighbourhoods. *Archives of General Psychiatry*, **55**, 393–401.

Swanson, J., Holzer, C. & Ganju, V. (1990) Violence and psychiatric disorder in the community: evidence from the Epidemiological Catchment Area Survey. *Hospital and Community Psychiatry*, **41**, 761–770.

Swartz, M. S., Swanson, J. W., Hiday, V. A., *et al* (1998) Violence and severe mental illness: the effects of substance abuse and non-adherence to medication. *American Journal of Psychiatry*, **155**, 226–231.

Thomson, L. D. G. (1999) Substance abuse and criminality. *Current Opinion in Psychiatry*, **12**, 653–657.

Williams, R. & Cohen, J. (2000) Substance use and misuse in psychiatric wards. A model task for clinical governance? *Psychiatric Bulletin*, **24**, 43–46.

World Health Organization (1992) *The ICD–10 Classification of Mental and Behavioural Disorders*. WHO.

CHAPTER 22

Literary and biographical perspectives on substance use

Ed Day and Iain Smith

Summary This chapter attempts to give a flavour of the influence that psychoactive substances have had on many authors and the literary process. It explores the idea of the narrative as it is applied to addictive disorders and gives a range of examples of writing about different substances that might enhance the reader's knowledge of current drug culture. The portrayal in literature of doctors with addictions is presented as a warning to psychiatrists. The authors hope to have demonstrated that literature can be a valuable tool in understanding the experience of drug and alcohol use and addiction.

The effects of psychoactive drugs have been closely linked to all forms of literature for as long as humans have been writing, but a review of the subject is currently very topical. Although the problems of alcohol have long been a theme covered by authors, other drugs have not been as well represented in mainstream publishing until the past few decades. However, the escalation of the drug problem in the Western world has had an influence on popular fiction and led to a rekindling of interest in an older literature that explored these themes. The work of the 19th-century Romantics and of the Beat Generation and counter-culture of the 1960s has been developed by the 'chemical generation', with ecstasy (methylenedioxymethamphetamine (MDMA)) joining the opiates, cocaine, cannabis, lysergic acid diethylamide (LSD) and amphetamines as a backdrop to popular fiction.

Writers and alcohol

Alcohol, in particular, has been strongly linked to creativity, and John Sutherland, a professor of English literature in London and a self-confessed 'recovering drunk', has written extensively in this area. His book *Last Drink to LA* (Sutherland, 2001)[1] provides some literary signposts on the path

---

1. All novels are referenced to their first editions.

to understanding alcohol addiction and describes his own experiences at Alcoholics Anonymous (AA). Through his attendance at AA meetings, Sutherland has come to see addicts primarily as storytellers, believing that 'telling tales (most of them tall, many of them self-serving) is one of the few things that booze makes you good at' (Sutherland, 2001: p. 73).

Analysis of the lives of many famous writers reveals evidence of heavy alcohol consumption, mental illness, physical disease, family breakdown, suicide and premature death (Post, 1994). There has been much interest in the link between alcohol and writing in the USA, particularly since the realisation that five of the first seven American-born writers awarded the Nobel Prize for Literature had alcohol-related problems (Sinclair Lewis, Eugene O'Neill, William Faulkner, Ernest Hemingway and John Steinbeck). However, it is the case of one name omitted from this list, that of F. Scott Fitzgerald, that illustrates some of the possible reasons for the link between writing and drinking alcohol (Box 22.1) – a source of speculation for academics and psychiatrists alike (Goodwin, 1988; Dardis, 1989).

There is a belief that creative people are expected to have a significant flaw in their character and that this is an integral part of their creativity. Baudelaire (Bold, 1982: p. 87) believed that intoxication was essential to creativity and Nietzsche agreed, stating that 'for art to exist, for any sort of aesthetic society or perception to exist, a certain physiological precondition is indispensable: intoxication' (Marks, 2001: p. 506). In the early 1920s, Fitzgerald was prone to introduce himself to people at parties as an alcoholic, a tactic apparently designed to shock. Many writers comment on their use of alcohol to help them to relax after an intense period of work. Ernest Hemingway, a close friend of Fitzgerald, had a regular routine each day whereby he would get up early, write in the morning, fish or hunt in the afternoon and drink to relax and unwind in the evening. Both he and William Faulkner said that they used alcohol to help them stop writing: to switch off the creative process.

Alcohol may give writers confidence and help them to overcome what Georges Simenon called 'stage fright': the doubts about their ability to write and the quality of their work (Goodwin, 1988: p. 186). Some writers have stated that alcohol improved their writing ability, and Fitzgerald felt that stories he wrote while sober seemed 'stupid' and 'all reasoned out, not felt' (Goodwin, 1988: p. 187). Other, more contemporary, authors have agreed with Stephen King, believing that 'a writer who drinks carefully is probably a better writer' (Goodwin, 1988, p. 187). However, sustained use of alcohol appears to have accelerated a decline in Fitzgerald's standard of both writing and health, as it did with contemporaries such as William Faulkner.

From a medical perspective, it is easy to view the life of Fitzgerald and others as being destroyed by alcohol. However, as Beveridge & Yorston (1999) point out, writers and artists have often seen the role of alcohol very differently. Alcohol has formed part of religious practices and customs for thousands of years and is often seen as an agent of mystical transport

Box 22.1 The case of F. Scott Fitzgerald

F. Scott Fitzgerald was both a creator and chronicler of the 'Roaring Twenties' in America and he achieved fame and fortune at a young age for his unique writing style. Born in 1896, by the age of 24 he was selling stories to a national newspaper for $2500 and his ability to turn out high-quality pieces enabled him to earn the money to maintain a lavish lifestyle of parties and drinking. Early in his career, Fitzgerald tried to keep drinking and writing separate and he abstained from alcohol while writing his most famous novel, *The Great Gatsby* (Fitzgerald, 1925). However, by the late 1920s, he was beginning to feel the pressure of producing a follow-up to *Gatsby* and rounds of all-night parties repeatedly forced him to abandon plans for writing a new novel in favour of producing short stories to sell.

From 1928 he was beginning to use alcohol to assist his writing, regarding it as a stimulant that would fuel his creative powers. However, it seems that he was aware of the problems that it caused him, writing that 'a short story can be written on the bottle, but for a novel you need the mental speed that enables you to keep the whole pattern in your head' (Dardis, 1989: p. 123).

In 1931 he moved to Hollywood to work as a scriptwriter and, although this earned good money, he was ultimately sacked for drunken behaviour at a party. He began to find it difficult to sell his stories and 1933 saw his first alcohol-related admission to hospital. Still he continued to drink and when his next novel, *Tender is The Night* (Fitzgerald, 1934), was finally published it fell below the standards expected of him. Critics agreed that the man who began the book in 1925 was not the same man that finished it in 1933 and Fitzgerald himself believed that alcohol had marred the work (Dardis, 1989).

In 1936, he wrote three short articles for a magazine that described his emotional collapse (which were ultimately published posthumously under the title *The Crack-Up*; Fitzgerald, 1945), but he avoided any mention of alcohol. The following year he took an overdose but managed to return to another job in Hollywood, which gave him the inspiration for his final (unfinished) novel, *The Last Tycoon* (Fitzgerald, 1941, posthumously).

In the last decade of his life, Fitzgerald experienced worsening physical problems related to alcohol and underwent frequent hospital admissions; insomnia and morning drinking became regular and disabling parts of life. He finally died of a myocardial infarction in 1940, aged just 44 (Dardis, 1989).

(Edwards, 2000). Writers such as Malcolm Lowry and Jack Kerouac have cited it as a means of spiritual exploration and a way of seeking enlightenment. Furthermore, bad behaviour by writers has been seen as a symbol of rebellion against contemporary values, and drinking has often formed an integral part of literary scenes. There is the added advantage that an alcoholic low-life is seen as especially conducive to the creative process and that some must experience degradation to produce great work. A striking example of this was Charles Bukowski who, in addition to his poetry, wrote a string of semi-autobiographical novels about his impoverished early life and his time spent drinking heavily in seedy bars. His ultimate elevation to riches and fame appears to have vindicated his life of excessive drinking and bad behaviour (Sounes, 1998).

Donald Goodwin (1988) believes in the idea that writers are introverted and lonely people, tortured souls who can express their overload of feelings only through writing. Artists have often been portrayed as individuals who are especially aware of the suffering of the world and need to numb themselves to cope. Such a perspective allows an unlimited licence for hedonistic excess, leading to a long list of writers who died prematurely, including Dylan Thomas, Brendan Behan, Jack Kerouac, Malcolm Lowry and Fitzgerald himself.

However, the final piece in the jigsaw may come from a study conducted by Nancy Andreasen (1987). She rated a group of writers attending a creative writing workshop and a control group of non-writers (matched for age, gender, education and IQ) using the research diagnostic criteria (RDC). The writers had significantly higher levels of bipolar disorder and alcoholism than the control group, 24 out of 30 having experienced an affective disorder at some point in their life.

Felix Post's work has also concluded that, in contrast to people showing other kinds of creative achievement, creative writers are excessively prone to depressive and perhaps to manic disorders, as well as to alcoholism (Post, 1994). In a study focusing on those writing poetry, fiction and plays, Post found evidence of psychopathology in the biographies of 93 out of 100 individuals (Post, 1996). These studies point to a link between creative verbal ability and affective as well as related psychopathology, and this might be the underlying basis that links creativity and alcohol dependence.

Addiction and the art of writing

The idea that psychoactive substances are linked to creativity goes beyond the writers themselves to the way in which they produce their work. From the Romantic poets of the 18th century to the Beat Generation of the mid-20th century, drugs have long been reputed to be central to the literary process. Several specific examples have been given of the direct role that opium played in the creation of literary works of the 18th and 19th centuries (Hayter, 1968). At this time, the drug was widely available throughout Europe and a variety of preparations could be bought over the counter. Laudanum, a drink consisting of opium mixed with alcohol, was particularly popular and many people used it as an effective means of pain relief. Opium carried with it a seductive air of Far Eastern mystique, and its 'specific power' to enhance dreams and memories appealed to many writers (Plant, 1999).

Perhaps the most famous example of opium-induced creativity is *Kubla Khan*, a poem written by Samuel Taylor Coleridge in the late 1790s. Coleridge called the poem 'a psychological curiosity' (Plant, 1999: p. 10) and claimed that it was a fragment of a much longer sequence that came to him in a dream induced by a dose of opium. Originally, the poem consisted of 200–300 lines, but when he woke up and began to write it down 'a person on business from Porlock' (Plant, 1999: p. 10) interrupted him. This was enough to break his flow and, on returning to the poem, he was left with only eight or ten lines and images. The fact that he later tried to recreate the situation without success did not deter others from experimenting with the drug.

In Sadie Plant's words, 'poets were enchanted by the possibility that such poetry could spring from the opiated edge of waking life' (Plant, 1999: p. 11). Mary Shelley's *Frankenstein* (Shelley, 1818) is another well-known story to have emerged in a similar way, and *The Bride of Lammermoor* by Sir Walter Scott is also reputed to have been dictated while he was taking large doses of laudanum for severe stomach pain. Alethea Hayter cites this and further examples in her book *Opium and the Romantic Imagination* (Hayter, 1968).

Wilkie Collins was one of the most popular authors of the mid- to late-19th century. For many years, he suffered from painful physical complaints, including gout and pains in the eyes, and had used laudanum regularly for at least 20 years before he wrote his novel *The Moonstone* (Collins, 1868). He is reported to have dictated the last part of the book largely under the influence of opium, and it is commented that when it was finished he was not only 'pleased and astonished' at the finale, but 'did not recognise it as his own' (Hayter, 1968: p. 259). The finale is particularly significant, as the plot has a central role for the drug. The book is about the theft of a large diamond (the Moonstone) by a man under the influence of opium who is left with no memory of his actions. Only when the scene is recreated does he find himself remembering what he has done. Opium clearly played a significant part in the author's life and it also appears in some of his other novels, including *The Woman in White*, *No Name* and *Armadale* (Collins, 1860, 1862, 1866 respectively).

Perhaps the most famous writer of the time using opiates was Thomas De Quincey. He wrote extensively about the use of the drug in his book *Confessions of an English Opium Eater* (De Quincey, 1822). Here, he described the magical effects that opium had on him, allowing him to slow things down and to enhance his dreams with his own fantasies.

He described a 'Dark Interpreter', a figure that allowed him to keep track of the thoughts that were arranging and rearranging themselves in his head. At first he was delighted by the drug's effects, but his deficit of dreams prior to using it became a surfeit and he found it difficult to cope with them. The sheer volume and complexity of these dreams became almost unbearable and his mind was invaded by 'flashback anticipations, sudden recollections and unpredicted twists' (Plant, 1999: p. 14).

Although De Quincey's descriptions of his dreams of oriental travel enthralled his readers, to him they became terrible nightmares. He lost the ability to distinguish between an increasingly hallucinatory waking life and the intensity of opiated dreams. He felt that his audience failed to understand the sheer intensity of these dreams, the terrifying worlds onto which his doors of perception could open.

More contemporary examples of the influence of psychoactive substances on writing include *On the Road* by Jack Kerouac (1957), which was apparently written in a 3-week burst of stimulant-fuelled creativity, and William S. Burrough's (1959) *The Naked Lunch*. Will Self's highly original and unusual work has been linked to his much-publicised problems with alcohol and drugs. However, further reflections on these legends of drug-fuelled writing often reveal them to be at least partly enhanced by fiction. Rather like the problems that Fitzgerald, Hemingway and others found in using alcohol, very little good work appears, in reality, to have been produced under the direct influence of drugs.

Careful analysis of the manuscripts of both *The Moonstone* and *The Bride of Lammermoor* suggests that they were largely completed before or after the authors' periods of illness (Sutherland, 1998). There is also evidence from their letters that both Kerouac and Burroughs preferred to write the bulk of their work while free from drugs, and the now-abstinent Will Self comments that he has 'always had to fight against them in order to get any serious literary work done' (Barber, 2000). De Quincey's florid descriptions of opium-induced behaviour certainly bear little resemblance to the experiences described by those who use the substance misuse treatment services that we run.

The narratives of addiction

An important question for the reader of any fictional portrayal of addiction is its plausibility. Qualitative studies have tried to make sense of the addicts' subjective experience of their own life history in relation to their problem (Hanninen & Koski-Jannes, 1999; McIntosh & McKeganey, 2000). One such example was based on the real-life stories of 51 individuals who had overcome some form of addiction, with the narratives influenced by the explanatory models for addiction that were available to each of them as they made their escape from dependence (Hanninen & Koski-Jannes, 1999). The authors identified the following five types of story.

The 'AA' story

This is the least surprising, given the worldwide influence of Alcoholics Anonymous (AA) and the extension of the organisation's explanatory model to all types of compulsive behaviour in our society. The trajectory of addiction is towards destruction, with individuals beginning to gain insight only when they reach their own 'personal gutter'. At this point, they can find salvation through applying the principles of AA, a process involving humility, finding the support of fellow recovering addicts and making amends where possible. Moral absolution and self-forgiveness follow from this disease model of addiction.

The 'personal growth' story

Here the addict has had his or her wishes and emotions disregarded as a child and the addiction has arisen as a denial of the individual's own emotional needs in favour of those of others. Recovery results from recognising and following these true emotions through self-discovery.

The 'co-dependence' story

The narrative is one where repressed secrets from childhood underlie the self-abusive behaviour of addiction, and the cure relies on becoming aware of and facing up to these memories.

The 'love' story

Addictive behaviour compensates for a lack of love in childhood and a cure comes through finding love.

The 'mastery' story

This was most commonly found in relation to addiction to tobacco. It was portrayed as a battle for autonomy during the different phases of the addiction, with 'giving-up' seen as part of achieving maturity.

Fiction's window on addiction

It is more difficult to get a narrative from someone who denies their addiction, and this may be where fiction can add to our understanding. As one author has observed, 'an addiction is held in place by an elaborate system of deceptions' (Beard, 1996) and a good fictional example of this is *The Legend of the Holy Drinker*, written in 1939 by Joseph Roth. This novella follows the fortunes of Andreas, an alcoholic vagrant who drinks as a response to external circumstances, but with little self-realisation. It is a simple story that engenders pathos and has parallels in Roth's own life story, although it is not autobiographical. Alternative narratives are also provided by the books *Junky* (Burroughs, 1953) and *Trainspotting* (Welsh, 1993), in which the addiction and its maintenance are seen as a matter of personal choice rather than something over which the individual has no control. This is no surprise when we consider the perspective of attribution theory outlined in the work of John Booth Davies. In *The Myth of Addiction* he suggests that 'most people who use drugs do so for their own reasons, on purpose, because they like it, and because they find no adequate reason for not doing so' (Davies, 1997: p. xi). However, the capacity to blame the properties of the drug or external circumstances for its repeated use seems to predominate in our culture and this is reflected in much of the writing cited in this review.

A further dimension brought out in literature is the polarisation that on the one hand warns against the dangers of drugs and alcohol and on the other

---

Box 22.2 Recently published drug anthologies

The Drug User (Strausbaugh & Blaise, 1991)

White Rabbit (Miller & Koral, 1995)

Psychedelia Britannica (Melechi, 1997)

Intoxication (Davidson, 1998)

Mindscapes (Melechi, 1998)

The Walls of Illusion (Haining, 1998)

Artificial Paradises (Jay, 1999)

Wildest Dreams (Rudgley, 2001)

The Howard Marks Book of Dope Stories (Marks, 2001)

---

argues that drug experiences are life-enhancing and so are something to be sought. In the face of this dichotomy, some of the more interesting literature, such as *Junky*, occupies a middle ground in taking a more matter-of-fact approach. The 'harder' drugs (heroin, cocaine) are mostly represented in the scare stories, whereas the psychedelic drugs (LSD, ecstasy) fall at the life-enhancement end of the spectrum. As an example, compare *Junk* (Burgess, 1996) and *Iced* (Shell, 1993) with *The Doors of Perception* (Huxley, 1994) and the recent anthologies about psychedelic experiences listed in Box 22.2.

It is perhaps no great surprise that most of the large number of autobiographical accounts of alcohol and drug dependence fall into the AA type of narrative. Anyone who has attended an AA meeting knows that it is based on the telling and retelling of life stories as a therapeutic tool. Furthermore, the fourth, fifth, eighth and ninth steps of AA's Twelve Steps (see chapter 2, Box 2.1 for a version of these) imply the need to examine your own life story. There are numerous examples of famous people recounting their stories in this way. They include *Addicted*, by the footballer Tony Adams (1998) and the critically acclaimed *Drinking: A Love Story*, by Caroline Knapp (1996). In the latter, Knapp takes the reader through the phases of her alcoholism and outlines the help she found in AA. A key to this process was a shift from thinking that she drank because she was unhappy to considering that she was unhappy because she drank. In contrast, Ann Marlowe's *How to Stop Time: Heroin from A to Z* (1999) does not follow the Alcoholics/Narcotics Anonymous story, with the author declaring that her addiction was 'chosen'. The narrative is disjointed as she takes the reader through a lexicon of relevant terms and, interestingly, she describes reading Burroughs and De Quincey at a young age. Her dependence seems to be predominantly psychological rather than physical and she gives a good account of the subtle thought processes that led to her eventual choice to be drug-free.

Current drug-related fiction

It is currently possible to find the whole range of drug-related experience related in fictional form on the shelves of bookshops and especially in the book sections of popular music shops. Heroin and cocaine are the drugs most often featured but, more recently, ecstasy has come a close third and much of the most recent fiction has been influenced by the relatively new 'rave' culture. In the late 1990s publishers appeared to be particularly drawn to novels with drug names in the title, with examples including *Junk* (Burgess, 1996), *The Story of Junk* (Yablonsky, 1997), *Cocaine* (Strongman, 1997) and *The Ecstasy Club* (Rushkoff, 1997). It would appear that such titles and their accompanying cover art are a selling-point. Anthologies drawing together work from a number of writers are a useful introduction to the topic and a number of examples are listed in Box 22.2. These books concentrate on drugs rather than alcohol and vary in the level to which they rely on fictional or semi-fictional sources alongside personal accounts and scientific writings on the effects of drugs. There is clearly a market for such anthologies in the era of 'recreational drug use', although they do demonstrate some of the difficulties of communicating in writing the intensity and personal nature of drug experience. Similar books about alcohol are harder to find but *The Faber Book of Drink, Drinkers and Drinking* (Rae, 1991) is broad in its coverage, with quotations from many famous literary works, and *Drink to Me Only – The Prose (and Cons) of Drinking* (Bold, 1982) covers the same ground more succinctly.

Few writers can have been as closely linked to the use of psychoactive drugs as William S. Burroughs, and his works such as *The Naked Lunch* (1959) and *Junky* (1953) openly reflect his addiction to heroin. However, it is less well known that his son, William S. Burroughs Junior, published two autobiographical novels (*Speed* and *Kentucky Ham*; Burroughs Jr, 1970, 1973) documenting his addiction to amphetamines and, later, heroin.

Burroughs Junior was clearly at high risk of developing problems of addiction as both of his parents were dependent on psychoactive substances. Indeed, in 1951, aged just 4 years, he was said to have been in the room when his father accidentally shot his mother. Burroughs Junior ultimately died of liver failure at the age of 34. Another important American author in this genre is Hubert Selby Junior, author of *Last Exit to Brooklyn* (Selby Jr, 1964). His novel *Requiem for a Dream* (Selby Jr, 1978) links four characters in a story of drug addiction that leads to imprisonment, death, prostitution and incarceration in a mental hospital. The main agent of destruction for the three younger characters is heroin, but this is ultimately seen as no different from the effects of prescription drugs used by the mother of one of them. In 2000 the novel was made into a compelling film of the same name, directed by Darren Aronofsky, with Selby Junior providing the screenplay and also appearing in a cameo role as a prison guard, laughing at the predicament of the two male characters. Much of Selby Junior's other work touches on issues related to addiction and degradation.

Doctors and addiction

How do addicted patients view their doctors? A literary insight is given by William Burroughs in *Junky* (1953), written at a time when doctors were the main source of heroin. He describes them disparagingly as 'croakers' and gives advice on how best to approach them in order to achieve the addict's goal of receiving a prescription. He prefers a convincing story that allows the doctor to save face in writing the prescription rather than a 'factual approach' and advises the reader that 'you need a good bedside manner with doctors or you will get nowhere' (Burroughs, 1977: p. 21). Although this account was written in the American context and before the current vogue for substitute prescribing, there are still lessons to be learned from it. Our patients who are addicted present us with stories that are designed to induce a desired response, whatever that might be.

There are few literary accounts of doctors who successfully help patients with addiction to overcome their problems, perhaps reflecting the reality that recovery is about self-discovery. Research suggests that the impact of treatment is modest in the long term and that recovery is about the individual constructing a new identity that does not revolve around drugs or alcohol and acknowledging the need to abstain. One exception is the writer Eugene O'Neill who, after many failed attempts at recovery from his heavy alcohol use, sustained prolonged abstinence after psychoanalysis (Ludwig, 1988).

In contrast, many accounts exist of unscrupulous doctors who produce addiction in their patients. An excellent example of this is the doctor in Hubert Selby Junior's *Requiem for a Dream* (Selby Jr, 1978). Not only does the doctor lead the mother whose son is addicted to street drugs into dependence on diet pills, but then he tries to counteract her descent into psychosis with tranquillisers, giving little time or thought to the consequences of the prescription.

Doctors who have themselves become impaired through the use of drugs and alcohol frequently appear in literature. Drug and alcohol misuse are, in fact, the most common reasons for doctors in the UK to come to the attention of the Health Committee of the General Medical Council, and perhaps this literary concern reflects not only reality but also an interest in the complexity of character found in such individuals. Although he was unable to accept his own problem with alcohol, in *Tender is the Night*, Fitzgerald wrote memorably about the psychiatrist, Dick Diver, and his descent into alcoholism. There are also some notable short stories on this theme, including Mikhail Bulgakov's *Morphine* in *A Country Doctor's Notebook* (Bulgakov, 1925–1927). This is a warning against the perils of self-medicating with drugs and the addictive process that might ensue, as the doctor, Polyakov, ultimately takes his own life. Finally, Verghese's *The Tennis Partner* (1998) is a personal narrative by an American physician who becomes aware of an addictive disorder in a junior colleague who is an ex-tennis professional. The author relates the problem of addiction in the medical profession to the expectation that doctors should conceal their own emotions and to the possibility that vulnerable individuals can be left in a position of isolation.

Conclusion

This short review is, by necessity, highly selective in its choice of examples, and space limitations have prevented us including other important addictive processes such as smoking, gambling and 'sex addiction'. However, we hope that we have shown that literature is capable of broadening our perspective on the phenomena of addiction and substance use. Modern diagnostic concepts and operational definitions of misuse and dependence tend to simplify a complex problem, and literary accounts help us to regain the perspective of the highly individual experience of using the different classes of psychoactive drugs. Furthermore, we have touched on new qualitative research on addicts' own narratives of their dependence which appears to complement this literary perspective. Finally, we have warned against taking too seriously the claims made by some authors of drug-enhanced creativity and also found literary warnings of our own vulnerabilities, as doctors, to addictive disorders.

References

Adams, T. (1998) *Addicted*. CollinsWillow.

Andreasen, N. C. (1987) Creativity and mental illness: prevalence rates in writers and their first-degree relatives. *American Journal of Psychiatry*, **144**, 1288–1292.

Barber, L. (2000) Self control. *The Observer*. 11 June (http://books.guardian.co.uk/departments/generalfiction/story/0,6000,330140,00.html)

Beard, R. (1996) *X20*. Flamingo.

Beveridge, A. & Yorston, G. (1999) I drink, therefore I am: alcohol and creativity. *Journal of the Royal Society of Medicine*, **92**, 646–648.

Bold, A. (ed.) (1982) *Drink to Me Only: The Prose (and Cons) of Drinking*. Robin Clark.

Bulgakov, M. (1925–1927) *A Country Doctor's Notebook*. Reprinted 1975 (trans. M. Glenny). Collins & Harvill.

Burgess, M. (1996) *Junk*. Reprinted 1999. Penguin Books.

Burroughs, W. S. (a.k.a. Lee, W.) (1953) *Junkie: Confessions of an Unredeemed Drug Addict*. Reprinted 1977 as *Junky*. Penguin Books.

Burroughs, W. S. (1959) *The Naked Lunch*. Reprinted 1986. Flamingo.

Burroughs Jr., W. S. (1970) *Speed*. Overlook Press.

Burroughs Jr., W. S. (1973) *Kentucky Ham*. Overlook Press.

Collins, W. (1860) *The Woman in White*. Reprinted 1999. Penguin Popular Classics.

Collins, W. (1862) *No Name*. Reprinted 1998. Oxford Paperbacks.

Collins, W. (1866) *Armadale*. Reprinted 1999. Oxford Paperbacks.

Collins, W. (1868) *The Moonstone*. Reprinted 1999. Oxford Paperbacks.

Dardis, T. (1989) *The Thirsty Muse: Alcohol and the American Writer*. Ticknor & Fields.

Davidson, T. (ed.) (1998) *Intoxication: An Anthology of Stimulant-based Writing*. Serpent's Tail.

Davies, J. B. (1997) *The Myth of Addiction* (2nd edn). Harwood Academic Publishers.

De Quincey, T. (1822) *Confessions of an English Opium Eater*. Reprinted 1986. Penguin Books.

Edwards, G. (2000) *Alcohol. The Ambiguous Molecule*. Penguin Books.

Fitzgerald, F. S. (1925) *The Great Gatsby*. Reprinted 1993. Wordsworth Editions.

Fitzgerald, F. S. (1934) *Tender is The Night*. Reprinted 1994. Wordsworth Editions.

Fitzgerald, F. S. (1941) *The Last Tycoon*. Reprinted 2002. Penguin Books.

Fitzgerald, F. S. (1945) *The Crack-Up. With other Uncollected Pieces, Notebooks and Unpublished Letters* (ed. E. Wilson). Reprinted 1965 in *The Crack-Up and Other Stories*. Penguin Books.

Goodwin, D. W. (1988) *Alcohol and the Writer*. Andrews and McMeel.

Haining, P. (1998) *The Walls of Illusion: A Psychedelic Retro*. Souvenir Press.

Hanninen, V. & Koski-Jannes, A. (1999) Narratives of recovery from addictive behaviour. *Addiction*, **94**, 1837–1848.

Hayter, A. (1968) *Opium and the Romantic Imagination*. Faber & Faber.

Huxley, A. (1994) *The Doors of Perception*. Flamingo.

Jay, M. (ed.) (1999) *Artificial Paradises*. Penguin Books.

Kerouac, J. (1957) *On the Road*. Reprinted 1998. Penguin Books.

Knapp, C. (1996) *Drinking: A Love Story*. Quartet Books.

Ludwig, A. M. (1988) *Understanding the Alcoholic's Mind*. Oxford University Press.

Marks, H. (ed.) (2001) *The Howard Marks Book of Dope Stories*. Vintage.

Marlowe, A. (1999) *How to Stop Time: Heroin from A to Z*. Virago Press.

McIntosh, J. & McKeganey, N. (2000) Addicts' narratives of recovery from drug use: constructing a non-addict identity. *Social Science and Medicine*, **50**, 1501–1510.

Melechi, A. (ed.) (1997) *Psychedelia Britannica*. Turnaround.

Melechi, A. (1998) *Mindscapes: an Anthology of Drug Writings*. Mono.

Miller, J. & Koral, R. (eds) (1995) *White Rabbit: A Psychedelic Reader*. Chronicle Books.

Plant, S. (1999) *Writing on Drugs*. Faber & Faber.

Post, F. (1994) Creativity and psychopathology. A study of 291 world-famous men. *British Journal of Psychiatry*, **165**, 22–34.

Post, F. (1996) Verbal creativity, depression and alcoholism. An investigation of one hundred American and British writers. *British Journal of Psychiatry*, **168**, 545–555.

Rae, S. (ed.) (1991) *The Faber Book of Drink, Drinkers and Drinking*. Faber and Faber.

Roth, J. (1939) *The Legend of the Holy Drinker* (trans. M. Hofmann). Reprinted 2000. Granta.

Rudgley, R. (ed.) (2001) *Wildest Dreams: An Anthology of Drug-Related Literature*. Abacus.

Rushkoff, D. (1997) *The Ecstasy Club*. Sceptre.

Selby Jr., H. (1964) *Last Exit to Brooklyn*. Reprinted 1987. Flamingo.

Selby Jr., H. (1978) *Requiem for a Dream*. Marion Boyars.

Shell, R. (1993) *Iced*. Flamingo.

Shelley, M. (1818) *Frankenstein*. Reprinted 1992 (ed. M. Hindle). Penguin Books.

Sounes, H. (1998) *Charles Bukowski: Locked in the Arms of a Crazy Life*. Rebel.

Strausbaugh, J. & Blaise, D. (eds) (1991) *The Drug User: Documents 1840–1960*. Blast Books.

Strongman, P. (1997) *Cocaine*. Abacus.

Sutherland, J. (1998) Turns unstoned. *Times Literary Supplement*, 30 October.

Sutherland, J. (2001) *Last Drink to LA*. Short Books.

Verghese, A. (1998) *The Tennis Partner: A Doctor's Story of Friendship and Loss*. Chatto & Windus.

Welsh, I. (1993) *Trainspotting*. Reprinted 1999. Vintage.

Yablonsky, L. (1997) *The Story of Junk*. Headline Publishing.

Index

Compiled by Caroline Sheard